The Curious Habits of Dr Adams

JANE ROBINS

JOHN M

First published in Great Britain in 2013 by John Murray (Publishers)
An Hachette UK Company

1

© Jane Robins 2013

A CIP catalogue record for this title is available from the British Library

Hardback ISBN 978-1-84854-470-3
Trade Paperback ISBN 978-1-84854-471-0
Ebook ISBN 978-1-8485-4473-4

Typeset in 12.25/15 Monotype Bembo by Servis Filmsetting Ltd, Stockport, Cheshire

Printed and bound by Clays Ltd, St Ives plc

John Murray policy is to use papers that are natural, renewable and recyclable products and made from wood grown in sustainable forests. The logging and manufacturing processes are expected to conform to the environmental regulations of the country of origin.

John Murray (Publishers)
338 Euston Road
London NW1 3BH

www.johnmurray.co.uk

For the Wilkinsons:
Carol, James, Kate, Harry and Freddie

Contents

Introduction

IN 1957 AN extraordinary trial took place at the Old Bailey. A family doctor, John Bodkin Adams, was accused of murdering a patient in the hope of inheriting her Rolls-Royce. It seemed inconceivable. People had such deeply held regard for doctors, such trust. As *The Lancet* reported: the family doctor 'enjoys more prestige and wields more power than any other citizen, unless it be the judge on his bench'. In 1950s Britain, when deference reigned, that was true. The doctor was uniquely placed 'to influence the physical, psychological and economic destiny of other people', and there was little doubt that – whether or not he was a murderer – Dr Adams was despicable in his exploitation of that powerful position.

His trial was a press sensation, covered all around the world – and the way in which it unfolded made gripping reading, with the advantage swinging back and forth between the prosecution and the defence. The judge, Patrick Devlin, wrote a book about it, as did the novelist Sybille Bedford. Both works were, in their way, quite brilliant but they told only part of the story of John Bodkin Adams, focusing on a single murder charge, that relating to the owner of the Rolls-Royce – a wealthy widow named Edith Morrell who owned a mansion in the seaside town of Eastbourne and a garden full of prize dahlias. But everyone knew that the police investigation into Dr Adams had been a far broader affair and that he had been suspected of murdering many more patients. Maybe dozens. Possibly hundreds.

After the trial, the police files were closed. All the details of the investigation – the mountain of witness statements, the forensic reports, Scotland Yard's internal documents – were to be hidden from the public for seventy-five years. Conspiracy theories started to take root and were later encouraged by the catalytic combination of the internet and the imposed secrecy around the case. Some thought Dr Adams was the most prolific serial killer in British history, worse than Harold Shipman, and suggested that dark forces were at work, keeping the terrible truth about the scale of his crimes hidden. Others were fiercely loyal to the doctor. For them, it was more likely that the mysterious closed files contained evidence of a witch-hunt, revealing that Dr Adams was a persecuted man, innocent all along, and the victim of an over-zealous investigation by Scotland Yard's Murder Squad.

Then in 2003 a local historian, Pamela Cullen, made a successful request under the Freedom of Information Act for the files to be opened before their due date. I bought the book that she wrote, thinking I might find a compelling narrative of the whole story of Dr Adams, informed by the new sources. But it was not that sort of book, and did not want to be. So I visited the National Archives at Kew and the East Sussex Record Office at Lewes to see the documents for myself and I found information that in its fine detail was quite different from anything already published. I started digging. I asked for permission to see the extensive archives of Dr Adams's solicitor and great friend, Herbert James. These, too, had been closed to the public, and when I learned that I would be allowed to see them I was thrilled – an inappropriate response to the subject-matter of murder, but new material is the adrenalin-hit that keeps introverted historical researchers focused on the task in hand. I bought another train ticket to Lewes.

At the same time, I tracked down the daughter of one of Dr Adams's alleged victims, someone who had known him and had been in the eye of the storm in 1957. Finding this daughter was not easy. Her surname had changed on marriage and the 19-year-old Patricia Tomlinson of then was now Patricia Piper, a sprightly senior citizen. There was also a grand-daughter named Judi, and I contacted Judi via email. She replied straight away and was keen to delve into the past, but her mother was reluctant. Then, after a few weeks, Patricia kindly agreed to meet me with Judi at her home, so I set off for Sussex. Both women were welcoming and generous with their time, and with their family photographs. I am immensely grateful to them − because it was this meeting that made the story of Dr Adams seem close and personal. Patricia's mother was the glamorous Bobbie Hullett, whose story I am about to tell, and it was the small details that Patricia remembered that made Bobbie and her family seem real to me − the games of tennis, the number-plates of the cars they had, the white chimneys on their house.

A few weeks later, I was once again travelling out of London in pursuit of Dr Adams. In the spring of 2011 I had been introduced to Virginia, the daughter of the judge Patrick Devlin. Devlin had died in 1992, but his beautiful Georgian country house, West Wick, was then still in the family and Virginia invited me to come and see the study in which her father had written his book on Dr Adams − *Easing the Passing*. His papers, she said, were still there. As a law student, long ago, I had fallen slightly in love with Patrick Devlin because of the intelligence and clarity of his writing. When you have to trudge through a dozen dull, obtuse legal judgements, trying not to fall asleep − one that is written beautifully, with a profound feel for words, is bound to win a place in your heart. So, with a heightened sense of anticipation, I drove down to Wiltshire.

The road to West Wick House curves elegantly through rolling fields, and the house itself appears gently but impressively, perfect in its proportions and sitting plumb in the landscape. Patrick Devlin's study was at the top, under the eaves, and

Virginia now took me up there. Many of his papers were packed up in cardboard boxes, but somehow the room seemed undisturbed, as though Devlin had been there yesterday – but not quite that. His presence was strong, but the room was dusty and a little ghostly, so you felt both the passage of time and the perturbing closeness of the past.

I spent some precious hours at Lord Devlin's desk reading a small part of the substantial collection of papers about John Bodkin Adams. Student notebooks were filled with his strange intense handwriting and his transcript of the trial was also there, with the sections that he had found particularly interesting underlined in red pencil. For me, this was treasure worthy of contemplation for months rather than hours, and after a while, with Virginia's blessing, I loaded all the papers into the boot of my car and drove them back to London.

At this point I was too deeply involved in the Dr Adams story to turn back. I was now on a quest to solve the puzzle of what really happened, but I also felt, quite keenly, the duty I have to the doctor's many patients, long since dead, whose experiences I am about to relate, and to their descendants. It is a duty of care of sorts and it will be hard to get it right because I know that whatever history I write, it has to be through a peculiar prism, piecing together moments in time using those fragments of evidence that have survived the passing of the years. I am collecting witness statements, birth certificates, marriage certificates, photographs, newspapers, interviews, police reports and any scrap of contemporary documentation that I can find. A story is emerging that, as it must, puts Dr Adams on trial again. And now I am the jury – and so are you.

I

Bobbie Hullett

As a girl, Bobbie Leefe was prettier than her sister Valerie and her half-sister Podge, and she knew it. Her real name was Gertrude, but her nickname suited her better; it was modern and had a bit of a kick about it. And, being unusual and charming, it recognised those aspects of her character that stayed in the memory: her ability to 'wrap people around her little finger' and her propensity to think of herself as special. It was obvious that somewhere deep inside Bobbie was a sense of entitlement. This may have been a gift from her mother, who had aristocratic pretensions though not much money, since the family fortune had been sunk into mines in South Africa and lost there. Or it might have been rooted in her beauty and innate sense of style. A 1920s portrait shows Bobbie as a young woman, gazing towards the photographer and looking like a movie starlet. Her eyes are wide-spaced and dreamy, her lips a perfect little bow and her skin creamy white and flawless. She stands in a way that is artfully relaxed, even sultry, showing off slender arms and subtle curves, and she is wearing a simple shift dress. We know that she is an expensive young woman from the jewelled buckle of the belt slung low around her hips, and the white fur of the cape that drapes her shoulders. She looks perfectly ripe, ready for love.

Happily, romance came her way and blossomed over games of tennis with a dazzling young man named Vaughan Tomlinson. Vaughan was clever, and had graduated in English from Cambridge, and he was sporty, being the wicket keeper for the

Surrey Seconds cricket team. Also, it was fortunate that he came from a wealthy family and, when Bobbie and Vaughan married, his parents financed the building of a smart house for them. It was called Wishanger and was at Willingdon, two miles inland from the Sussex seaside town of Eastbourne, on a lane that wound upwards out of the village and on to the South Downs. It was while the Tomlinsons were here that their daughter Patricia was born, and it is from Patricia that we know some aspects of Bobbie's early life.

She adored Vaughan, and loved being married. In her social circles, there was no expectation that a wife should work. Instead Bobbie became a housewife, a role that involved socialising with other mothers, or hosting dinner parties at Wishanger, or pottering about in the garden. She did not have much actual housework to do as the Tomlinsons employed a live-in maid, and it seems that she was not a particularly warm or attentive mother, reserving her considerable charms and nervous energy for Vaughan and her friends, and leaving Patricia to the care of a nanny. Bobbie drove, and had her own car – an American Essex.

During the Second World War she volunteered to help out on the home front, cutting a dash in her corduroy trousers and brown jacket, as with her friend Marjorie Hawkins she drove a YMCA van, taking refreshments to the men at the gun emplacements along the coast around Eastbourne. These were difficult times – the south coast of England was bombed heavily, and Eastbourne most of all. But Bobbie flourished then. She appeared to have a sense of purpose as a war worker, and as a wife and mother too. Patricia was about six years old when Eastbourne was bombarded by the Germans – but she wasn't afraid, because her mother was a trooper, never showing fear and keeping up the family spirits. She would take Patricia up on to the South Downs to watch the bombs falling on the town, and for her child's sake she made the occasion seem exciting, like a firework display.

Vaughan had become a teacher of English first at St Cyprian's school, and then at St Bede's at the Beachy Head end of Eastbourne, up on the cliff with views across the town and the English Channel. He fared exceptionally well at St Bede's and soon became headmaster. When the school was evacuated to Oxford because of the bombs, he went too. These were difficult times for the family, but not unbearable, since Vaughan spent the entire war in Britain, working at St Bede's and then the British Overseas Airways Corporation in Bristol. After the war, life soon returned to normal, and Bobbie and Vaughan settled back into their bright, sociable style of living at Wishanger. Then, in 1950, out of the blue, everything changed when Vaughan – still handsome and youthful – suffered a severe heart attack, was taken to hospital and died.

Bobbie was distraught. She 'appeared to lose grip on herself', said a family friend, and she fell into a deep depression. It was also a terrible time for Patricia who, at 16, had lost her father and now watched as her mother fell apart. Bobbie did not find the resources within herself to be a comfort to her daughter. Instead she was difficult and self-pitying, and Patricia just wanted to be out of the house. It was about this time that Dr John Bodkin Adams came to Wishanger. He was a round-faced, pink-skinned corpulent Irishman who, said Patricia, struck her as very unattractive. But his concern for her mother was obvious – he came to the house every day to check on her.

Dr Adams remembered his visits well. When Vaughan died, he said, Bobbie 'was heartbroken and asked, "what can I do to die?"' Her physical condition was poor and she lost weight, said the doctor. 'Her nerves were in a dreadful state, she couldn't sleep and was absolutely like a person demented.' So he treated her for her 'nerves'. Bobbie could not know it, but this was one of Dr Adams's favourite diagnoses. 'Nerves', he thought, were common in women patients – and could be treated very well with sedatives. Some nervous women might, like Bobbie, be deeply upset by something grave. Others might simply be a little out of sorts.

His views on the subject were not unusual. In 1922, when Dr Adams was starting out on his career in Eastbourne, many medical conditions had been put down to nerves rather than physiology. According to *The Lancet* of that year, it was widely accepted that an epileptic fit was, in essence, psychological, being 'a flight from undue stress into unconsciousness . . .' And pernicious vomiting in pregnancy was put down to 'nerves' by most doctors. Dr Carlton Oldfield of Leeds took that approach, and informed *The Lancet* of his treatment for the condition: 'I explain to the patient's nurses the nature of the disease and ask them on no account to place a bowl at the bedside. The vomiting usually ceases immediately and recovery quickly follows.' Since women were prone to nerves anyway, it was unsurprising that a shocking bereavement might make a nervy woman like Bobbie 'demented'.

Before the war, a lively debate on women and their nerves had been published in the medical press. In 1938 Dr Stephen Taylor made a big impression with his identification of an increasingly common phenomenon – 'the suburban neurosis'. Women were coming to him complaining of 'trembling all over' and jumping at the slightest noise. They might have a swollen stomach, stabbing pains over the heart, or buzzing in the ears, and be unable to sleep at night. 'On examination,' he wrote, 'there is definite but variable tremor . . . pendulous flabby breasts, poor abdominal muscles, very brisk reflexes and nothing else . . .' Looking closely at her condition, Dr Taylor could see that the woman's problem lay in her boredom in her modern labour-saving home, and her reliance on gossip magazines and the cinema for excitement. 'What wonder,' he wrote, 'that the underdeveloped, relatively poor mind of the suburban woman seeks an escape in neurosis? No doubt the roots of these neuroses lie buried in a heap of infantile adolescent manure.' For Dr Taylor the answer for such women was not sedation: 'A carefully graded reading list is perhaps more use than a bottle of medicine. Another baby, rather than a new wireless, if it can be afforded, may effect a permanent cure.' Visits to the swimming bath, the gymnasium and the public library would also help a good deal. Throughout the ensuing debate there is little suggestion that a misogynistic male doctor might not be a superb authority on such female matters.

In 1950, when Bobbie Tomlinson was struck low, female nerves were to be seen everywhere. That January it made front page news when Ingrid Bergman, the film star, became pregnant by her lover, Robert Rossellini. Ingrid had fled to a retreat in the hills outside Rome, reported the *Daily Mirror*. She was 'utterly ashamed by the publicity, [and] broke down with jangled nerves'. At the same time, advertisements in the paper made it clear that 'nerves' were a pernicious menace. Ovaltine was a night time drink that 'soothes the nerves', Nestlé's Milo drink was advertised under the banner 'Is this happening to you? Her children got on her nerves'. Bournvita, made by Cadburys, encouraged the 'right kind of sleep', in which 'body, mind and nerves are completely relaxed'. In the *Daily Express* an advertisement for the new quiet Electrolux vacuum cleaner proclaimed that: 'It's kind to your nerves . . . and his. It won't disturb baby or irritate the neighbours.'

When Bobbie was lying prostrate with nerves after the death of Vaughan, Dr Adams gave her sleeping pills – and possibly some daytime sedation too. He also recommended getting away from it all, and taking a restorative holiday in Switzerland. She took his advice and went away for a month, with a local vicar, the Revd Harry Copsey, as her companion. 'It was then that I noticed she was taking sleeping tablets and I tried to get her to give them up,' said Harry Copsey. 'It was difficult to get her up in the morning and on one occasion I went into her room shortly after 9 a.m. and found that she did not appear to be sleeping normally and I found it impossible to waken her. When she appeared at lunch time she appeared her normal self.' At the end of the holiday, she was 'wonderfully well'.

After Switzerland, Bobbie was in better spirits. She started to socialise again and became friendly with Jack Hullett, a wealthy widower who had built himself a fancy mansion called Holywell Mount, on the cliff right next to St Bede's School, where Vaughan had been headmaster. Holywell Mount was an impressive home, with fifteen rooms, a solarium and a terrace that had a fabulous view over the sea, and Jack Hullett was a swanky old gentleman, a retired stockbroker who was reputed to earn more than £60,000 a year, drove a Rolls-Royce and had his initials incorporated into the Holywell Mount gates – in gilt and 9 inches high. Dr Adams was a regular visitor, since Jack was both his patient and a friend, and he had also looked after Jack's wife, Theodora, in her final illness.

Jack's assistant, Nellie Caton, remembered Dr Adams's visits to the Hullett household, and recalled that he had excelled himself more as a friend than as a doctor. Sometime during the war, she said, the doctor had told Jack that he needed an operation, urgently. 'Fortunately Mr Hullett, on the advice of one of his partners, took a second opinion and it was found that the operation was completely unnecessary.' This episode, though, did not dent the Hulletts' relationship with Dr Adams, who continued to look after Theodora. 'Both Mr and Mrs Hullett thought there was nobody like him,' said Nellie. When Theodora died, it was revealed that she had left Dr Adams £100 in her will. Nellie Caton said that Jack was disgusted that the amount was so small, and told the doctor that he would put things right by mentioning him in his own will.

Jack Hullett's home was the hub of a lively social circle that included, along with his doctor, the singer Anne Ziegler, the actor Leslie Henson and his wife Martha, Marjorie Hawkins, who used to drive YMCA vans with Bobbie during the war, and Richard Walker – the chief constable of Eastbourne. According to Dr Adams, Jack's relationship with Bobbie began when, to help him, and to help her, he persuaded him to take her to dances at the Grand Hotel on Saturday nights. Jack was twenty years older than Bobbie – but they seemed to make a good couple.

One day Jack Hullett told Dr Adams that he was going on a cruise and wanted a travelling companion. The doctor replied, 'Why don't you ask Bobbie Tomlinson. She is a cheerful person, you know her more or less, why don't you invite her to go on this cruise? There is no reason why you shouldn't go together.' Another friend of Jack's, Hugh Hubbard Ford, remembered him phoning and saying: 'Believe it or not, I am going to take Mrs Tomlinson for a cruise. I shall probably shock Eastbourne, but I don't care.' It was after this trip, to South America and the West Indies, that Bobbie and Jack announced that they were to be married. This was at some point in 1952.

Bobbie had been saved from her wretchedness, rescued from miserable widowhood. For her, it was essential to be a wife – to be admired, provided for, and to have a place in society. Patricia confesses that she was relieved when her mother remarried, though she found Jack an odd old man. And Jack was delighted with his young pretty wife. 'There is no doubt that Mr and the second Mrs Hullett were ideally happy,' said Hugh Hubbard Ford. 'Mr Hullett often used to say to me that life had started for him again and that all the things that he longed to do, namely foreign travel and cruises, he was now able to do because Mrs Hullett was of one mind with him in this enjoyment of such recreation. They in fact went to Australia one year, South Africa the next year, New Zealand another year . . .'

According to Dr Adams, Jack Hullett took him aside several times to thank him for his matchmaking. 'He said: "I have never been so happy in my life. Life is one long dream of happiness. We are happy in every way". He also said: "She is going to break me with her minks and jewels." I said: "What's the good of money in the bank? You now have something to see for your money." He said: "That's true, you are right."' It was Dr

Adams's style to boast, but in this case his observations had much truth in them. For Bobbie, wealthy old Jack could never replace handsome young Vaughan, but she had found an acceptable, enjoyable second-best.

Bobbie was not entirely free of her nerve problems, however. 'I called each Sunday morning on Mr Hullett, as I had always done,' said Dr Adams. 'I called officially on him but I saw her because she developed a skin rash. It was all over her body but chiefly on the side of her neck . . . The fact that she had this rash was the only blot on the horizon and it worried her to pieces because of her inability to wear evening dress.' The doctor put this rash down to the continued effect of the death of Vaughan and also to nervous tension. After a while, he decided to send Bobbie to see a skin specialist in London. 'He took her over and gave her [an] x-ray and we got the thing cleared up in the end, but it was a tedious business.' Then Jack Hullett developed a similar nerve-based disorder. 'He was a nervous man,' said Dr Adams, 'and I treated him for various functional nervous illnesses.'

In November 1955, Jack's health problems took a more serious turn. One Sunday evening, shortly after a cruise to America, he sent for Dr Adams because he had a terrible pain in his stomach. He had experienced a similar pain when on board ship, but the ship's doctor had dismissed it as colic. 'I examined him and to my horror I found he had a sub-acute obstruction of the lower bowel,' said Dr Adams, 'and I thought it might be cancer.' Sadly, on this occasion, his diagnosis was correct. The doctor sent for a well-known London surgeon to operate on Jack at the local Esperance Nursing Home. He decided against having a partner in his practice, Dr Laurence Snowball, perform the operation, 'because I knew it was going to be fatal and I thought if I had a local surgeon to operate, his relations might say, "why didn't you get a London man?"'

In the event, when the London man performed the operation, something went wrong, and afterwards Jack was in great pain.

'These doctors have murdered me!' he told his friend Hugh Hubbard Ford – a cynical comment packed with anxiety that his life was in unsafe hands. About ten days after the operation, Jack's whole abdomen burst, said Dr Adams. 'Snowball and I were called at once, got him into the theatre at Esperance and operated immediately and repaired the burst. For some days we despaired of his life, but by constant attention we got him through and out of danger.' Dr Adams's role in the operation was as an anaesthetist – he had a diploma in the subject. His competence, though, was a matter of some discussion among Eastbourne medics – he had a reputation for putting patients under extremely deeply, and also for falling asleep during operations. On the positive side, this speciality meant, or should have meant, that when Dr Adams prescribed sedatives or hypnotics for patients – as he did very often – he would have an accurate and precise knowledge of their effects.

While Jack was in hospital, Bobbie became terrified that she was going to lose another husband. Dr Adams described her state as 'absolutely desperate'. She came in to see Jack, he said, sometimes twice a day and was adamant that he should be home by Christmas. 'She was in a great state of agitation – half hysterics.' So Dr Adams prescribed barbiturates – which was something he did quite regularly for his nervous patients. These were hypnotic drugs that were well known to be addictive. A full-page editorial in the *British Medical Journal* of Christmas Day 1954 warned of their 'sinister potentialities', and reminded doctors that an overdose would often lead to death. Most controversial, said the *British Medical Journal*, was the practice of 'sedating' during waking hours 'people whose symptoms are the result of anxiety and frustration'. The tone of the editorial was critical of the many doctors who continued to prescribe barbiturates at the drop of a hat. A 1951 study had found that barbiturates accounted for 10 per cent of all NHS prescriptions written in a single month in Scotland. That figure, thought the authors, could well have risen to 15 per cent. So Dr Adams's predilection for prescribing addictive hypnotics would have been frowned upon by the top doctors of his time, but it was not particularly unusual.

When Jack came home to Holywell Mount, he was looked after by a team of four nurses, and by Bobbie. 'Every improvement made by Mr Hullett seemed to have a reaction on Mrs Hullett's attitude,' said Hugh Hubbard Ford, 'as she seemed so relieved at every sign of recovering good health.' She wanted to stay with Jack all day, and to sleep in the same room at night – but Dr Adams felt that, as she was so highly strung, her constant and close attention was bad for Jack. He was a very poorly man and his cancer care included many doses of painkillers, and repeated high doses of barbiturates, as well as morphine and heroin.

One of the four nurses attending him, Audrey Goodchild, remembered that while the nursing staff would give Jack his tablets, it was the doctor who gave him injections of morphia. She did not like Dr Adams, she said, because 'he refused to co-operate and would not explain the names or types of drugs he was administering'. On one occasion, she asked what certain tablets were and received such a rebuff from the doctor that she never asked him again.

Hugh Hubbard Ford called in to see Jack Hullett on the evening of 7 March 1956. He found him in low spirits and 'very depressed'. He spent three hours with his friend, trying to cheer him up with talk about old friends and future plans. During their time together, Jack said: 'I don't think I am going to pull out of this. Now, you are my executor, I would just like to run through my affairs very briefly with you.' He took Hugh to his desk, which was full of index cards relating to his financial affairs, and of lists of people who owed him money. When he died, he said, he wanted Hugh to collect the sums due on the loans immediately.

Hugh Hubbard Ford saw Jack Hullett only one more time,

this time with Bobbie. They met at The Pilot, a pub across the road from Holywell Mount. Hugh said Jack seemed 'very frail and weak', although he was able to chat, but he said: 'I am too full of dope to say anything sensible.' Bobbie, he added, 'looked very strained and very worried'. A few days before this meeting, Jack had been examined by a heart specialist, as he had been very breathless, and struggled to walk up the stairs at home. Dr Roy Campbell Price concluded that Jack had been suffering from some type of heart trouble since childhood, and that his condition was now deteriorating. Because of the heart condition – never mind the cancer – there was a possibility that he might live only a few more months. He could die suddenly, at any time. However, he was not this direct with Jack, who came away from the consultation thinking his heart was functioning well.

Then, on 13 March, Jack suffered severe pains in his chest that looked very much like a heart attack. Dr Adams was summoned to Holywell Mount, and he escorted Jack up the stairs. One of Jack's nurses, Gladys Miller, thought it odd that the doctor steered Jack all the way to the top without a rest. 'During the three months I nursed Mr Hullett,' she said, 'I had assisted him to climb the stairs to his room on many occasions and he could only do this by resting at every second or third step.' About five or ten minutes after he reached the first floor, Jack once again had an acute pain in his chest and found breathing difficult. Nurse Miller thought this was a second heart attack – and later insinuated strongly that it had been brought on by Dr Adams.

Jack was put to bed, and at about 10.30 p.m. Dr Adams returned to check on him. He said later that Jack had suffered a bad headache that evening and 'I wasn't happy about him, so that is why I looked in last thing that night.' The nurse, Gladys Miller, was in Jack's bedroom, with Bobbie. 'I saw Dr Adams take from his case a small brown bottle,' she said, 'and standing in a darkened corner of the room draw up the liquid from the bottle into the hypodermic syringe and then inject the contents into the patient's left arm. I recognised the bottle used for the injection as a type which contains a highly-concentrated form of morphia . . .'

Gladys Miller stayed with Jack for the whole of the night. He was in a deep sleep, she said, and his breathing was stertorous – meaning that it was marked by a heavy snoring sound, or gasping. At six in the morning Nurse Miller drew close to Jack, and as she touched his bedclothes he woke up briefly, smiled and asked the time. She told him to go back to sleep for a couple of hours, and he settled down again. 'At about 6.45 a.m. I was in the dressing room making a cup of tea,' she said, 'when I suddenly realised I could not hear the patient breathing. I went immediately into the bedroom and found Mr Hullett was gasping his last, and in a matter of seconds he died . . .'

Dr Adams was summoned and soon arrived at Holywell Mount. 'He walked into the patient's bedroom,' said the nurse, 'and without looking at the body said: "Cerebral haemorrhage. In any case he was malignant. He complained of a headache last night."' So the official cause of death was not Jack's cancer, the botched operation, or his heart – but a cerebral haemorrhage, and although he had been so frail, friends described his death as sudden. 'Mr Hullett was a sick man,' said Nurse Miller, but 'I thought his death was unusual.' Jack Hullett was to be cremated – and so the doctor filled in and signed the required cremation form. In doing so, he declared that he did not expect to gain financially from Jack Hullett's will. There is no doubt that he knew this to be a lie.

It was Dr Adams who broke the bad news to Bobbie. 'Thank goodness we had the night nurse on,' he said, 'because if Mrs Hullett had been in the room when this happened I don't know what would have happened. I went to tell her and she jumped up and screamed and said, "Has Jack died?" I just looked at her and nodded and said, "Yes he is dead." She fell back on the bed and collapsed. Then she became quite impossible.' We do not know what words of comfort he offered Bobbie, but it seems that, because she was 'quite impossible', he gave her an injection 'to counteract shock'. At least, that is what the parlourmaid Mary Mayo told the housemaid Teresa Yogna.

For Bobbie, the next few days were horrendous. On Dr Adams's advice, she did not go to Jack's funeral, but stayed 'in bed, prostrate'. There was also a memorial service in London – but Bobbie was too distressed to attend. And from this point onwards, she was often in a bad way – emotionally unstable, sometimes desperate, and in poor health. Her housemaid, Teresa, noted that she had lost her appetite and smoked more than before. Her daughter Patricia said that: 'she kept saying she felt so ill. She looked awful and gradually, from March, got so thin.' The cook, Kathleen Durrant, commented on the contrast between Bobbie's happiness before Jack's illness, and her misery after he died: 'She changed very much, she was depressed for a long time and seemed to lose interest. Her moods varied. We would think, Oh, she is beginning to get better and then she would be going down. At first she cried a lot but not latterly. She seemed to be holding herself in.'

Sometimes, Bobbie found it hard to concentrate. At the best of times, she was not adept at paperwork. It was Jack who had taken care of all that, with his carefully maintained accounts books and perfectly filed index cards. But now she became altogether useless – which was a pity, because there was much to be done in winding up Jack's estate, valued at £94,644, and she was an executor, along with Hugh Hubbard Ford. Dr Adams was a legatee – receiving £500. But this was hardly noticed at the time, since the bulk of the work consisted of collecting money owed to Jack, and sorting out the death duties. Hugh Hubbard Ford said later that Bobbie's attitude was 'a very difficult one. She could not understand why death duties were payable at all, she could not understand her fate, and altogether she was in a very distressed frame of mind.' In fact, he found it easier to deal with the will without her help, and instead he sought the assistance of a local solicitor, John Dodd, and an old friend of Jack's and Bobbie's – Robert Handscomb.

John Dodd tried to include her in discussions about finances, but she 'gave me the impression of being unable or unwilling to grasp details or to concentrate on what was being discussed'. In general she was in an 'overwrought and nervous state'. Robert Handscomb commented on 'how awkward she was. How strange she was in her behaviour and what an anxiety it was to him . . .' Bobbie was not coping, not taking responsibility for herself. All her life she had been looked after and spoiled by men – and now when she was required to behave like a mature adult she found it impossible to summon up the resolve. The heroic spirit that she had shown during another crisis – the bombing of Eastbourne – had gone. Hugh Hubbard Ford was watching her closely and thought 'that she seemed to be under the influence of some sort of drug'.

The drugs in question were barbiturates, which Dr Adams continued to prescribe. Each morning he came to Holywell Mount and saw Bobbie in her bedroom, giving her two pills of high dose sodium barbiturate – 7½ grains (486 mg) each. These were to be taken at night, to ensure that she was able to sleep. He had a holiday planned from 1 to 18 May, so before he left he wrote a prescription for thirty-six tablets for her to take while he was away. During June and early July Bobby asked for a higher dose still but, said Dr Adams, he did not give it. Instead he tried reducing the dose to two 5-grain tablets, or sometimes 6. These lesser doses, though, were still extremely powerful.

Several people thought that Dr Adams was also giving Bobbie injections of some sort. Bobbie's friend Martha Henson said Bobbie had told her that the doctor was giving her injections, and that sometimes she gave herself injections. Another friend, William Galloway, came to stay at Holywell Mount for a few days in June. After the doctor had left the house, he said, Bobbie told him that he had given her an injection. Mary Mayo also thought that Bobbie was receiving injections, although Teresa Yogna said she did not find evidence of injections when she cleaned Bobbie's room – no 'ampules, cotton wool or anything that I expected to see . . .'

Everyone in the house agreed that Bobbie was sleepy, and sometimes dizzy in the mornings. Patricia described her 'occasional fits of giddiness' and the way 'she felt as if the floor was coming up to her'. Early in May, the Revd Harry Copsey accompanied Bobbie on a rare journey out of Eastbourne, when they went to Coventry to see the enthronement of a new bishop. 'Mrs Hullett had the greatest confidence in her doctor and spoke in glowing terms of his care,' he said. He noticed her take a tablet at dinner time. Very shortly afterwards she 'became pale and shrunken', and said that she would not be available until eleven o'clock in the morning. The Bishop, who knew Bobbie, 'was very distressed at her condition'. 'From the time of her husband's death,' said Teresa Yogna, 'Mrs Hullett began to appear drowsy and listless, and as time went on these symptoms increased and on one occasion when she came downstairs she looked like a drunken person. She had to walk by holding on to the furniture to steady herself, and I saw her on a number of occasions leaning against the wall for support.'

The staff at Holywell Mount – Mary, Kathleen and Teresa – were becoming suspicious of the treatment that Bobbie was receiving. Bobbie's friend Martha Henson visited her in April, the month after Jack had died. 'I saw the maid Teresa,' she said. 'She told me she wanted to tell the police that Mrs Hullett was being drugged by Dr Adams.' Teresa said that the cook, Kathleen, was willing to go to the police with her. When asked about this, Kathleen did not admit that she had been willing to bring in the police. 'Teresa is a nice girl, but rather excitable,' she said. But she did confirm that all the staff thought that Bobbie should get away from Eastbourne, and from the care of Dr Adams.

Martha Henson had her own concerns. Bobbie had told her that she always felt as though she were a long way off, and her head felt like cotton wool after the doctor's visits. 'It was common gossip in Eastbourne that Mrs Hullett was being drugged,' said Martha. In the end, Bobbie went to London with Martha – but would only stay one night. Bobbie had mentioned to Teresa that 'she did not like going away for long periods as Dr Adams did not allow her to do so'.

By mid-June 1956, said Teresa, 'Mrs Hullett had got weaker bodily and she became rather absent minded and . . . was forgetting things.' In early July, Bobbie attended the wedding of the daughter of her friend Marjorie Hawkins. Hugh Hubbard Ford thought 'she appeared most strained and strange . . . she gazed vacantly at us and didn't seem to know us, and many other friends remarked on exactly the same thing and we were given to understand that she was rather heavily doped for the occasion'. The Revd Harry Copsey agreed that she seemed 'very strained and unwell' at the wedding. Later in the day, though, he went back to Holywell Mount with Bobbie who suddenly perked up and 'appeared as well as I have ever known her'. This was the last time he ever saw her.

All of this – the mood swings, the muddled head, the giddiness, the drugs – was worrying, but most disturbing was Bobbie's talk of suicide. By the third month after Jack died, said the cook, Kathleen Durrant, she had lost the will to live. Her mother Gerty recalled visiting Bobbie, and looking around her bedroom, saying: 'How bright your brushes look.' It was small talk – the hairbrushes were mentioned just for something to say. But Bobbie's response changed the mood. 'Ask Patricia for those when I am gone,' she said. 'She had no interest at all in life,' said Gerty. Patricia remembered her mother saying, 'I wish I was dead.' The young woman found this hard to understand, and asked why they could not move out of Holywell Mount and 'have a little house somewhere – the two of us – and start again'. But Bobbie would not listen.

With Hugh Hubbard Ford, she was more direct. He noticed that sometimes she was well and cheerful one second, and then overwhelmed by gloom the next. She often turned to a favourite subject – namely, her despair about the future and her dismay that she did not have the courage to throw herself over Beachy Head. When she talked like this, Hugh would treat her remarks in a 'slightly jocular' manner, telling her that her attitude was a selfish one because of all the bother it caused other people. She brushed his views aside, he said, and on one occasion told him: 'I have got nothing to live for, if only you could get me a couple of drug pills, you could have the lot.' She was referring to her wealth, which she wished to trade for death. Hugh tried to reason with her, pointing out how much she had to live for – her daughter, her friends, her home and her 'lovely motor cars'. But, he acknowledged: 'I wasn't very effective in my arguments.'

Bobbie put the same proposition to the Revd Harry Copsey. On their return from the outing to Coventry she said to him: 'It is all yours if you will only put me out of the way.' But, of course, it was her doctor who had the means to deliver the drugs that she wanted. And, out of all her friends, he was the one who saw her most – every morning, when he came to the house bearing barbiturates.

When asked about Bobbie's suicidal state of mind, Dr Adams acknowledged that she had told him that she did not want to live. In reply, he said, he had tried to persuade her that she 'must live' because that is what Jack would have wanted, telling her: 'I have helped you through your troubles and I will help you always to get well. But pull yourself together.' According to Dr Adams, she had replied that she would not; that she did not want to.

She told him several times, he said, that she had taken a car and driven up to Beachy Head, but that something stopped her and she couldn't drive off the cliff. The doctor replied: 'That was Jack's influence, he would not let you do it.' She also talked about crashing her car, but worried that she might not be killed. On several occasions she said that she would swim out to sea. That, she thought, would look like an accident rather than suicide and would not be 'a blot on her daughter Patricia, and that was the only one she thought of'. If she asked Dr Adams for a fatal dose of drugs, as she had asked Hugh Hubbard Ford, he did not mention it.

On 12 July 1956 Bobbie made a trip to London to see her solicitor, in order to make a new will. Two days later, she saw the Eastbourne solicitor John Dodd, told him about the will, and confirmed that he was an executor. She asked him to reassure her that 'if anything happened to her' he and Robert Handscomb would 'see that Patricia was all right'. He did so. 'At this interview,' said John, 'I was favourably impressed with the change in her outlook,' he said. 'And she was more cheerful and more natural.' In this new will, she had left most of her estate to her daughter, and had decided that her Rolls-Royce Silver Dawn, worth close to £3,000, would go to Dr Adams.

The following day – Sunday 15 July – Bobbie's mood changed again, for the worse. She telephoned her doctor 'in a great state of agitation', having had no sleep. 'I gave her ½ a grain of Amytal to steady her,' he said. This was a small dose of a particularly strong barbiturate. Afterwards, he would describe her condition as a 'nerve storm' – a rather archaic description with no precise medical meaning, but his way of interpreting her extreme agitation.

The following day, Bobbie appeared 'cheerful and natural' again. 'I last saw Mrs Hullett alive on Monday 16 July 1956,' said Robert Handscomb, 'when she called at my home. She then seemed more determined than she had been of late. I gained the impression that she was more calm, as in the case of a person who has come to a decision about something.' On the evening of 17

July Dr Adams visited her and the conversation turned to motor cars. We do not know whether she mentioned that she had left the doctor her Rolls-Royce in her will, but Dr Adams did say that Bobbie told him she would like to give him some money for an MG sports car to add to his already impressive collection of motors, because this was something that Jack had promised him. She took out her cheque book and wrote him a cheque for £1,000.

On Wednesday 18 July the doctor took the cheque to his bank and asked for it to be given special clearance. This was the strangest thing. A 'special clearance' was a way of clearing a cheque far more quickly than the usual three days, and could be achieved within twenty-four hours. It was generally used if the recipient needed his money urgently – but Dr Adams did not, since he had tens of thousands of pounds in his bank accounts already, and was a wealthy man. Special clearance might also have been appropriate if Dr Adams had had doubts about Bobbie's financial credibility. But Bobbie Hullett was well known to be one of the wealthiest women in Eastbourne, and Dr Adams had daily experience of her affluent lifestyle – the big house, the servants, her furs and jewels, the Rolls-Royce. According to one account, when he asked the cashier Kenneth Pill for special clearance of the cheque, Dr Adams explained: 'This lady is not long for this world' – meaning that if she died before the cheque was cleared, he would not get his money. In any case, the bank allowed the special clearance.

On the morning of Thursday 19 July, said Dr Adams, Bobbie suffered another 'nerve storm'. This was around ten o'clock in the morning, when he came to visit. He said that the attack was similar to the one she had experienced on the previous Sunday, and she had told him that she 'just could not go on and she would not go on and that she was just going to swim out to sea and probably the next I would see [of her] would be her rotting body coming in about four days after'.

On Friday 19 July 1956 Bobbie's friend, Kathleen Reed, arrived at Holywell Mount. Kathleen had driven down from Yorkshire and was due to stay for a few days. She was one of Bobbie's oldest friends – they had been at school together and had known each other since they were eight years old; she was a practical, resourceful woman – a midwife and something of a feminist. The house was in desperate need of someone like her – mature and bright and sensible – to take control. As soon as she arrived at Holywell Mount that evening, she realised that something was wrong. 'I rang the bell and walked in as I usually did,' she said, 'and saw Mrs Hullett sitting in the study at the desk and she got up and came forward to meet me. I hadn't seen her since June and I thought she looked very much thinner on this occasion and she didn't seem to be well. When she greeted me, her walk was slightly unsteady. We talked about general things and for a few moments she would appear perfectly natural, but at other times she was very unhappy and depressed.' Kathleen Reed sensed that Patricia was anxious about her mother, and reassured her that she would look after Bobbie.

That evening Kathleen Reed and Bobbie had dinner together. They were warm and snug inside Holywell Mount, but outside a heavy thunderstorm was raging, and at ten o'clock Bobbie said that it had given her a headache and that she would go to bed. Kathleen had had a long journey, so an early night suited her well. Patricia was also in the house. She said that Bobbie looked tired, but that was normal: 'she said "goodnight" to me in the usual way and went to bed'. Before she went up, Bobbie stopped to chat to Mary Mayo, the parlourmaid. 'She didn't look unusually ill,' said Mary, 'she was quite her usual self and conversed about breakfast.' Bobbie had a drink of orange juice, which Mary had prepared. 'When she took her drink in my presence,' said Mary, 'she took nothing with it. No tablet or anything.' Mary Mayo said she went to bed at the same time, as did other members of the household. No one was disturbed during the night.

At eight o'clock the following morning Mary Mayo went up to Bobbie's bedroom, taking her a glass of orange juice. Bobbie was asleep, which was not unusual for that time of the morning, because of the sleeping pills she took; so Mary left the orange juice beside the bed and left the room. Bobbie did not stir. An hour later, Mary went up again, this time with Bobbie's breakfast on a tray. The orange juice was untouched, and Bobbie was still sleeping. Mary put the tray on a stand by the bed, left quietly, and went down to the servants' quarters to have her breakfast. At 8.30 that morning Patricia had left the house to go to her job as a secretary in Hailsham. Later, Kathleen Reed came down to breakfast. On learning that Bobbie was sleeping, she decided to go into town to do some shopping. Just before ten o'clock Dr Adams turned up, as usual. He went to Bobbie's bedroom door, saw she was sleeping, heard her breathing and, Mary stated, said something like 'Oh well, let her sleep.' He left, but said he might call back later in the day.

The household went about its business, the servants working downstairs preparing for the return of Kathleen and Patricia, and expecting a bleary Bobbie to emerge from her room. But as the hours passed, she remained in bed, lying perfectly still, slightly on her left side, sleeping deeply – and a day that should have been ordinary started to feel unsettled, faintly edgy. 'I shook her by the shoulder,' said Mary Mayo, but she would not wake. At lunchtime Mary went downstairs and came upon Kathleen Reed, who was returning from her shopping trip. Kathleen went up to the bedroom with Mary and said: 'Come on, Bob, wake up.' There was no response, so the two women decided to telephone the doctor.

They phoned at lunchtime, but Dr Adams was out and the call was taken by a receptionist, who said to phone again if Bobbie had not woken up by mid-afternoon. At three o'clock she was still sleeping, so Kathleen Reed telephoned again. It emerged that the doctor was at a medical conference in Lewes that afternoon, and according to Kathleen Reed, she asked if his partner would come to the house. Mary Mayo agreed that it was she and Kathleen Reed who suggested that a locum come. Dr Adams said that it was *his* suggestion that one of his partners, Dr Harris, go to Holywell Mount at once. Either way, Dr Vincent Harris now entered the scene, although it is uncertain whether, had he had his own way, Dr Adams would have liked him there.

Dr Harris said that until that day he had never encountered Bobbie Hullett – 'All I knew about her was purely from hearsay talk. I had heard that she was a rather neurotic type.' He arrived at Holywell Mount shortly after 3.30 in the afternoon, and examined her, and found that she had a slight squint, and that the pupils of her eyes were slightly contracted. Her pulse was 90 – and 'regular and full', respiration 24 breaths a minute, and her colour was good. Her reflexes were absent, and there seemed to be nothing wrong with her breathing or circulation. When Kathleen Reed mentioned Bobbie's headache of the night before, and a slight attack of giddiness, Dr Harris made the immediate diagnosis of a cerebral lesion, possibly a cerebral haemorrhage, cerebral thrombosis or cerebral tumour. As Bobbie was plainly in a coma, the doctor also wondered whether 'there was anything she might have taken, because the question of barbiturate or other sleeping drugs had entered my mind as a possible cause'. But he could see no signs of bottles or containers for pills in the room, empty or otherwise. And when he questioned Kathleen Reed she said she also had seen nothing, although she understood that Bobbie received sleeping tablets from Dr Adams.

Nobody mentioned to Dr Harris that Bobbie had, for the past five months, seemed drugged, or that she had been threatening suicide and talking explicitly about the ways in which she could kill herself – swimming out towards the horizon, until she lost her strength and drowned, or taking her car up on to Beachy

Head and driving into oblivion. And Dr Harris was not told that she had, more than once, offered all her money to someone who might give her a fatal dose of drugs or some other means of ending her life. But then, the women who happened to be in the house that Saturday – the staff, Kathleen, Mary and Teresa, the friend Kathleen Reed, and Bobbie's daughter Patricia – were only vaguely aware of the extent of Bobbie's anguish. Her more graphic threats had been made to men – to Robert Handscomb, John Dodd, Harry Copsey and Dr Adams.

At five o'clock that evening, Dr Adams arrived, and went straight to Bobbie's bedroom, where Kathleen Reed was keeping vigil. Kathleen remembered something about the doctor's arrival which was quite extraordinary in the light of subsequent events. When he entered the room, she stated: 'He said – "I don't know where she got them from and I am not touching anything" at the same time glancing around the room.' It was her impression that Dr Adams's first thought when he saw Bobbie in the bed was that she had taken an overdose. And, given that she had talked to him of suicide the day before, it was an obvious, logical conjecture. His words, though, are enigmatic: 'I don't know where she got them from and I am not touching anything.' Was he genuinely wondering where she might have got drugs from? Or did he know very well that she had a stash, but wished to distance himself? And that 'I am not touching anything' – it sounds as if he is anticipating an investigation.

His own version of what happened when he saw Bobbie in a coma and examined her rejects the idea of an overdose entirely. 'On Friday afternoon at 5 p.m. I didn't suspect poisoning in any form when I examined Mrs Hullett,' he said. He was put off 'any idea of drug causation' because of her squint (although a squint is, in fact, consistent with barbiturate poisoning). Also, her general condition was, in his view, good, her heart and her respiration being 'regular and normal'. He examined the room, he said, and saw no bottles on the side table. Dr Adams discussed Bobbie's condition with Dr Harris. He did not mention her suicide threats, or the fact that she had been taking heavy doses of barbiturates for at least five months. Instead, he favoured the diagnosis of 'cerebral lesion'.

When Robert Handscomb and his wife arrived that evening they accepted without question Dr Adams's view that this was a case of cerebral haemorrhage or something similar. When Patricia came home at six o'clock: 'It did cross my mind that Mummy might have done something to herself because she had been so miserable and unhappy.' But she did not mention the concern to Dr Adams because, like everyone else close to Bobbie, she completely trusted him. It was normal to trust a doctor, and not to question his judgement; and this particular doctor was the world expert on Bobbie and her health problems. Everyone knew that he knew about her professed wish to die.

He appeared to be utterly conscientious, and said he would stay the night at Holywell Mount. He also arranged for a night nurse to come to the house. Agnes Higgins arrived at 9 p.m., and was told that her patient was completely comatose and that nothing would rouse her. She asked the doctor about sleeping pills, but Dr Adams said Bobbie took only those he gave her each day, and there was no chance of her having more. He then told Nurse Higgins that she must not be moved 'because of her heart condition'. This was odd – as there had been no suggestion of a heart problem, and there was no subsequent indication of anything wrong with her heart. When Dr Adams left the room, she said, she checked the bedroom for medicine bottles – but found none. She didn't look inside cupboards or drawers, though. At first the night passed quietly. Bobbie continued to sleep; her breathing was natural. Her temperature and pulse did not give cause for concern.

That changed at three o'clock the following morning

– Saturday 21 July. Bobbie's breathing had become shallow and her pulse rapid. Nurse Higgins woke Dr Adams, who came at once and agreed that her condition was 'not so good', and he injected her with coramine – a stimulant that could be used to counteract the effects of barbiturates. At this stage it was obvious that Bobbie's situation was serious, and that Dr Adams knew it. Sometime during Saturday he told Robert Handscomb, who told John Dodd, that if she did not come out of the coma by Sunday evening then 'there would be little chance of recovery'. He also said that her chances of survival, overall, were fifty-fifty. And yet, Dr Adams did not think it right for Bobbie to be taken to hospital. She had told him, he said: 'Never remove me to Esperance [Nursing Home] or hospital whatever may be my condition.'

Later that Saturday morning, Dr Adams and Dr Harris called in a third doctor, Arthur Shera, who was a consultant pathologist to the Eastbourne Hospitals Group. Dr Shera came to Holywell Mount and took from Bobbie samples of cerebral fluid, urine and blood, in order to do some tests. By now, Bobbie was showing signs of pneumonia, and Dr Adams gave her a penicillin injection. That afternoon Dr Shera told Dr Adams that his tests showed slightly raised protein and sugar levels and some tinging of the blood. A cerebral haemorrhage could produce these findings, he said, but the results were inconclusive. Dr Shera then visited the local Princess Alice Hospital with the urine sample, which he gave to the chief laboratory technician for analysis. On the form he filled out, he wrote 'investigation suggested' and 'excess of barbiturates'. The technician asked if the examination was urgent and needed to be done that day – Saturday. Dr Shera replied that it was not urgent, and said, 'Monday will do.'

While Dr Shera was at the hospital, Dr Adams was back at Holywell Mount telling Patricia that her mother was suffering from a cerebral problem. But immediately afterwards he went to the Princess Alice Hospital and changed tack entirely, for the first time talking seriously about the possibility of an overdose. He spoke to Dr Peter Cook, a surgeon at the hospital, about a new drug called Megimide which could be used to treat barbiturate poisoning and, if administered early and properly, might save a life. Dr Cook remembered that he and Dr Adams had been discussing Megimide just two days previously (in the hours before Bobbie took her overdose).

Dr Adams acquired 100 ml of the drug from the hospital dispensary, which came with a pamphlet on its use. Dr Cook explained that Megimide was best administered through an intravenous infusion. If done by intravenous injection, then 'it should be done very slowly in doses of 10 ml every five minutes'. The instructions were perfectly clear. And it was also obvious that Megimide would be better administered in hospital. Peter Cook said he expected to see this patient during the weekend at the Princess Alice, but she never came.

Dr Adams returned to Holywell Mount that afternoon, he said, and gave Bobbie 10 ml of the Megimide intravenously, and then no more. The problem was – as was written in the pamphlet and then stressed by Dr Cook – she needed 10 ml every five minutes. One dose on its own was entirely useless. The doctor again spent the night at the house. Dr Harris looked in at about ten o'clock, and the doctors gave Bobbie more penicillin. Nurse Higgins asked Dr Adams about Bobbie's general condition, and he replied: 'It is something cerebral. It must be because of the temperature', thus reverting to the 'cerebral' diagnosis. He did not mention anything about an overdose, or the Megimide. Bobbie had another bad night – so bad, said Nurse Higgins, that she and Dr Adams both thought she would die that day.

At nine o'clock that Sunday morning Dr Adams telephoned the coroner for Eastbourne, Dr Angus Sommerville, and asked whether he could arrange a private post-mortem on Bobbie's body. Private post-mortems were unusual, and Dr Sommerville was taken aback by the peculiarity of the request. The phone call became odder still when the coroner asked the doctor for the time of death of his patient, and was told that she was not, in fact, dead yet. Dr Adams was told, in the plainest of terms, that if his patient were to die, he would have to go through the normal procedure and notify the coroner's office then.

Half an hour later Dr Harris met Dr Adams at Holywell Mount, and Dr Harris gave Bobbie an injection of crystamycin – a penicillin compound. Dr Adams now said that, rather than dying, Bobbie was responding well to the injections, and all that day everyone's hopes for her were raised. But in the evening, she took a sudden turn downwards. Her temperature shot up to 105 degrees, and her colour, her heartbeat and her breathing all became worse. Another crystamycin injection was given – and, once more, Dr Adams settled down to stay the night at Holywell Mount.

At 2.30 in the morning, Nurse Higgins saw that Bobbie's temperature had risen again. So she woke Dr Adams, who gave Bobbie an injection of coramine and antropine. 'The patient's reaction was nil,' said Agnes Higgins. 'In fact there was no reaction at all from that time onwards, her condition didn't improve.' She called Dr Adams again at 6.30 a.m. because she thought it was 'only a matter of minutes' before Bobbie died. 'He agreed with me,' she said, 'and he said "We will give her oxygen as a last resort."' But the oxygen had no effect, and Bobbie deteriorated further. At about the same time Patricia woke up, because she heard someone walking about. 'I opened the door and met Dr Adams outside,' she said, 'and he told me Mummy would probably only live an hour. I realised then that I had expected it really in a way since Friday.' Bobbie Hullett died at 7.23 a.m., on Monday 23 July 1956.

The news soon spread beyond the ornate gates of Holywell Mount, giving the gossips of Eastbourne much to talk about because, as anyone in the tea rooms and hotel lobbies would tell you, this was not the first time that Dr Adams had presided over the unusual death of a wealthy widow. Generally, when such deaths occurred, they had been examined only through the prism of insinuation and suspicion. But now, because of the disputed cause of death, there would be an inquest and, God willing, proper public scrutiny.

2

The Young Doctor

D R JOHN BODKIN Adams had always presented himself as a good Christian doctor, whose mission was to do God's work. He kept in his desk a long tract as 'a kind of aide-memoire to the good and proper life'. Part of it read:

Am I – kind, gentle, loving, meek, patient, thoughtful for others?
Helpful to those around? Not given to rashness, criticism, foolishness?
Am I wise, earnest, cheerful, prayerful, honest, fearless, determined?

A text on the wall above his bed read 'Rest in the Lord', and another in the surgery was framed: 'One Day, One Step'. His religion was an essential part of him and, as he would tell anyone who asked, that was because of his upbringing and the firm guidance of his parents, Samuel and Ellen Adams.

He was their first child. Born in 1899 in Randalstown in Northern Ireland, and raised there, he had a strong Ulster accent that marked him out as different when he came to live in Eastbourne. His particular branch of Christianity – the Plymouth Brethren – was also a distinctive marker, which could make him seem unusually pious and caring, or hypocritical, or strange, depending on your point of view.

In Plymouth Brethren communities, the head of the household played a particularly strong role and Samuel Adams conscientiously presided over the moral welfare of his family, leading prayers every morning and night, and a Bible class every Sunday. John's earliest memory, he said, was of disobeying his father, who then caused him to 'regret it'. We do not know what punishment the young boy received, but his offence is known, and it is very minor. A friend had offered him an apple, and he had refused it. Samuel bore down on this act of ingratitude. His father's reaction, said Dr Adams, 'taught me that you can never begin to train a child too young. If I had not been corrected then it would have had a grave influence on my future life.' Small transgressions were to be stamped upon, and that was good. His mother's approach to life was equally pious, and had earned her the reputation in some circles of being 'the most religious woman in Ireland'.

The constant prayers and this harsh first memory give an impression of an austere childhood, but there was occasional gaiety in the Adams household. Ellen, according to her son, was one of 'the pioneer lady cyclists of 1900', and Samuel cycled too. The image of him, all long limbs and bony, cycling around country roads on one of the first penny-farthings in the county is a happy one. 'We used to stand on the pavement in amazement and watch him fly past,' said a neighbour, Paddy Kane. 'He was very popular and was known to be a good man.' When motorcycles came to Ireland, Samuel Adams bought one; and after the motorcycle, he made his most daring purchase – a Wolseley open top motor car.

There was money in the family – Samuel had a jewellery and watch business, which did well, and Ellen had an eye for a good investment, particularly in property. So, when John was three or four, the family moved to a better house – at Ballinderry Bridge in County Tyrone. This was a proud and solid home, the best in the village, with fine views over Loch Neagh to the mountains beyond, and it was there that, in 1903, a second Adams child was born. He was named William. Friends later remembered that

William was the carefree, fun-loving boy, while John was more inclined to avoid other children and to stick close to his mother. And it was observed that John was 'a wee bit mean'. But these are isolated comments made to journalists long after John Bodkin Adams left Northern Ireland. Others may have had a different view.

When John was 12, the family moved again. This time to Coleraine, so that he might study at Coleraine Academical Institution; and it was about now that the pressure grew for the boy to pursue a career in medicine. He had been named after Ellen's brother, John Bodkin, a brilliant doctor and missionary, and there were other medics among his uncles and cousins. So doctoring was in the family – and it was an ideal occupation for a good Christian man, since it combined God's work in caring for the sick with a good income.

John was set on this course, and was on the point of entering the medical school at Queen's University in Belfast when tragedy struck – Samuel Adams died of a stroke at the age of 57. John, as the eldest boy, would now have the duty of leading the family both economically and morally, and success at Queen's became vital to him. He worked extremely hard, supported by his mother Ellen, who moved to Belfast to be near him. Also in the household were his brother William and his cousin Sarah Henry, who was John's age. Sarah had been taken in by her Aunt Ellen when her own mother died. It was at this time that Ellen asked her two sons to sign a declaration: 'In God's name and with His help I do promise to abstain absolutely from every form of intoxicating drink, also from gambling in every form knowing this to be the wishes of my father and mother . . .' As any good son would, the two boys signed.

It soon became clear that John Adams was not a particularly bright student, and despite his exertions he failed to keep up. He struggled socially too – and his anatomy teacher, Richard Hunter, noticed that he did not fit in. When the professor gave his class a body to dissect, he assigned three of his young men an arm, another three a leg, and so on. In general the students became friends, and stuck to their sets until the end of the course. But not John, who wandered around joining in where he could, first with one group and then another. It did not help that he was physically unattractive, being pinkish and on the chubby side, or that he possessed fat sausage-like fingers that were unseemly in a doctor. Thus a picture of him at Queen's emerges – he is slightly isolated but studying hard. His strength comes from his religion, and from his devoted family.

Then, in 1918, his younger brother William died of influenza – 15-year-old William, who was sunnier and more sociable than John, artistically inclined, more handsome, and probably the brighter son. This was a devastating bereavement for the family – and for John it brought an extra dimension. He was now the only boy left. If the family was to have a happy secure future, it fell to him alone to deliver it. All his subsequent actions, and words, make it clear that he saw himself as a provider for Ellen and for Sarah; and so he worked late night after night, however tired he felt. His efforts were admirable, but in the end the work-load overwhelmed him and one day he collapsed, and was forced to take to his bed. At first it was thought that he was suffering from tuberculosis, 'the white plague'. This proved not to be the case, and he later told people that his incapacity was due to a 'virulent septic infection'. It seems more likely that, exhausted by intellectual demands, the young man was on the brink of a nervous breakdown. His teachers were so concerned about him that they advised that he give up medicine altogether.

For some this might have been a relief, but for John it was a terrible prospect. He felt he owed it to Ellen and Sarah, to his dead father and brother, to Uncle John Bodkin and to the Plymouth Brethren, to succeed. At first, he stayed in bed and was nursed by the two women in his life. Both were devoted to John and had a high opinion of him. And, indeed, it was a striking characteristic of his personality that, whatever doubts he may have had in his heart, he appeared to others to have an excessively high opinion of himself. At home he was a hero, but at university he was facing the possibility of failure. The discrepancy was stark.

Faced with this crisis in his life John decided to give his studies one final push. After several months of his unexplained debilitating illness, he returned to university and worked even harder than before, doing whatever it took to catch up on missed lessons. To his credit, he did not crash out again and managed to obtain his degree – though it was without honours. This was not a glittering start to his career, but the achievement was none the less great. He had overcome adversity, and as a doctor he was now automatically entitled to considerable status within his family and society, and an unquestioned authority over patients. In future years, he was to demonstrate repeatedly that it was vital to him that other people recognised his hard-won status, and showed him deference. If they did not, it made him angry.

John's next task was to find a job. And this was achieved with the help of Professor Arthur Rendle Short, a fellow member of the Plymouth Brethren, who had met John at a missionary study class. The professor, who was a doctor at Bristol Royal Infirmary, invited the newly qualified Dr Adams to take up a junior post there. 'This I accepted,' said Dr Adams, 'and found myself on duty at Bristol within two weeks.' Once again he worked around the clock, both to fulfil his duties as a house assistant, and also to qualify for a diploma in public health. The one break he had was Sunday when, he explained, 'I went to church in the morning then took a 5-mile walk into the country, returned to Bristol for the Plymouth Brethren services in the evening . . . and then home to bed.' But, despite his diligence, he seems not to have settled in Bristol, being unhappy that Ellen and Sarah could not join him. And deep inside he must have known – how could he not? – that he lacked the brains and the flair for a brilliant career in hospital work. Not that he admitted that to others: 'I had excellent prospects of an academic career at Bristol,' he said. To someone who did not know him well, the comment might appear boastful. To those closer to him – except perhaps Ellen and Sarah – it was simply unrealistic.

Then, in the winter of 1921–2, Arthur Rendle Short handed Dr Adams an advertisement which had been cut out of a Christian weekly newspaper. A group of Christian GPs in Eastbourne was looking for someone to join the practice, with a view to a partnership. The young doctor took the hint and, in February 1922, on 'a filthy night' he arrived in Eastbourne to attend an interview. There was nobody at the railway station to meet him, and his first impression of Eastbourne was not good. But, after being interviewed the following day by Drs Gurney, Emerson and Rainey, he was offered a place at the 6 College Road practice – and he returned to Bristol to consider his options. For a while he put off a decision, then Rendle Short said to him: 'Adams, I can trust you to take that job. Go to Eastbourne. I can trust you to keep abreast of the times and not to sink into oblivion.' At least, this is Dr Adams's version of their conversation. 'I never go past the red light,' he added. 'I pray and wait. When the professor said "Go" . . . it was like the walls of Jericho falling. And so – in the spring of 1922 – I went to Eastbourne.' The truth was that general practice would allow him to fashion a life in which he did not struggle, in which he might set his own terms and receive the respect that he, very clearly, felt was his due. He could set up a home with Ellen and Sarah, and reinvent himself as a family doctor – a man who could go about his work generally unobserved by his peers, creating his own style, doing things his own way.

For a man whose sense of self-worth was both elevated and easily broken, it also helped that Eastbourne was a prosperous and fashionable town. There was a certain windswept grandeur about the lie of the land, from the drama of Beachy Head and the

South Downs to the west, and the long flat view towards Pevensey Bay and Hastings in the east. The regiment of Victorian villas and hotels that faced the English Channel was impressive too, particularly the palatial Grand Hotel, which in the first decades of the twentieth century attracted the smartest of visitors. The Kings of Spain and Greece stayed there, as did the Viceroy of India, assorted Lords and Ladies, and celebrities such as the ballerina Anna Pavlova, the singers Paul Robeson and Nellie Melba, the composer Edward Elgar, and the aviator Amy Johnson. The explorer Ernest Shackleton had long lived in Eastbourne – and the fact that great swathes of the town were owned by the Duke of Devonshire added to its cachet. Dr Adams was sensitive to such things, and he was to be marked out by the zeal with which he cultivated Eastbourne's in-crowd and by his high regard for the social rituals of the Home Counties – the charity dances, afternoon tea at the Grand and even, despite his promise to Ellen, sherry at noon.

But first the young GP had to establish his credentials by putting in long hours, making any number of home visits, and building up a sizeable, profitable practice. This Dr Adams did with alacrity. He purchased a bicycle, and then a motor-scooter, and zipped about Eastbourne working from early morning until late in the evening, and quickly earned a reputation as a doctor who could be called out in the middle of the night or at weekends. The treatments he provided were, in the main, basic. Antibiotics had not yet been discovered. Vaccines were few. On one occasion, he recalled, he applied leeches to an elderly woman with pneumonia. 'She did very well,' he said, 'and made a full recovery.' More conventionally, he could provide aspirin and morphine to alleviate pain, a referral to a surgeon when needed, and the valuable and comforting aura of the professional man. And sometimes he laced his treatments with a generous dose of Christianity, openly expressing his trust in the Good Lord for a favourable medical outcome.

The Plymouth Brethren remained a central part of his life – both in and out of work. When Ellen and Sarah arrived in Eastbourne, the household began the day with family prayers, followed by prayers at the surgery in College Road. With local dentist Norman Gray, Dr Adams set up the Eastbourne branch of the Young Crusaders Bible Class, and he quickly established himself as a prominent member of the local YMCA. But his overt Christianity and good works sat slightly awkwardly with his obvious leanings of a worldly kind. From the beginning, Dr Adams seemed to be very impressed by the lifestyles of the Eastbourne elite, and particularly attentive to those patients who possessed Rolls-Royces and large houses. There were plenty of these in and around Eastbourne, and one of the finest was a 500-acre estate called Ratton, near Willingdon, at the edge of the South Downs.

One day, sometime in the 1920s, Dr Adams was called out to attend a patient at Ratton – and the image of him arriving on his motor-scooter is an arresting one. He would have passed by the old gatehouse, driven through 'beautiful pleasure grounds' of 'gardens, park and woodlands', and arrived at an extraordinary mansion, newly built in the Elizabethan style. The outside was a fabulous confusion of half-timbering and mullioned windows, and the interior was magnificent, resembling a Scottish hunting lodge – all wood-panelling, baronial crests and mounted stags' heads.

Ratton undoubtedly impressed the young man. It was home to William and Edith Mawhood. William was 61, and had made his money as a steel man in Sheffield, manufacturing good-quality tools and cutlery. (Some ninety years later, Mawhood Bros bevel-edged chisels and beech-handled gouges still turn up on internet auction sites and at car boot sales.) Edith was younger. She was 43 when the couple moved into Ratton, and was a feisty, straight-talking person, the daughter of an East London warehouseman who had gone up in the world when she became William's second wife.

The couple had no children, and so shared the twenty-nine-bedroom house, in the main, with their servants. This was not the grandest sort of English household, the type that was still sometimes to be found at the country estates of the aristocracy. But it was a fine example of the middle-class upstairs-downstairs arrangement that was common in the life and literature of the time. Had a murder happened in the Mawhood home, detectives might have had an entire household of witnesses and suspects to interview – the cook, the maids, the gardeners, the chauffeur, the housekeeper, the valet. The maids would have been in uniform, though starched white caps were, by now, loathed by those who had to wear them. And housemaids and kitchenmaids who were addressed by their employers simply as 'Gladys' or 'Elsie' or 'Mary' were coming to resent the lack of respect. The dramatic decline of domestic service was beginning. But in the Eastbourne area this process was to be exceedingly slow, and the investigation that follows has in it a supporting cast of servants, watching and remembering. This was the world imagined by Agatha Christie, whose country house murder-mysteries had a reference point in real homes, in houses like Ratton.

In this sort of society, the family doctor played his part. The wealthier classes would not expect to join long queues of their poorer neighbours, in order to see a GP in his surgery. Instead, if someone became ill, a medical man would be called to the home, and it was not unusual for the family doctor to become a friend or adviser. So, when Edith Mawhood had an accident and broke her leg sometime in 1923 or 1924, she did not rush to a GP's surgery or a hospital. Instead, a search was made in Eastbourne to find a doctor who could come out to Ratton, and Dr John Bodkin Adams responded. He examined the broken leg, Edith said, and arranged for treatment. But it never mended properly despite three operations on it. Other than her leg difficulties – she and William were perfectly healthy.

Nevertheless, Dr Adams kept returning to Ratton. He was not

summoned by Edith or William Mawhood, but just turned up twice a week to check on their health. 'He always used to visit at meal times,' said Edith, who felt she had no option but to offer the doctor something to eat. On other occasions he arrived in the morning at sherry time, and often he brought with him his mother, Ellen, and cousin Sarah: 'he used to leave them sitting on the terrace outside my house whilst he visited. The servants always provided tea for all of them.' After a while, Dr Adams had become such a regular feature in the Mawhoods' life that they started to include him in their social events, inviting him to the pheasant shoots on their land. Dr Adams, it turned out, was a keen shot.

Edith noticed that the doctor could be rather pushy. She later told the story of how, when her leg started to improve, she had decided to recuperate at a house she owned in Lynton on the north Devon coast. Instead of wishing her well and offering a few words of encouragement, as might be expected, Dr Adams said that he too would like to visit Devon, and that he would make the trip as a passenger in her motor car. Despite his audacity, Edith agreed, and set off with the doctor and her chauffeur, with the two men sharing the driving. When they arrived, it transpired that Dr Adams had not arranged any accommodation for himself, and he announced that, in fact, he would stay with Edith in her house. Once again she agreed. It got worse. She noticed that he had not brought any luggage with him – so she loaned him some of her husband's pyjamas.

There were other quirks that stayed in the memory. William Mawhood had a brother who was also in the steel business. He mentioned this brother to Dr Adams, and said that he could get hold of good-quality medical instruments at wholesale prices. The doctor made it clear that he would like some of these instruments for himself. 'My husband got him a very nice case with all the medical instruments fitted into compartments,' said Edith. But the doctor never paid for them. Instead he used to tell Edith that he was hard up, and she would occasionally lend him a pound or a ten-shilling note. On another occasion, William Mawhood bought a mackintosh. Dr Adams admired it, then visited the shop that it came from, acquired an identical mackintosh for himself, and charged it to William's account. He never repaid the Mawhoods. Then he did the same thing again – this time with a new pair of boots.

If Dr Adams had been hard up in 1922, when he first arrived in Eastbourne, he did not intend to remain that way. As his private practice grew and he became wealthier, he stopped using his motor-scooter, and acquired a car, and then another. First there was a Renault two-seater coupé, next a Belsize, then came a Humber 15, after that a Hillman, then an Austin with a specially customised chassis for carrying medical equipment. It was noticed that he took immense trouble in caring for his cars – and that he constantly seemed to be seeking a model bigger and better than those he already owned. In 1920s Eastbourne, a motor car was a tremendous status symbol. Most people could not afford one, but the rich elite – the stockbrokers, retired businessmen and wealthy widows – owned fancy cars, and some paraded about in a Rolls-Royce, a Bentley or a Daimler. A few people employed chauffeurs, and in 1928 Dr Adams joined this special group, and took on a chauffeur of his own called David Jenkins, who ferried the doctor from one house call to the next, and when Dr Adams did not need him, he took Ellen and Sarah on shopping trips and outings to the countryside. The doctor 'never had less than two cars at any one time and he was frequently changing the make of cars he used', said Mr Jenkins.

The chauffeur also noticed that his boss was becoming increasingly interested in shooting, and was a guest at a great many shooting parties, not just at the Mawhoods' estate, but 'throughout the country and Scotland'. Mr Jenkins recalled that the doctor was on 'very friendly' terms with his next-door neighbour, Mrs Young. He said that on his birthday she bought him a very smart set of guns: 'I am almost certain it was a pair of Purdey 12 bore sporting guns . . .' He also remembered that Mrs Young was a wealthy woman who owned a Daimler car and had her own chauffeur.

Dr Adams next decided that it was time to move to a grander house and in 1930 he found a suitable property. It was called Kent Lodge and was in a road named Trinity Trees, in the centre of the town, just back from the sea and close to some of Eastbourne's best hotels. It was advertised as a 'four-square, superior, Victorian villa, adequate front lawn and spacious back garden' – and was quite spacious inside. A semi-basement could be used for the Young Crusader Bible classes. Half the ground floor became his surgery and consulting room, and there were eight bedrooms in total throughout the house, some of which were used for himself, Ellen, Sarah and the chauffeur. Others became storage rooms for his growing collection of guns and, in time, his fishing rods, golf clubs and cameras. The price of the house was £3,000, which Dr Adams borrowed from Edith and William Mawhood. Edith said that he did, in this case, pay up what was owed to her.

Even in these early days, Dr Adams divided people. Many were impressed by his hard work and close attention to his patients, and found him good-natured, even charming. Others described him as voluble and cocksure. Elsie Muddell was one of his detractors. 'I didn't like Dr Adams from the start,' she said, and told the story of being on the point of giving birth to her daughter when the doctor came to see her and gave her a 'mixture to ease my pains'. The medicine, she thought, made her worse and she refused to take any more after the first dose. 'Dr Adams was furious when he knew,' she recalled, 'and prescribed the hot water treatment for me – sitting on a pail of hot water.' After that, she loathed him, but could not avoid him, since they were both involved with the YMCA. 'I always put people against Dr Adams whenever I could,' she said.

Eva Carlyle also had doubts about Dr Adams. She had moved to Eastbourne with her husband in the 1920s, and consulted the doctor because she was run down. Consultants had told her she was suffering from tuberculosis, but on a visit to Switzerland the diagnosis had been disputed by experts there, leaving the cause of her poor health a mystery. Dr Adams now told her she was suffering from gall stones and 'suddenly suggested or rather ordered' that she have an operation, and with no further consultation he made arrangements for the operation to take place. 'The suggestion of an operation for gall stones was a complete shock to me and although I pointed out to Dr Adams that I never had any symptoms of gall stones, he still persisted and continued to make the arrangements . . .' said Mrs Carlyle. She then consulted her brother, Colonel M. W. Walker, who was a doctor, and mentioned to him that Dr Adams had not arranged for any X-rays to be carried out. The Colonel took his sister to London for a second opinion, and Mrs Carlyle's scepticism proved well-founded. No suggestion could be found of a problem with gall stones, and the plans for an operation were dropped.

Mrs Donnet, who was in her seventies, was another detractor. She was still in good enough health to enjoy a game of tennis, but some time in 1934 or 1935 a ball struck her in the eye with some force. Then she had a second tennis accident, and Dr Adams was sent for. The doctor told her that because of her damaged eye she would be unable to sign cheques, and announced that he would take over Power of Attorney for her. Mrs Donnet was upset by this unexpected turn of events. Elsie Randall, who lived nearby, visited her the same day and offered to see her bank manager 'with a view to forestalling the doctor'. Mrs Donnet thought that a good idea – and Elsie Randall hurried off to Barclays Bank in Terminus Road. Forms were produced, and Mrs Donnet signed them, giving Power of Attorney to Miss Randall and the bank manager. When Dr Adams returned and found that his efforts had been frustrated, he became 'very annoyed'.

Other patients thought the doctor utterly wonderful, and welcomed him into their lives. One of these was Matilda Whitton, a widow who in the 1930s was living as a permanent guest of the Kenilworth Court Hotel in Eastbourne. She had been born into a lower-class family in Warwick. Her parents' marriage certificate of 1860 shows that her father, George Chaplin, was a journeyman carpenter, and that her mother Elizabeth was illiterate, signing her name with a cross. Matilda, though, prospered when at the age of 37 she found a husband – Robert Whitton, who was a 56-year-old widower from Northampton. Robert, it seems, earned a good living as a manufacturer of shoe lasts in a town that was world renowned for its shoe factories. The couple had no children of their own, but Matilda inherited two stepchildren, Amy and Robert.

After her husband's death, Matilda, who was now in her seventies, moved south to Eastbourne, which at the time was reputed to be the 'healthiest town in England'. She was now a wealthy woman, owning shares in the Northampton shoe industry, the Northampton Brewery Company, Lever Brothers, *The Financial Times*, Rand Mines and Imperial Tobacco, and her income was quite sufficient to finance her new life at the Kenilworth Court Hotel, a central part of which was her daily visit from her doctor. There did not seem to be a medical reason for such close attention, but Matilda welcomed it, and came to regard Dr Adams with great affection.

The doctor regularly lent Mrs Whitton his car and also his chauffeur, David Jenkins, who would take her for drives in the country, and sometimes back to Northampton on business trips or to see her friends there. In the summer, she went for picnics at Beachy Head with the doctor's mother, Ellen, and his cousin, Sarah. And when Dr Adams suggested that Mrs Whitton send for a little two-seater motor car that she owned to be sent down from Northampton, she agreed, and told a friend that once the car had arrived in Eastbourne, she had given it to the doctor as a gift. Word went about that she had then bought him a second car – this one brand new.

During Mrs Whitton's time in Eastbourne she became increasingly ill, and in time her outings in Dr Adams's chauffeur-driven car became fewer – 'she seemed to have no energy and was always tired and spent many days, and sometimes weeks, in bed'. The doctor, of course, visited every day, and a chambermaid at the Kenilworth Court Hotel, Elsie Gander, said that she often found him in Mrs Whitton's room 'holding the patient's hand or with his hand on her knees'. Mrs Whitton would refer to him as 'my John', and her friend Beryl Buck said: 'She had two enlarged photographs of Dr Adams in her room. She was obviously very attached to him and at one time told me that she thought Dr Adams would marry her.' She was forty years older than him, but there is no evidence to suggest she found the age gap extraordinary, or the idea of marrying her young doctor implausible. Certainly, he seemed to have found his way into the intimate workings of her finances, and she told her friend Beryl that he was 'arranging her affairs and helping with her investments'.

Mrs Whitton's lawyer was Herbert James of Eastbourne, who also happened to be Dr Adams's solicitor. Mr James later confirmed that she made three wills while she lived at the Kenilworth Court Hotel. The first in 1929, the second in 1932, and the third in 1933. The first two wills were made with Mrs Whitton giving direct instructions to Mr James in person. The third will was different. It was Dr Adams who called into Mr James's office to tell him of the new instructions – Mrs Whitton, he said, wished to make a legacy of £500 to the doctor's cousin, Sarah Henry, along with another of £100 to the Mansfield Hospital. The doctor himself was to become the residual legatee. He was also the executor of the will. Mr James then visited Mrs Whitton at the Kenilworth Court Hotel, where she was laid up in bed.

She confirmed that all the changes mentioned by Dr Adams were correct, and she signed the new will.

About this time, some of the staff at the hotel became concerned about the effect they thought Dr Adams was having on Matilda Whitton's state of health. The chambermaid, Elsie Gander, noticed that she seemed drained of energy and lifeless when Dr Adams was around, spending many days or weeks in bed. When he was away on holiday, though, 'she seemed much better and would be up most of the time'. Lucy Atkins, the manager of the hotel, said that every time Mrs Whitton had been away from Eastbourne, she always looked in good health. But, on her return, would become ill again. 'I asked her once why she always came to Eastbourne,' she said, 'as I did not think the place suited her. I do not know, of course, whether she was ill in Northampton.'

Little is known of the medical treatment that Matilda Whitton was receiving other than the observation of a local chemist that her prescriptions were of a 'hypnotic sedative type'. And there were occasional injections. Beryl Buck remembered going to visit her friend one day and finding her very ill. Dr Adams had just visited and had given Mrs Whitton an injection. According to Beryl, 'she thought the injections upset her'. She also thought that Dr Adams was going to return that evening to give her another one, so she asked Beryl to leave a message with the hotel management saying she did not want to see him. 'I discussed this with her,' said Beryl, 'she was quite definite about it and I left a message to that effect at the hotel office. I wondered what the reaction of the doctor would be and I positioned myself to see him when he arrived.'

Dr Adams was in the habit of using a side door of the hotel which allowed him to go straight to Mrs Whitton's room without encountering hotel staff. On this occasion, though, the side door was shut and he was forced to use the main entrance. Beryl said: 'I saw him come in and having received the information he appeared very annoyed, threw his bag on to a chair with such force that it rebounded, he grabbed his coat, went out and really slammed the door.' On another occasion when Mrs Whitton seemed very ill, Dr Adams told the hotel manager that she might not last the night. The manager asked Dr Adams to communicate with Mrs Whitton's relatives, so that they might be at her side. Although he knew of her stepchildren in Northampton, he replied that she had no relatives. Whether he was following her wishes to keep her stepchildren away, or had some other motive for lying, it is impossible to know.

A state registered nurse named Bridget Monnolly remembered being called to the Kenilworth Court Hotel and attending an elderly lady who was confined to bed, and who had a photograph of Dr Adams in her room. It was obviously Mrs Whitton. 'She was quite conscious,' said Bridget, 'and asked me if I knew Dr Adams. I said I did and she passed some remark to the effect that she thought he was a very nice person . . .' Bridget noticed that the patient was restless and thought she must have a heart condition or be in danger of having a stroke. 'I went out of the room then to change and left Dr Adams in the room with the patient. I returned after five minutes and Dr Adams met me just outside the door. He said he had given the patient an injection and that she was sleeping comfortably.' Bridget asked if the lady had any relatives, and the doctor said that she had not, and mentioned that he was the sole executor of her will. 'He told me not to sit in the room as the patient did not like the light on.' Dr Adams had stayed for an hour and left at about 11 p.m.

After he left, Bridget sat outside Mrs Whitton's room, but went inside from time to time to check on her. An hour or two after midnight she noticed a change in her patient's breathing, which was heavy, and 'she appeared very ill to me and appeared to have had a stroke and was unconscious'. Bridget notified Dr Adams, who came at once to the hotel. 'He gave the patient a hypodermic injection and I was present in the room at the time.

He did not inform me of the type of injection given on either occasion.' He then left, and asked to be kept informed of Mrs Whitton's condition. 'The patient's condition got gradually worse, her pulse becoming weaker and she remained unconscious, but I could not say whether as a result of the drug or her general condition. She remained in that condition about two hours and then, quite suddenly, her breathing became shallow and her pulse much weaker. I notified the doctor, but before he arrived she was dead.' Dr Adams gave the causes as 'myocardial degeneration, high blood pressure, renal insufficiency'. These were all chronic problems and not actually causes of death – and they did not fit well with the treatment the doctor had given Matilda Whitton. The date was 11 May 1935.

Elsie Gander said that another chambermaid, Mrs Flint, had noticed Dr Adams put a bottle of Mrs Whitton's pills in his pocket. Mrs Flint had also said that the doctor had given her a pound note, and told her to keep the death quiet. The nurse, Bridget Monnolly, said that she had removed Matilda Whitton's watch after she died. She then saw Dr Adams pick it up and take it away with him, along with a small attaché case. 'We discussed this matter at some length,' said Elsie, 'as we were very suspicious and had been so for some time.'

The estate of Matilda Whitton proved to be a substantial one – some £11,465 (worth about £600,000 now). Her outstanding bills were few – she had purchased a red straw hat and blue purse from Bobby and Co, an Eastbourne department store, also a fur coat, five massage treatments and seven electrical treatments. The legacies she bestowed were £1,000 to the Northampton General Hospital to endow a bed in her name, another £1,000 for the upkeep of All Saints Church, Northampton, and a number of smaller bequests of £500 or £100 to individuals. Her stepchildren did not benefit from the will. The largest sum, which was £2,000 and also the residue of her estate, went to her doctor – John Bodkin Adams. In total he inherited about £5,000 (worth about £270,000 now). 'After her death, her car was brought to Kent Lodge, as also were some of her personal effects and belongings,' said Emma Benson, a relative from Ireland who was staying with the Adams's at the time. 'I do not remember what exactly these belongings and effects comprised, but I believe there was jewellery among them. I remember hearing that Mrs Whitton's false teeth were among the belongings which arrived at Kent Lodge, and I also remember hearing that the teeth were placed in the dustbin. Jenkins, the chauffeur, told me that he was going to retrieve the teeth and sell them, but I am not aware whether he did so.' The car, she remembered, was a small green touring car with a canvas hood, and was soon sold off by Dr Adams.

Matilda Whitton's stepchildren, Robert and Amy, made the decision to challenge the will. They assumed that they had been mentioned in Mrs Whitton's earlier wills, and that they had been excluded only after she became so friendly with her doctor. But Herbert James, the solicitor who acted both for Mrs Whitton and Dr Adams, testified that he had received clear instructions from her. The 1933 will was upheld, although a codicil which gave £500 to Dr Adams's niece, Sarah, was not.

About this time, rumours about Dr Adams and his influence on old ladies started to spread around the shops, tea rooms and nursing homes of Eastbourne, though it was not clear whether the doctor was aware of them. Then, one day at Kent Lodge, the housekeeper brought the afternoon mail into his office and put it on his desk. When he came to open his letters he found one that was written anonymously in a scrawling hand. It read: 'Keep your fingers crossed and don't bump off any more wealthy widows.' He tore it up and threw it in the wastepaper basket.

3

Inquest

MATILDA WHITTON HAD died in the Kenilworth Hotel in 1935 and Bobbie Hullett at Holywell Mount in 1956. During the long period between the two deaths Dr Adams had treated hundreds of patients, many of them wealthy widows who died under his care. Of course, the same could be said of all the family doctors in Eastbourne, as ageing wealthy widows were not thin on the ground and were to be found on every GP's list. But those who were inclined to dislike Dr Adams noticed the unusual zeal with which he accumulated such patients, his fondness for sedating them, and the unsavoury interest he appeared to take in their financial affairs, and particularly in their wills. It was remarked upon that he was becoming increasingly well-to-do – he now owned a Rolls-Royce and regularly went on shooting holidays to Scotland. In appearance, he was fatter and more well-heeled, and in manner, he sometimes appeared disgustingly pleased with himself. His chauffeur complained that the doctor would sit in the back of the Rolls, stuffing himself with expensive chocolates without ever offering one. And to ensure that he never ran out of chocolate, he had a regular order of violet creams and other staples sent from Charbonnel et Walker of Old Bond Street in London.

His cultivation of friends who owned large and fancy houses was a continuing occupation. He had worked his way into the Mawhoods' life at Ratton, of course, and also into the lively social circle at Holywell Mount. But, for gossiping types, his most interesting social climbing was with the set presided over by Roland Gwynne, at Folkington Manor (pronounced Fowington), a stately early Victorian house at the foot of the South Downs. Roland Gwynne was a handsome war hero who was well known throughout East Sussex, partly because he had been both High Sheriff and mayor of Eastbourne – but more because his lavish parties were legendary, and his lifestyle was said to be scandalous, even depraved. Homosexuality was illegal – but Roland Gwynne was gay, and flamboyantly indiscreet. It was observed that he was a very close friend of Dr Adams. He often visited the doctor at Kent Lodge, and sometimes he accompanied him on holidays.

Some of the whisperers of Eastbourne had it that the doctor and the magistrate were part of a 'homosexual ring' that also included a senior police officer. Whether or not he was, in fact, gay is a matter of dispute. From time to time Dr Adams walked out with lady friends, and in the 1930s he had become engaged to one of them – Nora O'Hara, 'daughter of Eastbourne's wealthiest butcher'. Nora's family bought the couple a house in Carew Road, Eastbourne – but they never moved into it, because for some unknown reason the engagement was broken off. Dr Adams never married, but he remained friends with Nora O'Hara – and his accounts show that in the mid-1950s he used to rent out his chauffeur to her at 10 shillings a time (a Mr White had, by now, replaced David Jenkins). The ambiguity surrounding his private life allowed the stories about Dr Adams to become juicier still – and packed with malice. Some people were saying that he was a gluttonous, widow-loving, money-grabbing pervert and – to top it all – most likely a murderer.

So it was not surprising that, as Bobbie Hullett lay in a coma at Holywell Mount, the rumours started up again. But, in the hours after her death, Dr Adams seemed unbothered by tittle-tattle. Instead, his attention was focused on covering his back as far as the Coroner, Angus Sommerville, was concerned, and he spent his time drafting a long and confused letter to him, justifying his actions. He explained that Bobbie had been married to 'a rich and adoring husband' who had died in March 'after a major abdominal operation. Since then has been ill generally and lost the will to live.' He said he had 'strictly doled out' her sodium barbiturates, giving her 10 grains a night. 'She could not possibly have secreted any of this,' he stated. 'She repeatedly refused to consult a psychologist or other physician.' He described her 'nerve storms' as being 'in a state of cerebral irritation, spasmodic twitching of face and limbs, and mentally excited'. And when he was rung up in Lewes on Friday because Bobbie would not wake up, he claimed he said 'Send Dr Harris at once', and later, when he visited her himself, he stated he had examined Bobbie's room carefully for any empty bottles or cartons 'and found none and nothing to suggest poisoning'. He described the tests conducted by the pathologist, Dr Shera, but did not explain that they had been done at a very late stage. He mentioned the Megimide injection, given 'in view of the remote possibility of barbiturate poisoning', but not that the dose had been wrong. He concluded that 'death was due to a cerebral lesion, probably involving the Pons with secondary complications in the lungs'. Finally, he wrote: 'Because of the pathologist's findings being inconclusive, and cremation requested, we are reporting the facts fully to you.' The letter was signed both by Dr Adams and Dr Harris, who added to the final sentence the words 'as we do not feel in a position to issue a death certificate'.

Before he received this unusual letter, Angus Sommerville was already expecting the involvement of the police in the case of Bobbie Hullett. He was unnerved by the telephone call that he had received from Dr Adams while Bobbie was in a coma, asking about the possibility of a private post-mortem. Now that she was actually dead, a conventional post-mortem was performed, but the pathologist 'was unable to find any natural cause of death'. So Angus Sommerville telephoned the chief constable of

Eastbourne, Richard Walker, and told him 'to obtain the aid of Dr Camps'. This was the famous Home Office pathologist Francis Camps, whose name – in the 1950s – was synonymous with murder. Three years earlier he had distinguished himself as the forensic pathologist at the trial of the 10 Rillington Place serial killer, John Reginald Christie.

Angus Sommerville was not the only person sufficiently suspicious of Dr Adams to call the chief constable. Bobbie's friends, Martha and Leslie Henson, were also extremely alarmed. Martha told the police that Bobbie's death was surrounded by 'some suspicious circumstances'. Leslie, who was performing in a show in Dublin at the time, said: 'Her death shocked me greatly. My wife and I saw her turning into a drug addict. It is a great pity as she was such a nice person. We invited her to our home in Harrow to get away from everything, but she rushed back after twenty-four hours to get her pills again. We saw her disintegrating mentally through them. I am certain the pills sent her nearly mad and through them she died.' He telephoned Richard Walker with these worries, and then gave a statement at Dublin police station.

The chief constable, Richard Walker, seemed unsure of how seriously to take the suspicions about Dr Adams. He knew the doctor very well, being his patient, and also as a friend of the Hulletts and a regular visitor to Holywell Mount. He was also aware of the increasingly malicious talk that was buzzing about Eastbourne. While the chief constable was still contemplating what to do, the Coroner Angus Sommerville started the inquest into Bobbie's death, and for some unknown reason held the proceedings in private. This was highly irregular, and Richard Walker decided to alert the press. He telephoned an Eastbourne journalist, James Donne, and read him a statement:

An inquest was opened today on Mrs Gertrude Joyce Hullett of Holywell Mount, who died yesterday. Only formal evidence of identification was given and the inquest was then adjourned to await the results of a post-mortem examination.

James Donne did not know what to make of this bland announcement. When he asked Richard Walker for more information, the chief constable said nothing. So the following day Mr Donne and a fellow journalist, John Bray of the *Brighton Argus*, visited Richard Walker at the police station. Still, he would not elaborate. But as they were leaving the station a policeman recognised them as pressmen and said: 'You on this Hullett job? Well it's about time somebody caught up with that bloody doctor.'

Richard Walker now despatched Detective Inspector Brynley Pugh to take statements from anyone who had been with Bobbie in the days before her death. Although the possibility of an overdose had been dismissed while she was in a coma, now that she was dead everyone seemed to think she had killed herself. 'After Mummy's death I did think it was possible that she might have been the cause of her own death,' said Patricia. Inspector Pugh asked her about the similarities between her mother's death and that of Jack – since, in both cases and within months of each other, Dr Adams had diagnosed the fatal problem as cerebral. But Patricia said she saw nothing strange in the coincidence. Kathleen Reed agreed that Bobbie had taken her own life, and Teresa Yogna, the parlourmaid, took the same view. Hugh Hubbard Ford said that his immediate reaction to Bobbie's death was 'that the whole thing was a planned suicide'. But he was surprised by suggestions of foul play.

Bobbie had been particularly close to her friend Robert Handscomb, who was a Lloyd's underwriter and had known Jack for thirty-five years. When the police interviewed Robert Handscomb on 24 July – the day after Bobbie died – he gave a detailed account of the events at Holywell Mount. He did not think that Bobbie was 'in any way addicted to drugs of any sort', and he said nothing about Bobbie having taken her own life.

But three days later, Robert Handscomb made a second statement, admitting that he had omitted 'certain facts' the first time around. When Bobbie died, he now revealed, he had gone to her deed box to find her will, and had found three letters which, according to the dates on them, were written in April 1956 – one to himself, another to Bobbie's half-sister Podge, and a third to her daughter Patricia. 'My darling Patricia,' she wrote, 'If I should die and you read this please be happy for me. I love you very dearly but I don't want to go on living without Jack. You will be unhappy at first but it will pass . . .' The letter to Robert Handscomb stated: 'If I should die please be happy.' Bobbie also requested that Robert 'make sure Dr Adams' MG is paid for from Jack. I know it was his wish . . .' This last request had been crossed through, with the words: 'Have done this 17.7.56'. 'These letters of course confirmed my previous conviction that there was no doubt that she had taken her own life,' Robert Handscomb told the police. He had, he said, not disclosed this information before because he was trying to 'shield, if possible, my dearest friend Mrs Hullett'. But, since he made his first statement he had gathered that the question of murder was in the air, and so had come forward.

Francis Camps, meanwhile, had conducted the second post-mortem on Bobbie's body, and had reached some conclusions. He had travelled down to Eastbourne on the evening after her death, and examined her body at the public mortuary in the presence of Inspector Brynley Pugh. Dr Adams had been invited to join them as an observer, but had declined. Dr Camps concluded 'that death was due to bronchopneumonia and respiratory failure due to barbiturate poisoning in the form of barbitone' and also that 'there was no other natural disease'. He had heard the history of the case, and thought that Bobbie's condition and background should have led naturally to an immediate suspicion of overdose.

Treatment of cases of barbiturate poisoning, he said, should be carried out in hospital. The blood should be oxygenated, and fluids were essential to eliminate the drug in the urine. Washing out the stomach might also have been a good move – though not necessarily so – but in any case was likely to be more effective if it was carried out early. His opinion read like a summary of all the obvious and sensible measures that Dr Adams, with Dr Harris at his side, had failed to take.

At some point – it is not clear when – Francis Camps also gave an opinion on the death of Jack Hullett. He noted Jack's attacks of breathlessness, and the fact that he had seemed well when he visited the pub on 13 March 1956 – the day of his death. He recorded, also, that Jack had complained of chest pain and head-ache that evening and that Dr Adams had been called. He mentioned the ushering of Jack up the stairs, without his usual rest on the way up, and the injection given by Dr Adams at around 10.30 p.m.

'In my opinion the treatment of this case was unusual,' he wrote. Jack was supposed to have had a heart attack, and yet no appropriate treatment was given. Instead 'the patient was submit-ted to an effort likely to produce a further attack. This, in fact, occurred. Again no treatment was given but later an injection of morphia was administered.' Afterwards, Jack 'slept', with ster-torous breathing. At 6 a.m. he opened his eyes and asked the time. 'This does not suggest a cerebro-vascular lesion,' he wrote (the cause of death assigned by Dr Adams). 'If the injection given at 10.30 p.m. was, in fact, ½ a grain or 1 grain of morphia, it is difficult to see for what reason. Hullett had no pain then. Such a large dose would seem unnecessary and even dangerous to life and might well contribute to his subsequent death. It is of note that he had never had such a large dose before.'

Richard Walker was trying to absorb these developments – the report from Francis Camps, the statements of the witnesses at Holywell Mount, and the letters written by Bobbie three months before her death. But most pressing was the context of the deaths of Jack and Bobbie. Taking a narrow view, the deaths could be natural, or might have resulted from incompetent or negligent doctoring. But the wider circumstances made everything more complicated and more serious – the fact that Dr Adams benefited financially from both deaths, his mysterious demand for 'special clearance' of the £1,000 cheque from Bobbie, the heavy sedation of Bobbie, and the allegations that, with an eye on their money, he regularly helped his patients to die.

At the same time, the chief constable found himself suddenly under pressure from the newspapers. The journalists James Donne and John Bray had quickly ascertained that Bobbie's doctor was Dr Adams, and that the police were at Holywell Mount. James Donne considered that he had enough information to file a short report, so he telephoned the Press Association and several London newspapers. Eastbourne police were inquiring into the death of the widow of a rich retired Lloyd's underwriter, he said. Her doctor was John Bodkin Adams, a fashionable local physician. Journalists at the Press Association and the *Exchange Telegraph* checked their cuttings, and found a reference to Dr John Bodkin Adams being the subject of the disputed will of Matilda Whitton, back in 1935. The doctor, it was reported, had received more than £3,000 under Mrs Whitton's will. The reporters sniffed a story that might involve murder and might span decades.

Percy Hoskins, the chief crime reporter of the *Daily Express*, wrote that 'the effect was electric. James Donne's telephone was jammed with scores of calls. Within two hours the vanguard of the press corps were disembarking at Eastbourne station. Immediate destination, James Donne's office. Then the police station.' That evening the pressmen toured the hotel bars and pubs of Eastbourne in search of local knowledge about Dr Adams, and were bombarded with salacious rumours that had been embellished, refined and polished over several decades. The chief constable's response to the situation was to hold a press conference the following morning, at which he did nothing to quell the excitement, telling the journalists of the possibility of foul play in Bobbie Hullett's death. When asked about the rumours in the town about the deaths of other women, Richard Walker said the gossip could not be ignored, and that his officers were now trying to get at the truth.

All the popular papers carried bold and prominent stories the following day, several of them on the front page and adorned with pictures of the 'attractive Mrs Gertrude Hullett'. The *Daily Sketch* splashed with 'Rich Widow Drama: CID Act'. The *Daily Mail*'s front page story was stronger still. Under the headline 'Rich Widow Murder Probe', it opened: 'Was rich Mrs Gertrude Hullett – the "Grande Dame of Eastbourne" – murdered at her luxurious 15-room home on Beachy Head? Detectives and Dr F E Camps, Home Office Pathologist, are tonight trying to establish the cause of the 50-year-old widow's sudden death . . . If inquiries show she was murdered investigations may be made into the deaths of several other wealthy women in Eastbourne.' To tie the name of Dr John Bodkin Adams to this murder story was to invite legal problems – if not libel, then the prejudicing of a criminal trial. But the *Daily Mail* none the less dropped an enormous hint. Towards the end of the article, it stated: 'Detectives saw her [Bobbie's] doctor, Dr J Bodkin Adams, a portly, balding man who owns three motor cars and has an extensive practice.'

The following day several of the newspapers signalled their belief that Bobbie Hullett's death was part of a far bigger story. The *Daily Mirror* of 27 July carried the headline: 'DEATH RIDDLE WIDOW, Now deaths of four women are probed'. The paper's crime reporter Harry Longmuir wrote that the police were investigating the deaths of other rich women in Eastbourne, and that 'exhumation of their bodies from local cemeteries may be considered'. And the *Mirror*, like the

Mail, hinted that the suspect in the case was Dr John Bodkin Adams.

The talk of 'probes' was widespread, and speculation about exhumations was too attractive to resist. More reporters were arriving in Eastbourne all the time, and by the end of July when Rodney Hallworth, a crime writer on the *Daily Mail*, showed up, so many hotel rooms were already booked that he was put up in the bridal suite of the Grand Hotel – 'a sumptuous boudoir of silks and brocades'.

In the midst of it all, Richard Walker decided that his investigation into the Eastbourne rumours was too hot, or too complicated, for the Eastbourne police alone – and so he called in Scotland Yard. A Scotland Yard man, it was decided, would attend the Bobbie Hullett inquest when it reopened on 21 August – this time in public – and immediately afterwards he would lead a thorough investigation into all the activities of Dr John Bodkin Adams. This development ensured that the pressmen felt justified in their hyperbole, and were ready to return to Eastbourne for the reopening of the Bobbie Hullett inquest.

From July onwards, the investigation into Dr Adams unfolded in the newspapers like a gripping drama serial – sometimes dominating the front page, sometimes set among the other happenings that contributed to British public life in 1956. On the lighter side, the actress Marilyn Monroe was in London that summer, filming at Pinewood Studios for *The Prince and the Showgirl* with Laurence Olivier. The papers were thrilled. 'MARILYN WIGGLES TO WORK', ran a headline in the *Daily Mirror*. The reporter observed that: 'In her dressing room, Marilyn was poured into a low-necked white satin dress, fitting as tight as the curves would allow. The seams, I was told, were reinforced . . .' And many papers carried photographs of the Queen's sister, Princess Margaret, looking lost and sad in the wake of giving up her relationship with the man she wished to marry, Group Captain Peter Townsend. The British actress and national glamour-puss Diana Dors was another celebrity of the moment. She was trying to establish herself in Hollywood and had – literally – made something of a splash when, wearing a sky-blue playsuit, she fell into a swimming pool at a party, conveniently in the presence of a dozen paparazzi with cameras.

Political news made a grim backdrop to the enjoyable froth, being dominated by a foreign affairs crisis which was becoming graver by the day and which, through some peculiar twists and turns, would eventually become part of the Dr Adams story. On 25 July the President of Egypt, Gamal Abdul Nasser, had nationalised the Suez Canal which linked the Mediterranean and Indian Ocean. Two-thirds of Europe's oil was transported through the Canal and the Western powers went immediately into a frenzy of concern, as did the British press. The front page of the *Daily Mail* of 26 July deemed Nasser the 'Hitler of the Nile', and the following day it ran the bellicose headline: 'TAKE THE CONSEQUENCES, NASSER – EDEN IS URGED TO SEND IN THE TROOPS'. Before long, it appeared that Britain was heading for war. The papers were split on the issue. 'War against Egypt means war against all the Arab states', warned the *Daily Mirror* on 15 August. 'Policing the Suez Canal means occupation of all Egypt . . . Britain would be saddled with a crushing burden.'

A few days later, though, the popular newspapers' main story was once again Dr Adams, and the events in Eastbourne. On 21 August – the day the Bobbie Hullett inquest was to be resumed – Rodney Hallworth of the *Daily Mail* led the way with a startling curtain-raiser for the event. On the front page he revealed: 'YARD STUDY WILLS OF 300 WOMEN IN £1M PROBE'. His article began:

A million pounds, that is the amount involved in an investigation of alleged fraud on wealthy women which Scotland Yard

men will start here tomorrow. And if a gigantic swindle is discovered, an immediate murder probe will begin. Yard detectives visited Somerset House today and took away copies of the
wills of 300 women who had died in the Eastbourne area since
1936. At least 500 people will be interviewed here, in London
and in the provinces to check on a chain of rumours, gossip and
suspicions . . . A townsman told me: 'I understand the Yard will
turn this town upside down during the next few weeks.
Forgotten incidents of the past may well become headlines of
the future.'

The inquest opened at the Town Hall in Eastbourne at 2.15,
packed with pressmen and local people keen to see what all the
fuss was about. The first witness to face Angus Sommerville,
the Coroner, was Bobbie's daughter Patricia, who confirmed
that Bobbie had suggested suicide 'in a vague way'. When she fell
into a coma, Patricia said, there had been no suggestion of a
second opinion being sought. Dr Adams's partner, Dr Vincent
Harris, next told the hearing that Dr Adams had never mentioned to him the possibility of barbiturate poisoning, and he had
not revealed that Bobbie had been very depressed, saying only
that 'she was very highly-strung – a nervy type of person'. Dr
Harris said that he had recommended that Bobbie be moved to a
hospital or nursing home, but that Dr Adams was against it,
because Bobbie had had an 'intense dislike' of such places. Dr
Alfred Shera, who had visited Bobbie when she was in a coma,
testified that: 'I said to Dr Adams and to Dr Harris: "I can't help
thinking this looks like a case of narcotic poisoning and don't
you think we should have the stomach contents?" They were
both strongly opposed to it and both strongly in favour of cerebral haemorrhage and I merely left the suggestion with them and
I heard no more.'

The Home Office pathologist, Francis Camps, confirmed that
Bobbie had ingested a fatal dose of barbiturates – she had 115
grains (7,450 mg) of sodium barbiturate in her body. He thought

it 'a matter for comment' that Dr Adams had not suspected barbiturate poisoning at once. The servants at Holywell Mount gave
their version of events there, as did Bobbie's friend Kathleen
Reed, and also Robert Handscomb, Bobbie's great friend. He
was very supportive of Dr Adams, telling the jury that he 'went
beyond a doctor's duties, that he took a personal interest in her
as though he were not a doctor. He did every mortal thing he
possibly could for her.'

If the pressmen were disappointed by the direction the inquest
was taking, they were now compensated by the appearance of
the object of their interest, as Dr John Bodkin Adams stepped up
to answer Dr Sommerville's questions. The account he gave of
himself was poor, but not sensationally incriminating. Yes, he
had given Bobbie barbiturates. Yes, she had told him she wished
to die. But, when she was found to be in a coma, he did not
suspect an overdose. 'Frankly and honestly it didn't occur to me,'
he said. 'I thought I had tied it up so well . . . ' He meant that he
thought she could not have hoarded tablets. His version of events
seemed unlikely, but not impossible. At no time, he said, had he
thought of calling for a second opinion. When he finally thought
of treating her for an overdose, and gave some Megimide, he
gave the amount that he thought was the right dose, and when it
had no effect, he stopped. This contradicted all sources of
information on the treatment – the written instructions, and
the instructions of the house surgeon who gave Dr Adams the
Megimide. But Dr Adams was not interrogated on the point.

On the £1,000 cheque he received from Bobbie two days
before she took the overdose, he confirmed that he had received
it, but was not asked why he had specifically asked for special
clearance.

The final witness was the man from Scotland Yard charged
with investigating Dr Adams. He was Detective Superintendent
Herbert Hannam. The Coroner, taking into account that
Hannam's inquiries had hardly begun, asked him whether he

would like the inquest to be adjourned. No, said the police officer, 'I have no application to make to you.'

In his final remarks to the jury, Dr Sommerville said that the options before them were verdicts of an accidental taking of an overdose, or suicide. A finding of criminal negligence should be ruled out. For such a serious finding: 'one must know and believe and have proof that the death of the deceased is directly caused by the doctor's negligence'. This, he said, was not the case here. There had, according to Angus Sommerville, been a horrifying level of ordinary negligence, but not criminal negligence. He pointed to Dr Adams's failure to tell Dr Harris of Bobbie's history of suicidal talk, to his failure to consider barbiturate poisoning from the outset, his failure to send her to hospital or at least get a second opinion, and the 'quite useless' treatment with a negligible amount of Megimide. He also mentioned the idea of motive – and talked of the £1,000 cheque, which might in some unspecified way have put a financial element into Dr Adams's mind when he was treating Bobbie. But 'motive', he said, 'does not convert negligence of a lesser degree into negligence of a more serious degree.' Because of his directions, it was not surprising that, after a short deliberation, the jury concluded that Bobbie Hullett had committed suicide.

When the inquest ended, Dr Adams left the court, and in the corridor outside came upon Angus Sommerville and Superintendent Herbert Hannam. Angus Sommerville introduced the police officer to Dr Adams, and the two men shook hands. The doctor seemed to be in good humour and said that he would help in any inquiries. 'Mr Hannam thanked him,' said the journalist Percy Hoskins. 'He joked that when it was all over they might have a champagne party.' It was a warm sunlit evening, and Dr Adams left the building, followed by newspapermen who trailed him home to Kent Lodge, where he rewarded them with a statement. 'I am glad that my name has been cleared at last,' he said. 'What started all the rumour that has been going around I just don't know . . .' He was glad to be able to tell the press that the rumours had not affected his practice '*that* much' – and he clicked his fingers, making it clear that through all the fuss, he had been working as normal. He didn't understand why people were critical of doctors receiving gifts, he said. He knew one doctor who had been left £27,000 and another £30,000. 'My conscience is clear,' he informed the reporters. He seemed relieved at the court's verdict, as though he believed that the commotion surrounding Bobbie Hullett's death would now subside.

4

Herbert Hannam

S COTLAND YARD GAVE the investigation a name – 'The Eastbourne Job'. Its scope was wide, being an instruction to see 'whether there is any truth in all these rumours about this doctor', and the officer in charge was suitably senior, but quite out of place in a genteel seaside town. Detective Superintendent Herbert Hannam was a Londoner, born and bred, and he was accustomed to breathing a different sort of air, gritty with exhaust fumes or thick with soot. The villains he had come across were usually of the urban lowlife kind, and his encounters with the criminal underworld had rubbed off on him. Photographs of Hannam record a don't-mess-with-me swagger in his walk, and a jut to his chin. They show a solid block of a man, who holds himself squarely as if ready to fight – he looks like a stevedore or a squaddie, a hard nut.

But Hannam's most noticeable characteristic was not his toughness – it was the way in which he presented himself as a toff. He had invested in a fabulous collection of well-cut suits, one for each day of the week; and when out and about, he liked to wear a bowler hat and yellow gloves and to carry a smart umbrella. As a young detective he had once strolled into Peckham Rye police station wearing spats, but his colleagues thought this an affectation too far and mocked him by fixing scraps of white paper to the tops of their shoes. Hannam took the hint and renounced spats for good, but his manner remained superior, and he broadcasted his taste for the good life by smoking Henry Clay cigars ('a favourite of aficionados with a more refined palate'). His nickname – The Count – was the sort you might give to a gangland boss.

His city seemed a thousand miles from Dr Adams's Eastbourne, being culturally diverse, and buzzing with new ideas and attitudes. By the mid-1950s immigrants from the West Indies were to be seen in the streets of London, 'queer pubs' in Soho were packed with men showing disdain for the law by cavorting in public, and a new self-assured youth culture was plain to see in clubs and coffee bars. Rock and Roll came to Britain in 1955 with the success of '[We're gonna] Rock around the Clock' by Bill Haley and His Comets. And in February 1956 Eastender Lonnie Donegan and his skiffle band had a massive hit with an upbeat version of Leadbelly's 'Rock Island Line'. Times were changing. It was obvious in London, but almost undetectable in the Eastbourne of mistresses and parlourmaids, of swanky hotels, bandstands, flower baskets and bowling greens.

In May 1956, two months before Bobbie Hullett died in a house full of servants, John Osborne's play *Look Back in Anger* opened at the Royal Court in London, shoving the uncompromising character of Jimmy Porter into the face of post-war British society. The play railed against the toxic effects of the British class system, and was an attack on everything that the Eastbourne set took for granted – gentility, deference and the hierarchy of the golf club. Jimmy Porter, played brilliantly by Kenneth Haigh, was scornful of the complacent, taste-bound middle classes embodied in the character of Mrs Redfern – 'an overfed, overprivileged old bitch', and her husband, the Colonel, who is 'just one of those sturdy old plants left over from the Edwardian wilderness that can't understand why the sun isn't shining anymore'. Through the prism of Osborne, the cream of Eastbourne society was obnoxious.

The *Sunday Express* writer Derek Monsey retaliated with a review that stood up for colonels, bank managers and the widows of clubbable men: 'Jimmy is supposed to represent the post-war generation,' he wrote. 'In fact, he is simply a rather nasty type of pretentious bore.' Kenneth Tynan adored the play – or, more accurately, the fact that it had been written. 'I doubt if I could love anyone who did not wish to see *Look Back in Anger*,' he wrote in *The Observer*. The debate was polarising.

Now it seemed that the contrast between angry young Britain and the sort of society represented by Eastbourne stretched beyond streetlife, music and theatre into the realm of murder. The Dr Adams case seemed like a murder story from the familiar past, not the turbulent present, a Home Counties mystery of the old school. Dr Adams, as prime suspect (indeed, only suspect), was of the type to be found in an Agatha Christie novel, where murderers were middle-class professional men, their motives rooted in wills and legacies. The perfect Agatha Christie murderer was the family doctor, a man with the means and opportunity to administer a fatal dose of some poisonous concoction without arousing suspicion. This was the sort of murder that was planned over a glass of sherry, and carried out discreetly in the orangery, the library or some other part of a desirable home.

By contrast, most of the murders that made the front pages of the newspapers in the 1950s were of a different kind entirely – hard-boiled, melodramatic and working class, and of the street rather than the drawing room. In 1952 the bleak and senseless story broke of Christopher Craig and Derek Bentley, two young criminals who set off to burgle the warehouse of a confectionery company in Croydon, and who climbed up on to the roof. The 16-year-old Craig was armed with a revolver, and his 'borderline retarded' assistant, 18-year-old Derek Bentley, was equipped with a knuckle-duster and knife. When Police Constable Sidney Miles appeared on the roof, Craig shot him dead – but it was Bentley who was executed for the killing, since he was, technically, old enough to hang and Craig was not. This was a messy sort of murder story – and Bentley's conviction was eventually quashed in 1998. There was nothing in it that was neat and tidy, least of all on the motive question. Nothing like the 'murder for legacy' theory about Dr Adams.

Six months later, another murder trial at the Old Bailey was more complicated – one infused with evil purpose, and extremely gruesome. The world's press followed the trial of John Reginald Christie for the murder of his wife Ethel at their flat at 10 Rillington Place in Notting Hill. Christie, it emerged, was predatory and depraved, and had killed at least seven women, and probably a child. He gassed his adult victims to make them drowsy, then raped them as he strangled them. The bodies were buried under the floorboards, or in an outhouse in the garden, or were propped up and papered over in an alcove in the kitchen. Number 10 Rillington Place was so packed with human remains that bones turned up casually in the ugly little garden – a thigh bone was used to buttress a fence, a skull was dug up by a dog.

The execution of John Reginald Christie on 15 July 1953 did not, in itself, stir up much agitation against capital punishment. But with his death came the realisation that another man, Timothy Evans, had been hanged in 1950 for the murder of his wife and young daughter, both of whom had probably been killed by Christie. The role of the Metropolitan Police in bringing Evans to court was far from exemplary – involving muddled confessions by Evans who, like Derek Bentley, had a very low IQ. Some said later that Evans's confessions were fake, that they had been made up by the police. There were officers at Scotland Yard who, though they did not actually manufacture confessions, believed that securing them involved a rare skill, and that nudging a suspect towards 'cracking' was an essential part of a murder case. Herbert Hannam was of this school, and had become known for the controversial confessions he secured from villains. When he arrived in Eastbourne, like an emissary from a rougher, dirtier world, he already had a reputation for the methods he used – methods that had been honed, and then questioned, in the famous Teddington Towpath Murder case of 1953.

On 31 May that year, John Christie was in Brixton jail awaiting trial, the young Queen Elizabeth was at Buckingham Palace preparing for her coronation on 2 June, and two teenage girls in Teddington decided to take an evening cycle ride along the towpath by the River Thames. But 16-year-old Barbara Songhurst and her 18-year-old friend Christine Reed didn't return home, and while the rest of the country was busy with bunting and fireworks, in Teddington a grim search of the river, the towpath and surrounding fields was begun. Barbara's body was pulled out of the Thames the following day, and two pairs of shoes were found near the towpath. Some days later, Christine's body was recovered from the river. Both girls had been savagely attacked and raped, and Herbert Hannam was assigned the task of finding their killer and bringing him to court.

He had little forensic evidence to guide him, and began his investigation by casting his net widely. The police files on the Teddington Towpath Murders show that he ordered house-to-house inquiries on an almighty scale. Officers called at nearly 4,000 homes, around 7,000 people were interviewed, and the number of written witness statements came in at 1,650. Hannam sent for the 'stop books' from police stations in west London, and looked for suspicious persons roaming the streets in the days after the girls' deaths. The stop book information remains in the police files and is an evocative record of the night beat in Shepherds Bush. Atwar Singh was stopped by police at 4.35 a.m. because he had 'bulky pockets', William Law was stopped at 1.20 a.m. for 'loitering near shops', Samuel Cooper was questioned about possessing army boots, and Theodore Bowser – a 'man of colour' – was stopped on the Uxbridge Road at 3.15 a.m. because he was 'in possession of plastic bag containing toilet requisites and negatives'. The mountain of documentary material on the case is testimony to Hannam's sweeping approach, and to a method that – in Eastbourne – would make him vulnerable to criticism. Some said his investigations became too wide-ranging, were too unfocused.

His critics were also irritated by his relationships with news-papermen. During the Teddington Towpath investigation, Herbert Hannam took time out to hold two press conferences a day, and it was said that he courted the press because he adored being on show, and was overly concerned about his public image. But he insisted that talking to journalists was useful, and that the press helped lead him to his prime suspect – a 22-year-old labourer named Alfred Whiteway, who was poorly educated and generally considered to be a bad lot. Whiteway was married, but had left his wife and was living with his mother, Ellen. When she spoke to the police about her son, she described a boy who had been wired-up all wrong, who had never seemed to get along with other people, was mean and cruel, and deficient in empathy. As a child, Alfie 'never had a mate and did not mix with other boys'. Rather, he was a loner, who took up petty thieving at a young age, and when he stole a bicycle he was sent to reform school. 'It would seem that he interprets leniency as weakness and kindness as an opportunity to be exploited. The general prognosis is very poor indeed . . .' wrote his headmaster, in a disheartening report. His mother also mentioned that he seemed to be fasci-nated by knives, forever throwing them about in the garden. Several other witnesses said they had seen him throwing knives at trees.

Alfred Whiteway admitted that he had attacked and raped a 14-year-old schoolgirl on Oxshott Heath on Whitsunday, a few days before the assaults on Christine and Barbara. His statement was taken at Chertsey police station and is a flat unemotional account. He said he had been out on his blue bike and just cycling around, when he saw the girl, who had her dog with her, go into the woods. She walked along the footpath, and he fol-lowed her in. 'I had a wood chopper in my saddle bag, and I lost her once in the woods and was looking around for her. I had made up my mind to seduce her, and I got the chopper out of my saddle bag. I caught up with her when she was on the footpath and I hit her on the head somewhere with the back edge of the chopper.' The girl survived.

It seemed that the attacks on Christine and Barbara had been similar – and the police found a Gurkha knife and an axe which they believed to have been the murder weapons. Forensics also found blood on the crepe-soled shoes that Whiteway had said he was wearing on the night of the murder. At this point in his investigation Superintendent Hannam went to Brixton jail to see Whiteway. The police report of the encounter is suggestive of Hannam's confidence in his skill as an interviewer. A fellow officer, Nipper Read, observed that Hannam had 'an ability in one sentence to create a situation which made things very sinister . . .'

'Are you quite sure you were wearing your crepe-soled shoes on the night of 31 May?' Hannam asked.

'Yes,' answered Whiteway, 'I know I was, I've said so all along.'

'Did you ever get any blood or bloodstains on either of your crepe-soled shoes?'

'No.'

'. . . A scientific expert will say that one of those shoes has been in a considerable quantity of blood, even over the uppers.'

'If they say that they are bloody liars. There's no blood on them.'

Herbert Hannam then produced the axe, and placed it on the desk without comment. His report implies that the shock of seeing the axe caused Whiteway to 'crack', saying:

'Blimey, that's it. It's been buggered about. It was bloody sharp when I had it. I sharpened it with a file.'

The Gurkha knife was then produced, again silently, and placed on the desk.

'Whiteway smiled broadly,' reported Hannam, and said: 'That's it, you got it out of the water did you?'

As the interview progressed, Whiteway, according to Hannam's report, accused the police of trying to 'put one over on' him by claiming there was blood on his shoe. Then he became self-righteous, telling Hannam to stop bothering Nellie, his pregnant wife. The interview came to an end on this note, and Hannam started packing up his papers and putting them into his briefcase, leaving the axe and the knife lying on the table. As he was about to leave, Hannam asked Whiteway if there was anything else he wished to say. Then, said Hannam:

> Whiteway said, 'were you kidding about blood on my shoe?'
> I said: 'I have explained that one of your shoes had heavy blood staining on it.'

In Hannam's eyes, it was now that the Whiteway cracking process reached its apex:

> He had been sitting down and at that moment stood up. He went very pale, which is unusual for him. He began to tremble and said, 'You bloody well know it was me don't you? I didn't mean to kill 'em. I never want to hurt anyone.'

Hannam now cautioned Whiteway, and took a further statement from him, which read:

> It's all up. You know bloody well I done it, eh! That shoe's buggered me. What a bloody mess. I'm mental. Me head must be wrong. I must have a bloody woman . . . Put that bloody chopper away it haunts yer . . .

It was a textbook 'It's a fair cop, gov' confession, which Alfred Whiteway immediately retracted.

His trial for murder took place in October 1953, three months after the execution of John Christie, and was reported against a backdrop of news about food rationing, the price of cigarettes and the thick, choking smog that had descended on London.

Alfred Whiteway was vigorously defended by Peter Rawlinson
– a gifted barrister who acted in many high-profile trials of the
1950s. Rawlinson observed that the forensic evidence was weak
and that Whiteway's confessions were the central plank of the
prosecution case – confessions that, according to Whiteway, had
never happened.

Rawlinson's cross-examination of Herbert Hannam became a
compelling piece of courtroom theatre – the 'duel at the Old
Bailey' being enhanced by Hannam's impressive physical presence in the courtroom. The *Daily Express* had him as 'the
immaculate man with the broad shoulders . . .'

'Dapper, grey hair carefully brushed, he gave his evidence in
a grave and solemn manner,' wrote Rawlinson, whose attack
was unsparing. He proposed that Whiteway's confession 'is a
statement manufactured by you'.

> 'That is absolutely untrue,' replied Hannam.
> 'I suggest that no such words were ever used by Whiteway
> on July 30 or at any other time when you saw him.'
> '. . . my answer is that they are in his own words from his
> own lips.'
> 'I repeat the suggestion – that that statement was invented by
> you.'
> 'I repeat, it is a shocking suggestion and I am pleased to deny
> it . . .'

Hannam continued to assert that the statement was exactly correct, exactly in Whiteway's own words, and that the suggestion
of police misconduct 'is a terrible one and is absolutely untrue'.
He was in the witness box for four hours.

In court, Alfred Whiteway said he had signed a piece of paper
without knowing what was on it, and had never made any confession. He denied rape, and denied murder. The jury believed
Hannam, the judge criticised Rawlinson for daring to question
the integrity of a police officer, and Alfred Whiteway was

sentenced to hang. But Hannam's Old Bailey clash with Peter Rawlinson had been a bruising one. He never forgot it.

From his prison cell, awaiting execution, Whiteway wrote Hannam a letter. '. . . Mr Hannam, you were wrong,' he complained. 'Why you made up that false confession I can't say, but you know your word would be more accepted than mine. Don't ever do a thing like that again, for it would go very hard for you if you slipped up . . . I played into your hands to [sic] easily . . . You were so possitive [sic] that it was me, that you risked a lot to have me hanged . . . It's a good job that I am finished or you would have to watch your step. I couldn't kill you but I could do the next best thing . . .' He was plainly guilty.

Alfred Whiteway was duly hanged and, beyond his immediate family, few people cared very much.

Two years later, in 1955, Herbert Hannam was once more in the news because of the confession that he had secured from a crook. He had led an investigation into police corruption in the Met – and on presenting a small-time criminal with evidence against him, the man 'cracked'. His words, as recorded by Hannam, were: 'If that is true, I am down. I don't care now what happens to me. They can give me time. I have had enough . . .' In this inquiry, too, Hannam briefed the press as he went along. His investigation was successful – several policemen and thieves ended up in prison.

But his style alienated some senior officers at Scotland Yard. They considered him too much of a bull in a china shop and did not trust him to handle 'the Eastbourne job' with any finesse or sensitivity. From Herbert Hannam's point of view though, his methods worked, and he intended to carry on in his usual manner. He would take hundreds of statements if necessary, sift decades' worth of evidence and, at the end of it all, conduct his customary skilful interview with his suspect. The expectation was that, like the others, Dr Adams would 'crack'.

5

A Cloud of Witnesses

HERBERT HANNAM AND his men set about interviewing anyone who could be found who had witnessed Dr Adams at work. At Hannam's side was a loyal cohort, Detective Sergeant Charlie Hewett, also of Scotland Yard, and Detective Inspector Brynley Pugh of the Eastbourne constabulary. Hewett was a cockney, a straightforward, no-nonsense officer who was a fan of Hannam's methods and his 'cracking' idea. Brynley Pugh was, as his name suggested, a Welshman. Like many in the Eastbourne force, he was sceptical about the Dr Adams rumours and not convinced that a major investigation was called for. The doctor had delivered Pugh's children, and it was hard to contemplate that a man so intimately associated with his own family, who had brought new life into the world, might also be a murderer.

An early priority was to talk to Eastbourne's nurses, and there were a lot of them. The hope was that the women who worked side-by-side with Dr Adams would know his secrets. It seemed a reasonable supposition but, from the murder point of view, the first interviews were disappointing. Nurse Grace Easter, who had worked with the doctor for fourteen years, told the police that his care for patients was 'beyond reproach ... He was most attentive, most kind and his one aim was always to get them well and more often than not he succeeded.' As for his motives: 'I cannot recall any occasion when patients informed me, or my staff, that Dr Adams was interested in their financial affairs.' Nurse Helen McSweeney thought Dr Adams the kindest man she had ever met, who 'gave every attention to his patients and would turn out at any time of the night'. Nurse Kathleen May was a patient of Dr Adams herself and had never seen anything in his behaviour to arouse her suspicions. He was a good doctor, she thought, and she liked his willingness to sit at a patient's bedside, and sometimes to hold her hand.

But another group of nurses was more than happy to tell the police of their misgivings. Nurse Marjorie Savage did not like the way Dr Adams ingratiated himself with patients, and thought his bedside manner 'far too friendly', and unlike that of any other doctor. Nurse Eunice Hitch was disgusted by the way he held patients' hands and commented on their clothes – and remembered that he would visit one old lady, a Mrs Coats, every night after 10 p.m. She had loved his attention, grown 'very fond' of him, and started to talk of leaving him money in her will. Her son became suspicious and had questioned the doctor about his bills, whereupon he 'became very irate'. Another lady, said Nurse Hitch, was blind and bedridden. When Dr Adams came to visit, he stole chocolates from the box that was in her room – a despicable act. She also recalled a patient named Mrs Hollobone who was given 'most unusual' injections by Dr Adams at noon every day that made her sleepy all day and unable to sleep at night. To round off her objections, she added: 'My experience of Dr Adams is that he is out for money and all he can get.'

Nurse Minnie Carey thought the doctor 'attentive and very kind', but there was one peculiarity that the police should know about. 'The only thing I noticed was his habit of administering sedatives or injections,' she said. 'He was generally inclined to give injections or drugs without disclosing what it was he was giving the patient . . . His attitude seemed to be that it was his concern what he was giving the patient, not a matter to concern the nurse. He seemed to keep things very much in his own hands and I know I was not the only nurse that felt that way. With some doctors one would feel quite in order in asking them what they had given the patient but I felt I could not do this with Dr Adams . . .'

Nurse Grace Osgood did not like the fact that Dr Adams gave his old friend Roland Gwynne pills that 'were too strong and made him drowsy'. And, in general, she found him dismissive of nurses and unwilling to answer questions about a patient's medication. She remembered a lady named Mrs Woolrych who had an extremely painful ear infection, which Dr Adams would not treat. Instead, he would sit and hold his patient's hand, reassuring her that she was 'getting along fine'. Mrs Woolrych had been scared of Dr Adams and his sudden 'terrible temper'. His general attitude towards Mrs Woolrych, said Nurse Osgood, 'was repulsive to me', and she resolved not to work with Dr Adams again.

Some of the nurses remembered that he had behaved strangely when a patient died. Nurse Blanche Goacher recalled that, after one death, Dr Adams had said to her: 'Don't worry about your fees. You want to charge – there's plenty of money there.' And Nurse Marjorie Savage told of the time Dr Adams had stood at the foot of the bed of a dead woman and said: 'The poor wee thing. I'll take the clock away with me now. Has the brandy bottle been opened? I'll take that too.' After that, he went off with the clock and the brandy, and instructed the nurse to have the rest of the dead lady's possessions packed up, 'and he would have them collected'.

Themes emerged. The doctor was dismissive and cold towards the nurses, while being over-friendly and ingratiating to patients. He gave the impression of being arrogant and hyper-sensitive to anything he regarded as criticism or a lack of respect, and was prone to fly off the handle if he was crossed or challenged. His behaviour was sometimes avaricious and unethical. Hannam found all this interesting, and it helped him build a psychological profile of his suspect – but in the litany of nurses' complaints, there was no clear indication of anything criminal. The matter of over-sedation was the most significant element; it fitted neatly with the heavy doses of barbiturates given to Bobbie Hullett and the odd last injection, thought to be morphia, given to Jack Hullett. But, again, there was no solid piece of evidence, no really grave accusation. It was as though the police had walked into a miasma of disapproval. Murder might be in there, somewhere in the mist, it might be all around. It was hard to tell. Hannam's response was to keep digging.

He anticipated that the doctors of Eastbourne would be more forthcoming than the nurses, and had heard that local GPs found Dr Adams – at the very least – an 'oafish bore', and 'inept bungler' and 'a disgrace to the profession'. During the war, they had excluded him from an arrangement to share out patients and income, and now most regarded him as a 'menace in their midst' who should be removed. But when Herbert Hannam approached the doctors for information, he met with an unexpected wall of silence. The BMA (British Medical Association) had intervened, sending a letter to all the GPs in Eastbourne reminding them of their duty of confidentiality to patients, including patients of a third party – meaning Dr Adams. The letter was designed to stop the doctors co-operating with the police and, for the most part, it was successful.

The BMA's action was frustrating, infuriating even, but also understandable. In 1956 British doctors were at war with the government, unhappy and angry about the low pay for GPs under the NHS, which had been set up in 1948, but was still bedding in, still regarded as a new idea. The BMA had been against the NHS in the first place – 84 per cent of GPs had voted against it – and now was so dissatisfied that it was threatening to pull out altogether, an act that would bring the system down, and probably the government with it. Many doctors felt jittery and under siege, and in the circumstances the fuss about Dr Adams seemed like one more attack on a beleaguered profession. Doctors had it hard enough, went the argument, without being accused of bumping off their frail and elderly patients.

But none of this was of much interest to Superintendent Hannam. As far as he was concerned, 'one avenue of most useful information in connection with Dr Adams's activities became greatly restricted'. It was annoying, but Hannam was not deterred, and his investigation now focused on the friends and relatives of Dr Adams's patients, and the maids, servants, lawyers and bank managers who knew them. The result was spectacular – a torrent of complaints and accusations going back decades. It was hard to know how far back the official inquiry should go, but Hannam started to build a dossier of cases, beginning with a patient of Dr Adams from twenty years ago – Miss Henrietta Hatton, who had died on 13 February 1935 at the age of 87.

Witnesses said that Dr Adams had visited Miss Hatton very frequently. She was in an extremely poor mental state; in fact, she was losing her mind. When the doctor came, he would order her maids out of her bedroom, and fall into whispered conversation about her finances (evidently, the maids were listening at the door). After a while, the doctor arranged for Miss Hatton to be moved into a nursing home, and at the same time took over the management of her money, obtaining Power of Attorney, and drawing cheques on her bank account.

Miss Hatton's relatives realised what had happened, and confronted Dr Adams about his unwarranted control of a vulnerable patient. He became angry, and 'insisted to the point of being extremely abusive' that Miss Hatton was perfectly compos mentis, 'fully aware of her surroundings', and had the 'clearest possible understanding' of the situation, and her finances. However, the relatives were so firmly of the opposite opinion that they arranged to go to the High Court, and they asked two independent doctors to assess Miss Hatton's condition. Both, without the slightest hesitation, said that the old lady was quite incapable of understanding matters put to her. At this point Dr Adams withdrew. It turned out that he had also been a beneficiary of Miss Hatton's will, though by the time she died, he was no longer in it. Superintendent Hannam thought Miss Hatton's case valuable as an illustration of 'the technique which this gentleman will adopt', but as it was so old, he left it there, and did not investigate further.

The 1940s, he thought, were of greater interest, in particular the case of a widow named Mrs Agnes Pike. Her treatment by Dr Adams was brought to Herbert Hannam's attention by Dr Philip Mathew – a local doctor who, despite the BMA letter, was determined to be helpful to the police. During the war, Mrs Pike and her daughter Nan had spent some time living at the Lathom House Hotel in Eastbourne. One day, Nan went on an outing to London and Mrs Pike, left to her own devices, 'commenced an orgy of drinking' which lasted for several days and culminated in her falling in her room and banging her head so badly that she was left unconscious.

Dr Adams was sent for. By this time, he was well-established in Eastbourne, a prominent figure in the YMCA, a founding member of the Bisley Rifle Club, a member of the André Simon Wine and Food Society, and the founder of a local camera club. Times were harder than usual because of the war. Even so, when Dr Adams arrived to see Mrs Pike, he seemed well-heeled, successful. Fat, pink, expensively dressed, and in possession of a fancy car.

His first act, on seeing the patient, was to say that she must stay in bed, and he arranged for two nurses to look after her. One of these was Nurse Edna Baldock, who told the police that on her first night with Mrs Pike, Dr Adams visited. He took a syringe from his bag, she said, filled it with liquid, and injected it into Mrs Pike's arm. After that she was quiet until between three and four in the morning, then she became restless and irritable and tried to get out of bed. Dr Adams subsequently visited often, and always gave Mrs Pike an injection, the contents of which came from his doctor's bag. When Nurse Baldock asked him what the injections were, he was abrupt and refused to tell her.

Nurse Baldock did not know what was supposed to be wrong with Agnes Pike. She said that during the whole of the time that she nursed her – about six weeks – Mrs Pike 'never appeared sensible' and could not manage a conversation 'because her mind always appeared a blank'. She always appeared to be in a stupor, but not from drinking, there was no smell of alcohol. It was something else – presumably the injections. Edna Baldock also indicated there was something creepy about the doctor's behaviour. She told Inspector Brynley Pugh that when Dr Adams visited, he always gave Mrs Pike an injection immediately, and then would sit at her bedside and stare at her.

The proprietor of the Lathom House Hotel, Gladys Parker, told police that 'the continued drugged stupor that Mrs Pike remained in alarmed me'. Mrs Parker summoned a friend of Mrs Pike's, who was similarly shocked. And the daughter, Nan, was so distressed by her mother's stupefied state that on one occasion she had gone upstairs to a hotel bedroom and screamed. Mrs Pike's friends now decided that something had to be done. They suggested to Dr Adams that she be removed from the hotel, possibly to a nursing home, and that a second opinion be sought on her condition. But Dr Adams would not listen, and dismissed both ideas out of hand.

So Mrs Pike's supporters brought in Dr Philip Mathew. Dr Mathew examined the prescriptions Dr Adams had written for Mrs Pike, 'all of which to the best of my recollections contained hypnotics'. He then visited Mrs Pike at the Lathom House Hotel, where he found her in bed being attended by Dr Adams. When Dr Mathew examined her, he 'found no actual disease but came to the conclusion that she was very deeply under the influence of drugs'. His opinion was based on the pinpoint pupils of her eyes, and her confused and incoherent speech. She had no idea what her own name was, he said, and gave her age as 200 years. She didn't know where she was, how long she had been there, or what the year was.

While Dr Mathew was examining Mrs Pike, Dr Adams suddenly, with no warning, gave her an injection, which he said was morphia. 'I asked why he thought it was necessary to give morphia,' Dr Mathew told Herbert Hannam, 'and I think he said, "because she might be violent".' It was a ludicrous answer, and Dr Mathew now took over the care of Agnes Pike, stopping all the hypnotic drugs she had been having. Over the next eight weeks, she regained all her faculties, and was well enough to go out and do her own shopping. Dr Mathew considered her to be in good health for a woman of her age. By this time, he said, 'she knew who she was, her age and that she came from New Zealand'. 'This was, in Dr Mathew's view, a case devoid of any reason other than ulterior in its method of medical treatment,' wrote Herbert Hannam.

A second case from the 1940s was more disturbing still. Irene Herbert was a wealthy divorcee who had a home in Surrey, but often came to Eastbourne for long visits. Until her divorce Mrs Herbert had been a happy enough person, but afterwards she became deeply depressed and started drinking heavily. There is something about her that is similar to Bobbie Hullett – she was younger than many of Dr Adams's patients, being close to 50 years old, and she was devastated at her changed status in life, at her lack of a husband. To be a divorcée was worse still than being a young widow – an object of pity and disdain.

Like Bobbie, Irene Herbert had material wealth. She possessed a fine beaver and ocelot coat, worth £500, as well as an ermine coat, and a silver fox cape. She owned diamonds and pearls, and expensive furniture. But there is nothing to suggest that her wealth did her any good at all. She could not have been more desperate. It did not help that she seemed isolated, having few friends and no family close to her. She had no children.

For long periods of time, Irene Herbert stayed at the Lathom House Hotel where Dr Adams treated her for her nerves. And he did this in his usual way, with bucketloads of sedatives – her prescriptions showed that she was sedated all day long. 'She was a neurotic type,' said the proprietor Gladys Parker. But Mrs Parker did not think that her condition was helped by the 'quantity of drugs' that she received from Dr Adams. She told Inspector Pugh that when Mrs Herbert came to Eastbourne, and saw the doctor, she would always experience a 'rapid decline in good health'. But Mrs Herbert did not blame Dr Adams; instead she described him as the only man who understood her condition. After a while Dr Adams arranged for her to stay in the Southfields Nursing Home. But, said Mrs Parker, Irene Herbert escaped, and took herself to the Eastbourne Railway Station where she attempted to throw herself on the live rail. Someone stopped her, and returned her to the care of her doctor.

In April 1943 Irene Herbert made a new will, making Dr Adams her executor, stating that she wished to be cremated, and increasing the amount she was leaving him to £1,000 from £500, 'as a slight token for all his kindness, which I can never repay'. Then, in January 1944, Dr Adams had a legal document drawn up which allowed him to take over her finances. He was to look after her house in Surrey, collect any rents, and also collect dividends on her shares. From her bank accounts he wrote cheques for 'the maintenance of the patient', with the largest sums going to the practice of Adams and Snowball – £170 that March, and another £42 in July. He also paid her housekeeper and gardener and arranged for the storage of her many furs.

Irene Herbert's health quickly deteriorated. In December 1944 she was admitted to the Brighton Borough Asylum in Haywards Heath, and then, in the spring, to the Otto House home for inebriates at Sydenham Hill in south London. When she first arrived she was well enough to go out for drives – and sometimes Dr Adams made his chauffeur available to her, at £2 a time. But by the summer she was in a terrible state, and on 5 August 1944 Irene Herbert died at Otto House. She was 50 years old.

Dr Adams was not attending her at the time – she was in the care of the hospital doctors, so there could be no question of murder. But it was a case that brought into sharp relief the central conundrum of Dr Adams. His treatment of Irene Herbert with heavy sedatives, while he took over the micro-management of her finances and secured a place in her will, was unethical, to say the least. But those who admired the doctor, including Mrs Herbert herself, regarded his actions as compassionate. For the police investigation, it was essential to discover his motives. It was possible that he was actually a kind man, motivated primarily by religious belief and a commitment to the Christian ideals of the Plymouth Brethren. It was possible that he made enemies because he was socially awkward, was edgy when challenged, and was physically unattractive. It was conceivable that he became so closely involved in his patients' private lives because he was lonely. But it was equally likely that Nurse Eunice Hitch's view of his motives had been the right one: Dr Adams 'is out for money and all he can get'.

During August and September 1956, Superintendent Hannam recorded several more suspicious cases from the 1940s, one of which was Mary Mouat, an 89-year-old wealthy widow, who had suffered a horrible accident in 1946. She had been standing too close to an electric fire, and her nightdress caught fire and burned her legs. Dr Adams was called. He bandaged her legs and put her to bed. 'Mrs Mouat owned a small Morris Minor car, and when attending her Dr Adams tried to induce her to sell the car to him,' wrote Hannam. When she declined to part with her car, he tried to get his hands on some fine pieces of furniture that she owned. Again Mrs Mouat refused.

A nurse, Marian Richards, was called in. Nurse Richards said Mrs Mouat was in fairly good health, apart from her burns, and was mentally alert. One day, Dr Adams came to visit, and she saw him in Mrs Mouat's bedroom, sitting next to her, with a blank piece of paper on his attaché case, which was resting on his knee.

He had a pen in his hand and was trying to make Mrs Mouat sign her name on the paper. Nurse Richards went into the room, but the doctor waved her out again. Later, Mrs Mouat told the nurse: 'Doctor wanted me to sign my name, but I can't, I'm too ill.' All that day, she kept saying, 'I'm sorry I couldn't sign the paper for the doctor this morning.' A few days later, she died.

Dr Adams wrote out a death certificate giving the primary cause of death as cerebral thrombosis. As he wrote out the certificate, he observed: 'It's lucky she died of thrombosis because otherwise there would have been an inquest on the burning accident.' As he was leaving the house, the doctor told Mrs Mouat's niece that he still wanted her Morris Minor. 'A callous remark I thought, at such a time,' said the niece. After the funeral, he again said he wanted the car, and in the end the niece sold it to him for £215.

It was possible that Mrs Mouat had been given a helping hand through death's door because Dr Adams was angry at her refusal to give or sell him her car. His attempt to have her sign something just before she died was odd, as was his comment about an inquest. And his diagnosis of cerebral thrombosis (or stroke) was emerging as his favourite fatality. Herbert Hannam noted that the Mouat case fitted with the general pattern of Dr Adams's behaviour but, because possibilities were not enough and there was a shortage of hard evidence, he decided not to take the case further.

Another patient, 75-year-old Emily Mortimer, died in 1946. Mrs Mortimer was a wealthy widow who had made a will that disinherited her close relatives, but left Dr Adams more than £3,600. When the police looked for her prescriptions, they found the usual mix of barbiturates and other sedatives and hypnotics. And when they inquired into the cause of her death, Dr Adams had once more diagnosed cerebral thrombosis – and not the heart condition for which she was being treated. After her death, he submitted a large medical bill, some £234. The circumstances were suspicious, but the case was too old, the details too few, and the surviving witnesses too vague.

Instead, Hannam turned his attention to Ada Harris, a wealthy widow in her eighties who had met Dr Adams at Plymouth Brethren meetings. At one point, the doctor gave her sleeping pills of such strength that Ada's sister Edith had threatened to report him to the General Medical Council. Ada, though, was unperturbed and over time allowed Dr Adams to take over the management of her daily life. First he advised her to move out of her house in Hailsham, and to come and live in Eastbourne, where he could treat her better. Then he told her to move into the home of Sarah Henry, the doctor's cousin (Miss Henry had moved out of Kent Lodge). Ada did as she was told, and also allowed Dr Adams to organise the sale of her Hailsham house, which fetched £1,901. When the money arrived, he told her to endorse the cheque, which he promptly paid into his own bank account. At the same time he sold the stair carpet from her house and seven lampshades to another of his patients and kept the proceeds, £12. Two years after the sale of her Hailsham house, Mrs Harris wrote to Dr Adams asking for her money back. He replied that he had decided to keep the money since the large amount the house fetched was entirely due to his efforts. Also, he regarded the payment as recompense for Mrs Harris's accommodation when she was living with Sarah Henry. Ada Harris now consulted a solicitor.

Letters flew back and forth. In one, Dr Adams said he regarded the money as a gift that recognised his kindness in looking after Mrs Harris as she was incapable of looking after herself. Her lawyers stood firm and eventually he started to cave in. He would return the money, he said, but would deduct a charge for Mrs Harris's accommodation with Sarah Henry. The lawyers replied with a threat to go to court. Dr Adams now returned the money in full – including the £12 for the stair carpet and lampshades. At one stage, Mrs Harris had included Dr Adams in her will – but now she cut him out again. The case was hard on evidence, in that there was documentary proof of Dr Adams's behaviour – but it was evidence of an attempt to defraud only, not of something more sinister. In her final years, Ada Harris lived in relative peace, free from the attentions of her doctor.

The case of Leslie Cockhead, who died in 1947, was also all about money. Mr Cockhead, 86, was a wealthy widower whose fortune came from custard, since he was connected to the Pearce Duff custard company. Dr Adams was treating him for a heart condition and he also brought in a nurse named Gertrude Gardner. Nurse Gardner, who was thirty years younger than Mr Cockhead, soon became romantically involved with him. The valet sometimes saw them kissing and 'embracing'. He also noticed that Dr Adams and Nurse Gardner seemed to be jockeying for position with Mr Cockhead and his money. Mr Cockhead's niece, Irene, agreed. 'I realised he had parasites around him,' she told the police, and she thought Dr Adams 'a very greedy man'. Her uncle, she added, had told her that the doctor seemed to expect to be mentioned in his will – 'why, I do not know'.

It soon became clear that Dr Adams was furious that Nurse Gardner was gaining the upper hand, and when Mr Cockhead was briefly in a nursing home, the doctor ordered that he should have no visitors – a diktat designed to exclude Nurse Gardner. Then, while the nurse was out of the way, Dr Adams attempted to find his patient a new flat to live in – but he was rebuffed when Mr Cockhead insisted that he be allowed to see Nurse Gardner – or Gee Gee as he called her – then chose to move to a flat that she had chosen.

When Leslie Cockhead died, a copy of his will was in his flat and Dr Adams learned immediately that he had received only £500, while Nurse Gardner had inherited £20,000. The niece, Irene, remembered the doctor behaving strangely, wiping a tear from his eye, and saying that he would like Mr Cockhead's gold pen 'as a little reminder of the dear patient'. Irene did not give him the pen, but when she told Superintendent Hannam about it, he thought it significant – the doctor had a habit of taking 'tokens' from his dead patients. Overall, though, it was the same story. The doctor's behaviour had been peculiar and greedy, but not convincingly criminal.

The case of Mrs Ethel Hunt stood out because she quickly got the measure of Dr Adams, and challenged him. Unlike many of Dr Adams's wealthy widows, Mrs Hunt had friends and family around her, including two supportive sons, one of whom was Sir John Hunt, war hero and leader of the historic Everest expedition of 1953. In 1944 the doctor had treated Ethel at home for a minor complaint, and she had been quite satisfied with the service he provided. Then, afterwards, even though she had no need of him, and certainly had not summoned him, he turned up at her house to check on her. 'On this occasion he told me he knew I was a widow and hoped my affairs were in good hands,' she told Herbert Hannam. The doctor wanted to know whether her finances and securities were being well managed and said he could help her with them.

Ethel Hunt did not regard Dr Adams's concern as thoughtful or kind. Instead she was instantly suspicious, and assured him that her Indian Army Pension of £350 a year would cease to be paid on the day she died, along with a small allowance from her two sons. 'It was made quite clear to Dr Adams,' she added, 'that my financial position was not attractive.' But, like a bad penny, he turned up again, this time at a particularly inconvenient moment. She was playing bridge with some lady friends, and her maid informed the doctor that Mrs Hunt was busy. None the less, he insisted on seeing her, so she broke away from her bridge game and met him. 'Dr Adams said he had come to tell me I was a most unsatisfactory patient, that I had not carried out his orders and he thought I was slightly mentally deranged.'

Mrs Hunt, sharp as needles, responded that she realised she was senile, but she had retained one grain of sense – she knew that once she had paid her doctor's bill she was quite free to open her door and show him out: 'I told him that was my proposition at that moment and I did it. He was furious and bounded out of the house and into his car,' slamming the gate and the door of his car as he went.

She was not the only widow to show him the door. A letter received at Eastbourne Police Headquarters alerted Superintendent Hannam to the story of Edith Mawhood, the wife of William Mawhood – whose mackintosh and boots Dr Adams had coveted and then ordered for himself on William's account. By 1956 Edith was a widow, and no longer the mistress of the splendid 500-acre Ratton estate, presiding over a multitude of servants. Instead she lived in a more modest house, in an ordinary road, in Rottingdean near Brighton. Over the years, she had become increasingly annoyed with Dr Adams – and the younger Edith, who had allowed him to hijack her holiday to Devon and had loaned him the money to buy Kent Lodge, was gone. These days she described the doctor as 'a real scrounger' and was disgusted by him.

She was no longer in good physical health but, according to Hannam, she was 'a remarkably intelligent and alert lady for her age' (she was 77 in 1956). And she was still extremely wealthy – William had left her £50,000 in his will. Edith was more than happy to co-operate with the police, and tell them all about Dr Adams's early days in Eastbourne and his peculiar attempts to acquire things without paying – not just the mackintosh and the boots, but also the Sheffield steel medical instruments. In the late 1930s and early 1940s, she said, he had tried to benefit from William's will by offering to be an executor, at a price – £3,000. William regarded that as too much, and gave Dr Adams a legacy of £1,000 in wills that he made in 1938 and 1942. Later, though, he cut him out altogether.

In 1949 William Mawhood had been diagnosed with cancer,

and his health had deteriorated rapidly. Just before William died, Edith happened to be passing the bedroom where he was resting, and she overheard Dr Adams's voice. The doctor was telling William to leave him all his money and was assuring William that he would see to it that Edith was 'well provided for'. When she heard this, Edith snapped, and charged into the bedroom. 'I chased Dr Adams around the bedroom with my stick,' she said. 'He ran down the stairs. I threw my stick at him and it smashed a valuable flower pot which was standing in the hall. Dr Adams drove off in his car.' Edith, astounded and infuriated, returned to the bedroom and asked William if Dr Adams had made him sign anything. William, who was extremely frail, said yes, he had. 'Dr Adams had written something out on a paper and my husband said he had put a cross on it. He was too weak to sign his name.' Edith immediately told her solicitor not to accept anything signed by William, and to make sure that any cheques written by him were stopped. She heard later that Dr Adams had gone, in person, to her bank and had enquired about William's will.

When William died, the doctor discovered that he was no longer in the will. He came back to the house, said Edith, and 'kicked up a fuss' about being left out. He also attended William's funeral, and shouted out at a fellow mourner about being cut out of the will. Then, said Edith, 'some time after my husband's death, Dr Adams came back to my house while I was in bed unwell. He had not been invited or sent for, and he just walked into the bedroom. I said I would have nothing to do with him. He saw on the dressing table a 22-carat gold pencil which was my husband's. He said he would have something of my husband's and took it away with him.' Afterwards, Dr Adams submitted a colossal medical bill to the executors – £1,102. This, he said, was to cover his work with the Mawhoods over the eleven years before William's death. Although the bill was grossly inflated, the executors decided to pay him £876.

Herbert Hannam added Edith Mawhood's strange encounters with Dr Adams to his file. Like so much of the information he had accumulated, her case was disturbing but not damning. But there was a sense that a breakthrough in the investigation was imminent; that with a little more digging some vital piece of information would be unturned; something that would remove the haziness from the allegations against Dr Adams, and make them solid and provable. Hannam was optimistic that he was on the right track, and this was the message that he passed on to the cabal of reporters who followed him around like hungry hounds; who, at the end of the working day, would join him for a beer in the New Inn, the pub across the road from the police station.

6

Police and Press

ONE REPORTER STOOD apart from the pack, choosing to keep his distance from Hannam and his gang. Percy Hoskins of the mighty *Daily Express* was, at 52, in his prime. He was a Fleet Street luminary – the chairman of the Crime Reporters Association; a crime expert who was consulted by the BBC; an author whose books inspired the popular television drama *No Hiding Place*. He was also a regular at Fleet Street bars, renowned for schmoozing his impeccable police contacts. On the side, he worked for the police as an adviser 'on the value of press guidance', gaining the nickname 'Scotland Yard's Dr Watson', and his flat in Park Lane was an open house for senior policemen who wanted to stop by for a drink. His friends said that if you were in trouble in high places, best to call Percy, even before you called your lawyer. In character, he was humorous and amiable, in appearance, portly and jowly, and he was pleased that he resembled Alfred Hitchcock, whom he knew. At the *Express*, he had a certain cachet, since he was on good terms with the owner, Lord Beaverbrook.

While the rest of the press went mad about the events in Eastbourne, Hoskins stayed calm or, as some saw it, aloof. He scorned his fellow reporters who were taking their lead from Hannam, and instead was in cahoots with the most senior officers at Scotland Yard – a relationship that led him to the view that Superintendent Hannam was not handling matters well at all; instead he was treating seriously every piece of malicious gossip in Eastbourne, giving credence to every poisonous rumour. At the same time, thought Hoskins, Hannam was shaking up Eastbourne society with unseemly clumsiness. It was as though he were marching along the promenade up-ending the flower-pots or storming the tea rooms and smashing the china.

Then, just as Hannam was getting into the swing of his investigation, Hoskins was summoned to Scotland Yard. The Assistant Commissioner, Joe Jackson, informed him that he was worried that things in Eastbourne 'seemed to be getting out of hand'. The chief constable of Eastbourne – Dr Adams's friend Richard Walker – had been on the phone to Scotland Yard, complaining that Herbert Hannam was going beyond his brief. 'Would Hoskins help out?' asked the Assistant Commissioner. Would he go to Eastbourne *immediately* and keep an eye on the situation? Hoskins was more than willing. He was driven by the police to his flat to pick up an overnight bag, then on to Victoria Station. When he arrived in Eastbourne, the chief constable's car was waiting for him at the station. Very soon, Hoskins was in conversation with Richard Walker and Herbert Hannam, and it was made clear to Hannam that Hoskins had been authorised by his superiors. In effect, Scotland Yard had sent Hoskins to Eastbourne as a spy.

Later, Hoskins wrote that he was dismayed by the 'rising flood of distortion' in Eastbourne, and the 'wild rumours' that were being printed daily in rival newspapers. And he was disgusted by Hannam's off-the-record press briefings in the New Inn. 'Information was not being leaked,' he wrote. 'It was gushing like lava from Etna in eruption', with the gravest of consequences for Dr Adams – 'In my many years as a crime reporter I had never seen a man so neatly trussed up and ready for the scaffold as John Bodkin Adams.'

His stand made him a lone figure among the journalists, save for one unexpected ally in Michael Foot, the Labour Party politician. In 1956 Foot was editor of the left-leaning *Tribune* magazine. In the issue of 31 August, he wrote:

One of the most appalling and shameful examples of newspaper sensationalism and persecution in the history of British journalism has occurred in the last ten days. The result has been that a man charged with no crime and against whom no evidence is available to base any charge, has been made the victim of the wildest gossip and rumour. The worst offender in this ugly competition is the *Daily Mail* . . .

Hoskins and Foot were writing in ignorance of the details of the unsavoury facts about Dr Adams that were quickly being collected by the police – his taking over of the finances of vulnerable patients like Henrietta Hatton, Irene Herbert and Ada Harris, his bold attempts to become beneficiaries in the wills of wealthy patients such as William Mawhood and Matilda Whitton, and his extraordinary willingness to sedate patients of all types, including those who were not actually ill. None the less, they had a point. Led by the *Daily Mail*, the newspaper headlines portrayed the 'Eastbourne probe' as the biggest mass murder investigation in British history – with dozens, or maybe hundreds, of suspicious deaths; exaggerations which were hopelessly out of proportion to the tawdry and inconclusive nature of the facts so far.

Percy Hoskins intimated that his wariness of Herbert Hannam had its roots in his handling of the Teddington Towpath investigation three years earlier. Peter Rawlinson, the lawyer who had defended the Teddington murderer, Alfred Whiteway, also happened to work as a legal adviser at the *Daily Express* – and he had told the paper's journalists that he distrusted Hannam's methods. 'It was not that Hannam was lying, Rawlinson said. It was the method he had adopted to secure the self-damning confession. A piece here and a piece there. A juggling of context. A clever manipulation . . .'

Hoskins was also critical of what he saw as Hannam's fixation on cornering and unsettling suspects until they 'cracked', and observed that he was now employing his cracking technique in the Adams case. The approach seemed to be to leave the doctor alone for the time being – unquestioned by the police – while all around him the investigation continued. The strategic cracking moment, the point of confrontation, was scheduled for later.

He set about persuading his bosses at the *Express* of the 'agitated concern among the most senior officers at Scotland Yard' about Hannam's methods and the paper took his advice to tread carefully. The senior executives 'had agreed, somewhat reluctantly, to adopt a low key while all the rivals were playing it double fortissimo,' he wrote. In an article bearing the headline 'THE TRUTH ABOUT EASTBOURNE', Hoskins proclaimed that he was sorting the facts from the rumours:

ALLEGATION: That four hundred wealthy widows were murdered. Untrue.

ALLEGATION: That the murderer has been at work twenty years. Untrue.

ALLEGATION: That a million pounds was involved. Untrue.

At the same time he argued that it was entirely natural that Dr Adams should have looked after so many wealthy patients who died. After all, a quarter of the Eastbourne population were pensioners and the death rate was high – 15.75 per thousand, to the national average of 11.7. And when old people were lonely, it was unsurprising that they should remember in their wills the doctor who had befriended them, and could give them some comfort and consolation. It was, he said, an accepted pattern. Even the death of Matilda Whitton seemed, to Hoskins, unsuspicious. (He knew that Dr Adams had looked after her, and that she left him £5,000 or more when she died in 1935. He did not know that she had been scared of the mysterious injections he gave her.) The doctor was already wealthy, Hoskins reasoned, so why would he murder for money?

Though his newspaper accepted his arguments and was prepared to back him, there was one condition attached – that Percy Hoskins be right. Supporting Dr Adams was a huge risk. If the doctor turned out to be a mass murderer after all, then the *Daily Express* would look ridiculous and wrong-headed. The proprietor, Lord Beaverbrook, was particularly uneasy about the stance, and he summoned Hoskins to a meeting at his house in London where he subjected him to a 'restless, probing interview'. Beaverbrook had started by being all but certain that Dr Adams was a master criminal. But Hoskins was persuasive, and in the end the proprietor agreed to back his journalist. 'I knew one thing for certain,' wrote Hoskins, 'I had put my professional head on the chopping block.'

Then, in late August 1956, Percy Hoskins met Dr Adams face-to-face for the first time. The two men came upon each other in the first class carriage of a morning train from Eastbourne to London, and fell into conversation. Hoskins was struck by the doctor's unprepossessing appearance – round and 'fleshy'. But his manner was friendly enough and, said Hoskins, Dr Adams spoke to him in an avuncular way, addressing him as though he were a patient. As they chatted, Hoskins gradually realised that the doctor was utterly 'unaware of peril threatening him. His unconcern was as massive as his physical bulk. At first, I thought he was masking his apprehension. Hiding his fear behind a front. But as we talked it became clear to me that his unconcern was genuine.' Dr Adams seemed to think that the fuss would blow over, and so Percy Hoskins warned him of the jeopardy of his situation. He might very well be charged with murder. If found guilty, he might hang.

Hoskins gives the impression that Dr Adams was cut off from reality to a bizarre degree. Practically everyone else in the country knew of the immensity of the allegations against him, while he was in a world of his own, believing it would all pass. His optimism appeared to come in part from the support that he was receiving from some of his friends and patients. 'I never discussed the rumours with my patients,' Dr Adams said, 'and they never mentioned them to me. They stayed loyal to me.' He claimed that he received more than 500 letters offering sympathy and good wishes. That may or may not have been so, but the number who wrote to the police on his behalf was no more than a handful. They included Lady Bertha Prendergast who condemned 'the wave of mass hysteria which has swept through Eastbourne', and said how very distressed she was at 'some of the innuendoes' against her excellent family doctor. 'Legacies left to doctors are by no means unusual,' she pointed out, 'and it is one of the only ways in which a patient is able to show gratitude for considerable kindness.'

Lady Prendergast was a vocal ally. But many of Dr Adams's society friends, including those at the rifle club and the YMCA, did not know what to think, and did not write in to the police. Though Adams socialised a great deal, attending prominent dinners and dances, having tea with lady friends in Eastbourne's grandest hotels, his circle of close friends was a small one. Roland Gwynne counted as a bosom pal, as did his former fiancée, Nora O'Hara, and there was a dentist named Norman Gray who was connected to the Plymouth Brethren. The other significant friend, who was at his service throughout his ordeal, was Herbert James, the solicitor who had drawn up many of the wills that featured Dr Adams, and who was convinced of his innocence. It was a small band of supporters, set against a much larger number of detractors in Eastbourne. The town was divided.

Many of his patients stayed loyal, and this was particularly important to Dr Adams since his close family were no longer around. His mother, Ellen, had died during the war, and his cousin, Sarah Henry, had died of cancer in 1952. She was only 51 years old and, by all accounts, Dr Adams had looked after her with great tenderness in her final weeks, which were spent at Kent Lodge. She had been in severe pain and he had made sure that hypodermic syringes containing morphia were always on hand. Another cousin, Sara Watson, had stayed at Kent Lodge while Sarah was ill. 'I would say from my experience of Dr

Adams, and my close association with him, that he was the kindest man I ever knew, both to his mother, his other relatives, and to me,' she said. Dr Adams gave the last morphia injection to Sarah Henry. In this case, Herbert Hannam was prepared to believe that the doctor was acting in a caring and professional way.

This was the side of Dr Adams that Percy Hoskins chose to see, and he continued to plough his lonely furrow, publishing articles designed to counteract the sensational reports in the rest of the press. But, with each day that passed, the Hoskins view of events seemed, to those in the know, more other-worldly, more risky. The truth was that Superintendent Hannam's dossier on Dr Adams was expanding rapidly, and – though Hoskins did not know it – the cases from the 1950s were looking more sinister than those from the previous decade. The statements relating to a wealthy widow named Annabella Kilgour, for instance, were causing Herbert Hannam to think seriously about seeking permission for the exhumation of her body.

Mrs Kilgour had died on 28 December 1950 at the age of 89. She had suffered a stroke that July, and was in the care of Dr Adams. She had 'the greatest confidence in him', her housekeeper Dorothy Badham told the police. But she was not sentimental about him and did not regard him as a close friend. Around Christmas-time, Mrs Kilgour went into a decline, and Dr Adams visited her twice a day. At night, she was sometimes restless, and would get out of bed – which was a bother for Miss Badham, whose sleep was disturbed. This was mentioned to the doctor, who gave Mrs Kilgour a hypodermic injection.

The following morning, which was Christmas Eve, a day nurse named Margaret Methren arrived and found Mrs Kilgour in a condition that she described as 'very unnatural'. She was in a deep coma, but her pulse was fairly good. 'Her colour was pale,' said Nurse Methren, 'she was quite warm, but it was impossible to arouse her.' She was alarmed, and when Dr Adams arrived,

she asked him what had been in the injection that he had administered the night before. She thought she remembered – she
could not be certain – that he told her it was morphine.

Mrs Kilgour remained in a deep coma all that day, and in the
evening had some 'cerebral spasms' which caused her body to
become rigid. On Boxing Day she was still comatose, and a night
nurse, Marguerite Roberts, was called in. Nurse Methren told
Nurse Roberts that she thought 'Mrs Kilgour would never come
round again', because of the injection Dr Adams had given her.
During the following two days Mrs Kilgour remained comatose.
'It was a most unusual case in Nurse Roberts' view,' wrote
Superintendent Hannam, 'because the patient never stirred
during the whole of the time she was with her.'

When Mrs Kilgour died two days later Dr Adams wrote the
death certificate and gave the cause, as he did so often, as 'cerebral thrombosis'. Nurse Methren told the police that 'she was,
and always has been concerned about the death of Mrs Kilgour,
particularly the manner in which she died'.

Mrs Kilgour's will had been made two years earlier. The gross
value of her estate was £47,600. 3s. 0d. Her diamond arrow
brooch and £2,000 went to the housekeeper Dorothy Badham.
Diamonds and pearls and £3,000 went to her sister Florence, and
all her furs and her wireless set and £3,000 to her sister Edith. All
her furniture and £3,000 went to a third sister, Elizabeth, and her
brother William received £500. Her doctor, John Bodkin
Adams, was to inherit her hall bracket clock and the sum of
£200. Her bank manager was the subject of a similar bequest –
the dining room clock, and £200.

So there was nothing unusual about the will. Indeed the way
in which it portioned out the estate was a perfect example of the
phenomenon that many of Dr Adams's supporters cited. Family
doctors, they said, were often mentioned in wills along with
other professionals whose role straddled the business and personal
– bank managers, for instance, or solicitors. This was natural.

And, in most of the cases in the police files, the inheritances received by Dr Adams were relatively minor – a small part of the total value of the estate, and certainly not enough to be a convincing motive for murder.

None the less, in the eyes of Superintendent Hannam, the Kilgour case was highly suspicious because it was a particularly sharp example of a combination of circumstances that was becoming familiar – a small inheritance, an injection that sent the patient into a coma from which she never recovered, and a cause of death recorded as cerebral thrombosis. Hannam mulled over the idea of requesting permission to exhume the body of Mrs Kilgour, who was buried in the Ocklynge Cemetery in Eastbourne, but in the end decided against it. After her body had been six years in the ground, he thought, it might not be possible to show that she had died from an excess of morphine. 'If ever there was an investigation in which caution should be exercised it is this one,' he wrote, 'and no sensational move could be justified unless the clearest credible facts support it.' In the fevered atmosphere, he wished to be perfectly sure of his ground before ordering exhumations. There would, he believed, be stronger cases.

In the meantime, he took statements relating to another wealthy widow who had been looked after by Dr Adams in the 1950s. Margaret Pilling was 81, and had lived in Eastbourne's swankiest hotel – the Grand. Unlike many of his favourite patients, Mrs Pilling had a close relationship with her family and was visited regularly by her three daughters. Mrs Pilling was a cheerful, positive person but, early in 1951, was confined to bed with a condition that Dr Adams diagnosed as influenza. Her daughter, Elaine, visited her several times while she was ill, but 'did not like the look of things as she was always partly unconscious'. She consulted her sisters, and they decided to ask a friend of the family, Nurse Clara Brierley, to come to Eastbourne and look after Margaret. When the nurse arrived at the Grand Hotel, she found Mrs Pilling in bed and 'seemed to be very ill, was drowsy and was very weak and helpless . . . She appeared to have lost considerable weight.' The nurse saw no symptoms of influenza.

Clara Brierley said that when Dr Adams arrived he 'gave me no idea what diagnosis he had made or whether one had been made'. He would not tell her what medicines Mrs Pilling was having, but insisted that the treatment should continue. During the following weeks, the nurse became increasingly concerned that Mrs Pilling was 'under the influence of drugs'. Mrs Pilling's daughter, Elaine, was also worried. 'I saw Dr Adams,' she told the police, 'and asked why mother was being kept under the influence of drugs and he told me she would otherwise be in great pain.' Elaine asked why this would be so, but he refused to answer.

The family decided to move Mrs Pilling to a new home in Ascot in Berkshire. But Dr Adams told Nurse Brierley that the patient was not well enough to travel, and would not be for some time. The nurse then said she had been asked to arrange for a second medical opinion on Mrs Pilling's health. Dr Adams answered that he was making his own arrangements for a specialist from London to see her. But no specialist ever came, and Mrs Pilling's condition did not improve.

Her family now decided to smuggle her out of Eastbourne, without Dr Adams's knowledge, never mind his consent. A private ambulance was booked to take her to Ascot, and on the night before she left Nurse Brierley did not give her the tablets that Dr Adams had insisted upon. The following morning – 28 March 1951 – 'she was brighter and less drowsy' and she seemed to thoroughly enjoy the trip in the ambulance. 'She arrived at Ascot that afternoon and seemed well and happy,' said Clara Brierley. That night, she vomited a brown-coloured liquid, and was sick the following day – which everyone took to be a reaction to the discontinuation of Dr Adams's medicines, all of which were now thrown away.

Margaret Pilling made a rapid recovery and soon became 'her old natural self'. She was lively and in good health at her grand-daughter's wedding that June – which was a sharp contrast with her condition while under Dr Adams's care. Back then, said Nurse Brierley, 'the treatment did not vary but she seemed to be in a continuous coma and a demented state I have never been able to account for'. After her rescue, Mrs Pilling continued well and happy until a final illness which struck her nearly two years later. She died in December 1952.

The case of Mrs Harriet Hughes was more murky. At the age of 66, Mrs Hughes was relatively young in 1951, and a wealthy widow. She lived at a fashionable apartment block called Kepplestone. In May 1951 she had made a will in consultation with her solicitor, Mr Perkins, and her bank manager, Mr Privett. Her estate was valued at £20,502.

In November 1951 she felt unwell, and Dr Adams attended her at Kepplestone. She was diagnosed with 'a thrombosed leg' and a heart condition, and was confined to bed. It seemed that Mrs Hughes was very fond of Dr Adams, and she told her house-keeper that when she was better he was going to take her out to dinner in London. During one of his visits, said the housekeeper, the doctor had kissed Mrs Hughes on the forehead – and after-wards Mrs Hughes had said she thought she would make Dr Adams the executor of her will. From then on the doctor visited often, and prescribed some white pills for her. Sometimes he brought her presents – on one occasion some fresh eggs; another time a wireless.

The other people on the scene were Mrs Hughes's old friends Elsie and Harry Thurston – who had known her for twenty years, but who had not been mentioned in her will. Two nurses were also appointed to help out. Around 22 November 1951 the nurses noticed a sudden flurry of activity around Mrs Hughes which involved Dr Adams arriving with documents for her to sign. On 24 November Mrs Hughes told her sister that Dr Adams had been advising her about her will, which she had changed, with Dr Adams and his solicitor, Herbert James, at her bedside to help her.

Her usual solicitor, Mr Perkins, and the bank manager Mr Privett, told the police that Dr Adams had informed them that Mrs Hughes was 'quite incapable of undertaking any business transactions for some time to come in view of the state of her health'. On 24 November, he had turned up at Mrs Hughes's bank and asked Mr Privett for a copy of her will. Mr Privett gave it to him, but was alarmed by the strangeness of the situation and wrote to Mrs Hughes saying he would call in and see her.

As soon as Mrs Hughes had signed her new will, her health dramatically worsened and the doctor started giving her injections. It was impossible to say which came first, the bad health or the injections. Either way, she quickly became comatose, and never saw the letter from Mr Privett saying he was on his way to see her. Harriet Hughes died on 29 November 1951, five days after signing the new will. Dr Adams signed the death certificate, giving the cause of death as 'a. cerebral thrombosis, and b. cardio vascular degeneration'.

The new will, it turned out, did not include the doctor. But there were two new legacies in it – £1,000 to Elsie Thurston and a further £1,000 to Harry Thurston. Superintendent Hannam was by now so suspicious of Dr Adams, and so well-acquainted with his behaviour, that he thought it probable that he had cut a deal with the Thurstons, and would receive a pay-off in return for securing their windfall. 'Both Detective Inspector Pugh and myself share the view of the solicitor Perkins and Mr Privett, the bank manager, that there is something highly suspicious about this matter,' he wrote, 'and it seems most likely that there was a conspiracy here between Adams and the Thurstons to share out part of the proceeds of a dying woman.'

The Thurstons denied any conspiracy. The police considered

checking their bank accounts for clues, but in the end they did not do so. It was the same story – a suspicious death, but no vital piece of evidence that would prove foul play.

Another particularly disturbing death was that of Julia Thomas, a wealthy widow who was the recipient of Dr Adams's closest attentions in the winter months of 1952. Mrs Thomas was 'a peculiar-tempered lady' with a large fortune. Dr Adams visited her often, even though she was not ill, usually staying for about an hour, and sometimes stopping for tea. Mrs Thomas's cook, Elizabeth Bryant, told the police that her employer sometimes discussed her private affairs with the doctor, and sought his advice on matters of finance. She always referred to him as 'Bobbums', said Miss Bryant, and always gave him chocolates.

On 6 November 1952 Mrs Thomas's cat was run over, and from that date 'she slowly deteriorated and became wandering in her mind'. Dr Adams now visited most days, and when the conversation turned to financial matters, he told her to change her lawyer. But she refused his advice, and stuck with her usual solicitor, Michael Davis. She was highly aware of the number of legacies that Dr Adams was receiving, she told Mr Davis. And she informed Dr Adams that he would never get one out of her. Instead, she said, she would leave him her new portable typewriter – worth £27 – as a keepsake.

On Tuesday 17 November 1952, Mrs Thomas was feeling poorly, and Dr Adams was sent for. He saw Mrs Thomas in her study and, said Miss Bryant, 'I heard the doctor say to her: "I want you to have a good night's rest, you must take the medicine and you will feel all the better in the morning." After she took the medicine, the doctor said to Rose, the parlourmaid, "We will get her to bed quick." Rose and Dr Adams helped Mrs Thomas up the stairs to bed. She fell asleep immediately and did not wake up until 2 a.m. on Wednesday morning, when she had a drink and fell asleep again. She slept all day Wednesday, and woke up briefly that night. Then she was asleep again. On

Thursday, said Miss Bryant, 'I saw Dr Adams preparing a hypodermic syringe to inject Mrs Thomas.'

The police heard another version of the same events from Julia Thomas's solicitor, Mr Davis. His information came from a lady named Gwendoline Werge, who had been staying in Mrs Thomas's house at the time. Dr Adams had told Mrs Thomas that she must go to bed, said Mr Davis, but she had been unwilling. The doctor insisted, and said 'that he was going to give her an injection and that she must be in bed to have it as she would probably want to go to sleep, and she went to bed and had the injection'.

Everyone agreed that Julia Thomas now went into a coma. On Friday night – three days after her illness began – Dr Adams was in the house and said to the cook, Miss Bryant: 'I don't think she will last much longer, it will all be over soon.' Before he left the house, he added: 'Mrs Thomas has promised me her typewriter. I will take it now.' Miss Bryant said: 'I went into the drawing room to fetch the typewriter, and left Mrs Werge with him. I know Mrs Werge was taken aback by this remark.'

Michael Harris told the police: 'Mrs Werge was more than surprised at the suggestion that the typewriter should be removed, because of course Mrs Thomas was not then dead. She made some excuses to the effect that the typewriter might well still have a letter in it, although its case was closed. But Dr Adams insisted and told her to open the typewriter and see whether in fact there was a letter there partly written. There was no letter and the doctor took the typewriter and walked off with it.'

Later that night, Mrs Thomas died. Dr Adams gave the cause of death as cerebral thrombosis. As an executor of the will, Michael Davis thought about asking Dr Adams what authority he had to remove the typewriter. However, because it was such a trivial thing, in the end he did nothing about it. Mrs Thomas was true to her word, in that Dr Adams was not mentioned in her will and inherited none of her £50,000.

When Superintendent Hannam came to write up the case of Mrs Thomas, he found it interesting because it 'further laid bare' Dr Adams's style. The taking of the typewriter, he thought, fell into the same pattern of behaviour as his taking of a gold pencil from Edith Mawhood and a gold pen from Leslie Cockhead. Also, he stated, 'we are assured by several people that Dr Adams frequently took cameras from houses, saying they had been promised to him by the patient who died. One of his hobbies is photography.' Once again, the death had followed an injection and a coma. Once again, the cause of death was given as cerebral thrombosis. However, in the eyes of Superintendent Hannam, in the case of Mrs Thomas, there was no motive. Dr Adams was not mentioned in her will. And he thought it unlikely that anyone would murder for a £27 portable typewriter.

The case of Annie Norton-Dowding raised different questions. It suggested that Dr Adams was not always 'on the make' or 'out for money and all he can get' – and so, for the police, it muddied the waters. Mrs Norton-Dowding was a wealthy widow who died in the same month as Julia Thomas. For years Dr Adams had visited her once a week, at 8 a.m. This was before she got up – so he would go straight to her bedroom, and would generally stay about ten minutes. As was so often the case, his visits were part-professional, part-social. And they fitted his pattern of making calls at any hour of the day – from first thing in the morning until eleven at night. Nobody could accuse Dr Adams of being a slacker.

Florence Sankey worked as a companion for Mrs Norton-Dowding. It was her impression that, until her final days, her employer was generally well but, none the less, 'always seemed to be having medicine of some kind'. It seemed to Mrs Sankey that the main purpose of the doctor's visit was for Mrs Norton-Dowding to discuss all her problems – financial and otherwise. Whenever she was troubled about something, she would say,

'The doctor will advise me what to do.' Witnesses said she 'simply adored him'.

Nurse Marion Stuart-Hemsley came to see Annie Norton-Dowding from time to time. She told the police she detested the doctor. She had first heard of him, she said, when she came to Eastbourne in the 1930s, and was looking for a good GP. She asked a local matron about Dr Adams. 'You don't want that pig,' was the reply. Then the matron told of a 'time when she had remonstrated with him for damaging some flowers in the front of the nursing home by throwing his bicycle among them, and he said, "if you live in this town long enough you will see me riding in my Rolls."'

More recently, Dr Adams had been the anaesthetist when Nurse Stuart-Hemsley's husband had an operation at the Princess Alice Hospital. Everyone seemed to have an anecdote about Dr Adams's behaviour during operations – of him falling asleep, or eating cakes and meringues and drinking tea. Nurse Stuart-Hemsley's complaint was that he had given her husband too much anaesthetic. When she came across the doctor in a shop, she accused him of giving enough to 'sink an ox', and asked, 'did you want to kill him?' She told the police: 'He spun round and said "what?", then he said, "He was a very nervous man and took a lot of getting under." Then he just told me to give my husband his compliments and out he went.' It was clear from everything she said that by the time Nurse Stuart-Hemsley came to talk to the police about Annie Norton-Dowding, she had a lot to get off her chest.

When she nursed Mrs Norton-Dowding in late 1952, she found her patient had no idea what was wrong with her. 'I told her that while she paid good fat bills to the doctor she would stay ill,' said Nurse Stuart-Hemsley. 'On one occasion I was visiting her in the Esperance [Nursing Home] when Dr Adams came in and threw a bed-jacket on the bed. I said to her: "What, is he making you presents now?" and she said, "No he has the keys to my house and he is most helpful in looking after my affairs and getting my linen."' On another day, when Nurse Stuart-Hemsley was busy criticising Dr Adams, Mrs Norton-Dowding said: 'Oh you misjudge him. He's really a very good doctor and if he doesn't know how to treat you he kneels down and prays for guidance.' Nurse Stuart-Hemsley added: 'Not so very long after that she died.'

Towards the end of her life, Mrs Norton-Dowding complained about abdominal pains. Dr Adams visited every day and gave her injections and pills. The housekeeper, Gertrude Boston, thought she suspected a malignant growth. A neighbour, Eva Barham, was not so sure. She thought Mrs Norton-Dowding was 'slowly slipping away' but had no idea what was wrong. Mrs Barham phoned Dr Adams because she was so concerned, but 'his attitude gave me the impression that he thought I was worrying unnecessarily'. At this time, Mrs Norton-Dowding was sleeping an awful lot.

While she was ill, Dr Adams went away on holiday, and his colleague Dr Snowball came to the house. When he examined Mrs Norton-Dowding, he recommended that she have an X-ray on her abdomen. She was most annoyed at this suggestion and said she was sure that Dr Adams would not allow it. Sure enough, when the doctor returned from his holiday, he told his patient that an X-ray was not necessary – and he continued with his treatment, coming to the house daily, or twice a day, to give her injections in her arm. By November she was asleep most of the time. On one occasion, said Mrs Boston, 'I was in her bedroom when Dr Adams came in. She was then in a comatose condition and Dr Adams gave her an injection in the arm. He sat with her for some time after giving her the injection. He rearranged the pillows himself and sat her up in bed and sat talking to her until she fell asleep. I heard her say, "when I get better we will take a cruise round the world together". The doctor's last words to her were, "I'll meet you at the airport."'

Before he left the house, Dr Adams asked Mrs Boston whether – given that Mrs Norton-Dowding was now comatose – she would like some nurses brought in to look after her, or alternatively for her to be removed to a nursing home. Mrs Boston chose the nursing home option, though Dr Adams said that if she were removed, Dr Snowball would want to operate on her. Mrs Norton-Dowding was taken by ambulance to the Esperance the following morning. Dr Adams told Mrs Boston that on no account must she write to Mrs Norton-Dowding's relatives, since it had been her express wish that they should not be informed of her condition.

For two days, Annie Norton-Dowding remained unconscious. Dr Snowball did then perform an operation to remove 'an acute obstruction' in her abdomen – but his efforts were unsuccessful, and she died within twenty-four hours. On the death certificate, Dr Adams wrote 'Toxaemia/Carcinoma of sigmoid colon'. He also arranged for a telegram to be sent to Mrs Annie Norton-Dowding's relatives, telling them she had died, and saying that the funeral would take place the following day. Mrs Norton-Dowding, it turned out, had made a new will three months before she died. She left an estate of £11,325, and Dr Adams received £500.

The case was intriguing. Some argued that, if Dr Adams was killing old ladies, then it was out of compassion – he was simply helping them die peacefully and without pain. While this theory did not fit easily with the circumstances of the deaths of most of his patients, it did seem to apply to Annie Norton-Dowding. She had cancer. But Dr Adams's preferred treatment was to keep her comatose, to spare her the ordeal of an X-ray, and to avoid any distressful operations. There was the troubling detail of the £500 legacy in a will made just before she died. But, in the circumstances, Superintendent Hannam decided his best course of action was to record the case, but not to investigate further.

He now turned to the case of 76-year-old Mrs Amy Ware, who had died on 23 February 1950 after being treated by Dr Adams. He had given the cause of death as 'a. cerebral thrombosis and b. cardio vascular degeneration'. Mrs Ware left an estate of £8,993 and Dr Adams inherited £1,000, under a will dated 16 February 1950, just seven days before her death. In November 1949 Mrs Ware's friend, Margaret Sumpter, had received a letter from Amy saying she was lonely. Margaret, who lived in London, replied saying she would visit the following Saturday. But before she had a chance to go to Eastbourne Margaret received a telegram from Amy saying: 'Not well. Dr says no visitors. Writing.' Soon afterwards Margaret received a letter from Amy Ware's brother-in-law James Priestley Downs, explaining that Amy was confined to bed suffering from 'nervous prostration', her illness being 'purely a nerve condition'. The doctor, he wrote, had ordered complete immunity from social activities and said that the intended visit on Saturday 'will have to be postponed indefinitely'.

On 1 December 1949 Margaret Sumpter went to Eastbourne to see what was wrong. Amy, she thought, looked vacant and seemed to be in a trance. A few weeks later, Mrs Sumpter wrote once more, inviting Amy to London. A reply was received, seemingly from James Priestley Downs, but unsigned, saying that 'we are advised that Amy is not to be troubled with correspondence or visitors'. Mrs Sumpter's husband now wrote to Dr Adams expressing his concern. The doctor replied, saying that Mrs Ware was very ill and he had forbidden her to be troubled by business matters, especially those of a distressing character. On 16 January 1950, he wrote again, saying Mrs Ware was now in a nursing home and a visit might be possible at some time. Then on 23 February the doctor sent a telegram saying simply: 'Mrs Ware passed away this morning. Adams.' Margaret Sumpter was upset and telephoned Dr Adams to say she would come to the funeral. He replied that Mrs Ware did not want anyone to come to her funeral, adding that Mrs Sumpter should not worry since both she and her husband were mentioned in Amy's will, a comment that, at the time, Margaret thought 'very strange'. Superintendent Hannam's records state that, while she was in the nursing home, Amy Ware's symptoms had included paralysis of her left side – a condition suggesting that she had had a stroke. He did not intend to investigate further, but noted that Dr Adams lied when he signed the cremation certificate for Mrs Ware, stating that he was unaware that he would benefit from her will, when in fact he knew perfectly well that he would receive £1,000.

Superintendent Hannam now turned his attention to Mrs Ware's brother-in-law, James Priestley Downs, who had died on 30 May 1955 at the Esperance Nursing Home, aged 88. Dr Adams gave the cause of death, once more, as 'a. cerebral thrombosis and b. cardio vascular degeneration'. Mr Priestley Downs had been admitted to the Esperance in February 1955 after fracturing his ankle as he rushed out of the house to catch the post. In the nursing home, under Dr Adams's care, he received sedatives, but he was a troublesome patient who often tried to get out of bed. By April, he was in a poor way, and Dr Adams was evidently very concerned about his will. The doctor visited Mr Downs every morning, and was heard to talk to him about legacies. One morning Nurse Gladys Miller was in the patient's bedroom when the doctor arrived. She told the police that he said to Mr Downs: 'Now, look here Jimmy, you promised me on the day Lily [his wife] was buried and on the return journey in the car that you would look after me and I see you haven't even mentioned me in your will.'

Nurse Miller said that, at the time, Mr Downs was very confused, and she heard him tell Dr Adams: 'Well I don't know. I can't remember what happened. I must have had a blackout.' Dr Adams then said: 'You haven't signed your will. Your nieces will get the lot and you don't want them to have it, do you? They have never done anything for you.' He added: 'Jimmy, I have looked after you all these years and I have never charged you a fee'. This was not true. A day or so later, said Nurse Miller, Dr Adams said he wanted Mr Downs to be more awake and that he was to be given a tablet to prepare him for the signing of his will.

On the morning of 7 April 1955, after the tablet had been given, Dr Adams visited Mr Downs and found him to be more alert. He telephoned Mr Downs's solicitor, James Heath, and asked him to come to the Esperance. Mr Heath asked for another doctor to be present, and Dr Adams's junior partner Dr Barkworth also came, as did Mr Downs's housekeeper, a Mrs Lavender. The police now took a statement from Mr Heath, and Superintendent Hannam wrote that when Mr Heath arrived at the nursing home at 11 a.m., he took with him a draft will in which Dr Adams was not named. Mr Downs then directed that the doctor should receive £1,000, and Mr Heath made the alteration. The will was signed at 1 p.m. the same day. It was read out twice, with Dr Adams listening. Mr Downs signed with a cross, as he was too weak to write his name, and Dr Adams and Dr Barkworth were witnesses. When James Priestley Downs died a few weeks later, Dr Adams signed the cremation form – answering the question: 'have you, so far as you are aware, any pecuniary interest in the death of the deceased?' with the words: 'of this I do not know'. 'This is another example,' wrote Superintendent Hannam, 'as clear as can be, that Dr Adams has made a false statement on the Cremation Act form.'

At the same time, he wrote up another incident which, though strange and incomprehensible, did not merit a criminal investigation. A solicitor named Edward Tilley wrote to the police to tell them about a client of his named Constance Brierley, who had lived at the Grand Hotel. On 19 December 1953, said Edward Tilley, he had received a telegram from Dr Adams which said simply: 'Mrs Brierley died this morning.' Mr Tilley then telephoned the Grand Hotel only to be told that Mrs

Brierley was very ill, but not dead. In fact, Constance Brierley died one week later – on 26 December 1953. Dr Adams gave the cause of death as uraemic coma and chronic nephritis. He did not benefit from the will, and the nurses who attended her did not report any suspicious circumstances surrounding her death. There was nothing for the police to pursue. However, wrote Superintendent Hannam, it 'adds to the peculiar circumstances surrounding so many of this doctor's cases'.

So much was weird and unpleasant, so much was ambiguous, and so little could be described as hard evidence of serious crime. But Hannam was not discouraged or deterred, as he had three further deaths under investigation which went beyond peculiar or disturbing, and which appeared to be highly suspicious. So much so that he was contemplating exhumations of two of the bodies. The third had been cremated.

7

Julia Bradnum

J ULIA BRADNUM WAS not a typical Dr Adams 'wealthy widow'. She did not live in a fancy hotel, or a grand house, and she did not employ a retinue of servants – in fact, she did her own housework. Her husband, Chapman, had been in service as a coachman when they married in 1890, and money had always been tight. In the early 1950s she was a one-woman embodiment of austerity Britain – she cooked a meal for herself only once a week and ate very little food the rest of the time. She never drank alcohol, so no sherry at noon, or thimbleful of brandy before bed. When she travelled, she took the bus or a coach. No chauffeur-driven outings in a Rolls-Royce for her. No dolling herself up in mink and sable. She had a few jewels that she kept in a safe at Barclays Bank, and some linen she thought worth putting into a will, along with a dinner service, the remains of a pink tea service, a cane chair and a glass clock. Her one big possession was her home, a three-bedroom house with rose beds at the front, and splendid views across to the South Downs. And it was because of 24 Coopers Hill, Willingdon, that her sudden death in 1952 came to the attention of Superintendent Hannam.

Mrs Bradnum was 84. Photographs show her to be an attractive old lady, there is prettiness and delicacy in her features and, of course, she is thin. But her face has something pinched and hard about it – a tension in her lips, an intensity about the eyes. When people described her character they said she was strong-willed. They were unlikely to report that she was cheerful, open-minded or generous. She was a devout Methodist, and subscribed to missionary magazines such as *News from Afar* and *Christian World*; and she had been close to her local minister, Harry Ingram, since the death of her husband in 1940 (his gravestone bore the inscription 'called to higher service'). Harry Ingram was an executor of the will that she made after Chapman died. The other executor was Percy Muddell, a manager at Barclays Bank.

Mrs Bradnum told Harry Ingram on many occasions that she would leave the majority of her estate – namely, the house – to her adopted daughter. Lily Overall's parents had died in a railway crash when she was 4, and Julia Bradnum had taken her in and brought her up. But she was not always a good guardian. She had a temper, and on one occasion had slapped Lily so hard about the head that the result was a 'life affliction of deafness'. When Lily grew up she married a man named Bertie Love, and it was Bertie who told the police that Lily had been treated 'unkindly' by Mrs Bradnum, being put to work in the house, and made to sleep in a lean-to greenhouse outside. After a while, Lily was sent out to service, and took a job as a parlourmaid. Her income was only £18 a year, and yet Mrs Bradnum had demanded a portion of her wages 'in payment for her upbringing'.

As Mrs Bradnum grew older Lily – now Mrs Love – and Bertie made an effort to look after 'auntie', as they called her. When called upon, Bertie helped with household jobs such as laying carpets and fixing curtains, and Lily visited once a fortnight. In the circumstances, it seemed right that Lily should inherit 24 Coopers Hill. The other person who could expect to be mentioned in Julia Bradnum's will was Mabel Onion, a niece on Chapman Bradnum's side of the family, who had worked as a housemaid for Julia and Chapman when, earlier in life, they had run a boarding house. Mabel Onion continued to visit Mrs Bradnum often, right up until the day she died, and had been assured that she and Lily Love would be the two main beneficiaries of her estate.

As Julia Bradnum grew older, though, members of the wider family started to take an interest in her will. On her husband's side, there was a nephew called Bertie Bradnum who thought he might stand to inherit. On her own side of the family – she was a Potter, from Leytonstone – there were brothers and a sister, who also had their eye on her house. However, Julia Bradnum told anyone who would listen that she would leave nothing to the Leytonstone Potters because they drank. She would not allow her money to be squandered on drink.

To complicate matters, she had taken into her house at Coopers Hill two lodgers – 'maiden ladies' of a certain age – named Emmeline Worthington and Mary Hine. Being penny-pinching and controlling, Julia Bradnum imposed rules. Miss Worthington was required to work in the garden, and Miss Hine was forbidden from entering the kitchen. Mary Hine, it seemed, conducted most of her life in one room – cooking on an oil stove there, and also doing her washing and drying in her bedroom. Over time, Lily and Bertie Love became rather antagonistic to Miss Worthington and Miss Hine – worrying that they were among the growing number of people who wished to inherit 24 Coopers Hill.

Given all the jostling for position around Mrs Bradnum, there was one element that was relatively stable – she had already made her will, with the help of the clergyman Harry Ingram and the bank manager Percy Muddell, so that was that. But in the summer of 1951, Julia Bradnum indicated that there was a change afoot – and the change involved Dr Adams.

Lily Love told Inspector Pugh that the doctor visited auntie once a month, on a Monday afternoon. There was nothing wrong with her – but Dr Adams said that, because Chapman had died, he would like to keep an eye on her. 'Auntie and I discussed his visits,' said Lily 'and we both thought that it was a waste of time and expense. I think auntie was afraid, or didn't like to tell him not to call, but I think Dr Adams appeared to have her round his little finger. I have seen Dr Adams during these visits sitting by the fire for a long time and holding auntie's hand. Auntie told him all her troubles.'

Mabel Onion confirmed that Dr Adams was a persistent caller. 'Mrs Onion considered Dr Adams made much more fuss of Mrs Bradnum than one would expect a professional man in his capacity to do,' wrote Superintendent Hannam. 'She has seen Dr Adams sitting beside Mrs Bradnum and in fact, kneeling beside Mrs Bradnum and holding her hand.' Most agreed that while she did not see the point of paying him, Julia Bradnum did confide in Dr Adams. One of the drinking Potters used a phrase that the police were to hear many times during their investigation: 'She thought there was nobody like him.' During his visits, Dr Adams wrote prescriptions for Mrs Bradnum – but she was not interested in taking pills, and after he left she threw the prescriptions in the fire.

In the winter of 1951, Mrs Bradnum had told Lily and Bertie Love that she wished to alter her will. Bertie Love offered to help, and set up a meeting with an Eastbourne solicitor. On 25 November 1951, while she was at Lily's and Bertie's house, Mrs Bradnum wrote out and signed a codicil to her existing will – establishing that 24 Coopers Hill would go to Lily Love and determining that, when she died, anyone living in the house – meaning the Misses Worthington and Hine – should kindly leave immediately.

But before the meeting with the Eastbourne solicitor could take place, Dr Adams became involved. He started advising Mrs Bradnum on her will, and she made him the sole executor. That December he came to the house with the paperwork for a new will, and Mary Hine was asked to be a witness. Miss Hine said the doctor pointed to where she should sign, but covered up the paper so that she could not see the writing on it. As soon as she had signed: 'Dr Adams opened the door and ushered me out.' So, the new will was completed under the solicitous, ushering guidance of the family GP. There was no need to fuss about visiting solicitors in Eastbourne.

But Miss Emmeline Worthington sensed that something was wrong. She said that during the flurry of activity it seemed to her that Mrs Bradnum did not really want to make a new will at all, but that 'someone was trying to force her to'. She did not say who this someone might be – it could have been either of the Loves, or one of the Potters, or Dr Adams. The minister Harry Ingram, who was an executor on her old will, had no idea that she had made a new one. Julia Bradnum told Lily Love that Dr Adams had persuaded her not to leave the house to Lily after all, but instead advised that it should be sold so that the proceeds could be divided among 'those that she loved'.

In May 1952, Lily Love was in hospital. At that time, Lily told Inspector Pugh, Mrs Bradnum seemed in very good health, and she came to visit three times, walking quite a distance from the bus stop to the hospital. Emmeline Worthington said that in the evening of 26 May Mrs Bradnum had appeared to be in good spirits, spending time in the garden and chatting to her neighbours. The following morning she was due to go on a coach trip with some friends, but seemed unwell. Miss Worthington returned home from the hairdresser around 10 a.m., and noticed that the curtains in Mrs Bradnum's bedroom were still drawn. This was unusual, so she went to the bedroom door and knocked, but got no reply. She knocked again, then heard the door being unlocked on the inside. Miss Worthington went in and she saw Mrs Bradnum walking back to, and getting into, her bed, and she thought she looked rather ill. Mrs Bradnum did not speak and Miss Worthington thought she had not recognised her.

The other lodger, Mary Hine, said she had also seen Mrs Bradnum that morning. She was in bed and complained of pains in her stomach. 'She asked for a glass of warm water and bicarbonate of soda. I thought she was not looking well.' The lodgers decided that Mary Hine should go to a friend's house nearby and telephone Dr Adams. He was out, said Miss Hine, but his secretary said he was visiting the Willingdon area and she could contact him quickly.

He arrived at 24 Coopers Hill very promptly, in fact before Mary Hine returned. Miss Worthington said he went straight to Mrs Bradnum's room and gave her an injection with a hypodermic syringe. As he did so, he said: 'I'm afraid she's going, it will only be a matter of minutes.' He was right. Mrs Bradnum died very quickly, with Dr Adams by her side. The doctor then left the house – he had been there only a few minutes. One minute, Mrs Bradnum had a stomach ache, the next she was dead.

Mary Hine returned as he was leaving. 'He said she was dead,' she remembered. 'I was completely shocked. I had only been out of the house for about a half-hour.' That same day, Dr Adams went to the Loves' house, and saw Bertie. 'Mrs Bradnum passed away this morning,' he said. 'I am the sole executor and have made arrangements with Haine's the undertaker and all concerned.' Bertie Love said he was flabbergasted at the news and couldn't understand it. Like all those who knew her, he had thought that Julia Bradnum was perfectly well. On the death certificate, Dr Adams wrote that the cause of death was 'a. cerebral haemorrhage and b. cardio vascular degeneration'.

The will had been made five months before she died. When it was read, it emerged that Mrs Bradnum's house was to be sold, and the proceeds were to be divided into six equal parts. These turned out to be worth £661. 1s. 0d. each. The legatees included Lily Love and various members of the drinking side of the family – namely Julia's brothers Frank and Bert Potter, and her sister Lily. Dr Adams was also among the beneficiaries of the proceeds of the house. There was no mention of anyone on the Bradnum side. Muriel Onion, the Bradnum niece who, with Lily Love, had been close to Mrs Bradnum for decades, was not included.

Mabel Onion was surprised about the will, not just because she got nothing, but also because Dr Adams had received so much. Frank Potter, who did benefit, was also surprised that Dr Adams was to get as much money as the close relatives, and had not known that he was the sole executor. As for the Bradnums, they were infuriated that the Potters, whom Julia Bradnum had always rejected, had inherited and they had not. The nephew, Bertie Bradnum, wrote to Dr Adams saying that he had 'heard with considerable surprise of the contents of my late aunt's will, under which none of my late uncle's side of the family received legacies'. This was so contrary to the conditions of her former will, he said, and so much the opposite of her 'declared intention' that 'I propose to institute an enquiry into the circumstances of the execution of the present will and the state of her health at the time'. He added that he would come to Eastbourne to visit his aunt's bank, to make inquiries.

Bertie Love also attempted a challenge. He cited the codicil that Julia Bradnum had signed stating that Lily Love was to receive the house, and wrote to Herbert James, Dr Adams's solicitor, who had handled the making of the new will. Herbert James's reply informed Bertie Love that the codicil had no legal force, since it had not been witnessed. The Misses Worthington and Hine also wrote in, saying that they would like to buy 24 Coopers Hill. Emmeline Worthington stressed that she and Miss Hine had lived in the house for ten years, and would like to buy it cheaply because of its 'bad state of repair and decoration'. Altogether, the scramble for Julia Bradnum's possessions was an unseemly affair. In the event, the 'Dr Adams will' was executed in full. He received his £661, the Bradnums and Muriel Onion got nothing, and the house was sold to the misses Worthington and Hine.

Superintendent Hannam regarded this as a particularly suspicious case. One thing that preyed on his mind was the fact that Mrs Bradnum, on the morning of her death, had got out of bed to unlock her bedroom door and then returned to bed unassisted. Was this, he wondered, consistent with Dr Adams's diagnosis of cerebral haemorrhage? (In fact, it was hard to say, since cerebral haemorrhages can have a wide range of symptoms, depending on where in the brain they occur.) Once again, it was the case that Dr Adams's patient had died shortly after he had overseen the changing of her will. Again, he had been there with his hypodermic syringe, though on this occasion death came more swiftly and dramatically than usual. It was fortunate that Julia Bradnum had not been cremated. Her body lay in Ocklynge Cemetery, and Hannam's thoughts turned to exhumation.

The second of Hannam's top three cases, and his other candidate for exhumation, was Clara Neil-Miller, who had died in February 1954, nine months after Julia Bradnum. Miss Neil-Miller had lived with her sister Hilda in Eastbourne. They were both spinsters, very close in age, and were always to be seen together. When they went shopping, they walked arm in arm. When they took a taxi to the seafront to listen to the band, they dressed alike, in old-fashioned navy-blue coats, and coloured straw hats decorated with imitation cherries and flowers. In the early 1950s the sisters were in their eighties, and not particularly wealthy, but they managed to get by in rented accommodation that had been found for them by Dr Adams, and lived in a boarding house called Barton run by a friend of his named Annie Sharpe. Clara had included the doctor in her will, and it was this that alerted Herbert Hannam to the deaths of the sisters – Hilda died in January 1953. From the probate documents, he discovered that Clara had been nursed by Sister Phyllis Owen who ran a small nursing home in Eastbourne, so, with Inspector Brynley Pugh, he called in on Sister Owen and took a statement from her.

She was one of the many Eastbourne nurses who thought Dr Adams was a dreadful physician. She had a friend, she said, who had gone to Dr Adams with a heart condition, but he had 'insisted it was only nerves' and given her medicine for 'nerves'. When the friend sought a second opinion, it was confirmed that she had a problem with her heart, and that her nerves were fine. Since then Phyllis Owen had looked after several of Dr Adams's patients and considered him to be 'a doctor who used sedatives very excessively. He always believed and said that his patients were nervous cases and sedative treatment was essential.' She knew that he had 'kept patients completely under sedatives for long periods, so that they quite frequently could only go about in a dazed condition'.

She told Superintendent Hannam that it was because of the extraordinary amount of sedatives he gave that old ladies returned to him 'for similar comforting treatment'. She believed, wrote Hannam, that 'he has a great influence over his patients and that it was mainly because he kept them in that dazed and doped condition'. Phyllis Owen had two comments to make about Dr Adams's relationship with the Misses Neil-Miller. When Hilda had died, she said, 'I saw Dr Adams pick up one or two articles about the room, look at them and put them in his pocket. This rather horrified me at the time.' As for the sister who lived another year, Miss Clara Neil-Miller, she remembered that each time she saw her, 'she was comatose and I am satisfied the condition was due to sedatives'.

On 1 September 1956, Inspector Pugh interviewed the only surviving relative of the Misses Neil-Miller, their sister-in-law Isabel Neil-Miller who had married their brother, and who lived in Bournemouth. The story Isabel told was unedifying. Hilda and Clara had been eccentric old ladies, prone to picking themselves up and going to live in different places, mercurial in temper, and sometimes difficult company and melodramatic. Hilda had been 'given too many pills which made her dizzy', by a doctor based in Eastbourne. Eventually, she had consulted a Bournemouth doctor who gave instructions that the pills were to stop. After that she got better.

The sisters had an odd relationship with their Eastbourne landlady, Dr Adams's friend, Annie Sharpe. Hilda hated her, but

Clara would not hear a thing said against her. When Annie Sharpe tried to get £5,000 out of them, and have them invest it in the Barton boarding house, Isabel advised very strongly against it, and the deal did not go ahead. Sometimes, when they were away from Eastbourne, Hilda told Isabel that 'there were people there she was frightened of', and said she did not wish to go back. On another occasion, Clara sent Isabel a telegram from Eastbourne saying: 'In great trouble. Can you come,' giving a telephone number. Isabel rang immediately, and arranged to meet up with Clara at Brighton Railway Station. 'She seemed frightened and worried,' said Isabel, 'and at several times during the day she appeared to be on the point of telling me something but each time stopped herself and said, "no I mustn't tell you. I must not give you all my worries." I implored her to confide in me but was unsuccessful.' Isabel never found out what had so disturbed Clara that she had sent the telegram.

Isabel was worried about the sisters, and she wrote to them often. In late 1951 her husband Thomas – their brother – became seriously ill, and she wrote saying he might be close to death. She received no reply. Then, one day, she received a letter from Clara which did not mention Thomas's poor health. Isabel realised that the sisters had not been receiving her letters. She wrote again, this time by registered post, so her letter had to be signed for. Clara replied immediately, saying how distressed she was to hear of Thomas's illness, and stating that the sisters would come to Bournemouth immediately. It was evident that their mail had been intercepted – and it seemed to everyone that the culprit was Annie Sharpe. Shortly afterwards, Isabel's letters once more disappeared, so she agreed with Clara and Hilda that, from then on, she would address all her correspondence to a family friend who lived in Eastbourne.

Clara and Hilda, said Isabel, were not wealthy at all, and in the 1930s she had persuaded her husband, Thomas, to lend them £2,000. The money was to be invested, and the sisters were to benefit from the interest – but the original £2,000 was to come back to Isabel when they died. But the capital was run down over the years, and when Thomas died in January 1952, Clara and Hilda told Isabel that only £1,000 could actually be returned to her. That summer, they made their wills – but did not make any mention in them of the money owed to Isabel.

At Christmas 1952 Isabel sent a Christmas present, and she received a thank you letter at the end of January 1953, signed 'Love from us both, Clara'. This was extremely strange, because Hilda had died on 15 January, at the age of 86. On the death certificate Dr Adams had given the cause of death as cerebral thrombosis. Clara told her friend Dorothy Wallis that Dr Adams was 'a wonderful man'. He had done everything he could for Hilda, she said, and then had arranged the funeral and the burial site at the cemetery. But Isabel, who had known Hilda for twenty years, was told nothing of her death, let alone the funeral – and she continued to address her letters to both sisters.

In the past, Clara had always been rude and unpleasant to Dr Adams, but after Hilda's death she became devoted to him. It was also about this time that she appeared to be almost constantly heavily sedated. Clara's friend Dorothy said that she received a telephone message from Annie Sharpe asking her to come to Eastbourne and see Clara as 'strange things were going on'. She said that Dr Adams was 'locked in Miss Clara's room for 20 minutes at a time, and she appeared to be under the influence of drugs'. Dorothy arrived at Barton – but did not notice that Clara was drugged. In fact, she seemed to be her normal self – 'indignant and annoyed' that Mrs Sharpe should be so interfering. From their conversation, Dorothy 'formed the opinion that Miss Clara was completely under the doctor's influence and prepared to listen to any suggestion he made'. When Dorothy asked her about being locked in the room with Dr Adams, Clara replied that her meetings with Dr Adams were her business and nobody else's. She added that the doctor was very helpful to her and had 'assisted her in many personal matters such as pinning on her brooches and adjusting her dress'. His hands were 'very comforting to her'. Dorothy found the conversation embarrassing.

By October 1953, wrote Superintendent Hannam, 'Dr Adams had Miss Clara Neil-Miller completely under his domination and a victim of hypnotic medication', and it was now that she decided to make a new will. The solicitor, Herbert James, prepared the final version, and Dr Adams was the sole executor. Clara's usual solicitor was unaware of the change, as was her banker, who had been the executor of previous wills. A few months later, in February 1954, Clara was taken ill. Mrs Sharpe said she had had a heart attack, and was treated at home by Dr Adams. When questioned by the police, Mrs Sharpe was reluctant to give too much information about Dr Adams, and she appeared to be 'scared – very frightened'. Hannam suspected that Annie Sharpe was in league with the doctor, and that he had sent many of his elderly lady patients to Barton. Dr Adams 'recommended clients to Mrs Sharpe', Sergeant Charlie Hewett told the journalists Rodney Hallworth and Mark Williams, 'and she recommended victims to him – not perhaps in a calculating or deliberate way, but by providing information . . . Mrs Sharpe was the key to the whole case. She had been involved with many of the victims. She was ideally placed, running this sort of twilight rest-home for the elderly and she knew so much about their personal and financial backgrounds.'

When Annie Sharpe was questioned for the second time by the police some unsettling facts about Clara Neil-Miller's final days emerged. 'Just over a week before Miss Clara died,' wrote Superintendent Hannam, 'Dr Adams was with the patient for some time and then came down to the semi-basement of the house into Mrs Sharpe's sitting room and asked if she could spare a minute. Dr Adams said to her: "My dear, I have got a nice surprise for you. Miss Clara wants you to have £200 and it can't be put into her will for you, for that is all arranged." Either the next day or the day after, Dr Adams came down to Mrs Sharpe's sitting room once more and gave her a cheque for £200, which Miss Clara had apparently just signed and Mrs Sharpe paid it into her bank account.' This information, said Superintendent Hannam, 'had to be dragged out of her'. From another source, the police established that Clara had written a second cheque just before she died; this one was for £500 and payable to Dr Adams.

Another disturbing account of Clara's last illness came from Dr Estcourt – a GP with the White House partnership in Eastbourne, where Dr Adams was held in low regard. Dr Estcourt had a patient named Miss Welsh, who was now dead, but who had lived at Barton at the same time as the Neil-Millers. Miss Welsh had said that a few days before Clara's death, Dr Adams visited. 'He was in the patient's room for over 40 minutes and Miss Welsh was perturbed about it. She opened the door of Miss Clara's room and was horrified to find that all the bed-clothes had been stripped from the bed and were lying over the footrail, and that the patient's nightgown had been pulled up around her chest, the windows in the room were open top and bottom, and Dr Adams was sitting reading a book.' Superintendent Hannam wrote that: 'it will be recalled that this lady was 87 years of age and the month of this occurrence must have been February, perhaps the coldest of the year'. When Clara died on 22 February, Dr Adams certified the cause as 'a. coronary thrombosis and b. myocardial degeneration'. He arranged for Clara to be buried in the same grave as Hilda and organised the funeral. Dr Adams and Mrs Sharpe were the only mourners.

Clara's sister-in-law, Isabel, learned of her death from a notice in the *Daily Telegraph*, and immediately wrote a letter of condolence which she addressed to Hilda. A few days later, she received a reply from Dr Adams telling her that Hilda had died a year earlier. When Isabel enquired about the money that she was owed by Clara, she learned that she was not mentioned in the will at all. The sum of £1,000 had gone to Clara's friend Dorothy – but the beneficiary who received most was Dr Adams, who was the residual legatee. He got £1,275. 12s. 2d.

It was the usual story – a heavily drugged patient, a new will featuring Dr Adams, and death following quickly afterwards. Superintendent Hannam decided to see what could be discovered about the medication that Clara had been receiving, and he seriously considered exhuming her body. 'Surely doubt must exist as to whether the death of Clara Neil-Miller was from coronary thrombosis,' he wrote, 'and the whole circumstances of her death are unsatisfactory.' He anticipated that Annie Sharpe would be a vital witness – he thought she was money-grabbing and in collusion with Dr Adams, but might well turn against him if he were facing a murder charge. Most significantly, he thought the cases of Julia Bradnum and Clara Neil-Miller would be useful in the 'cracking' process, and the time was approaching for Superintendent Hannam to question Dr Adams directly. First, though, he wished to finish investigating one remaining case, a death that appeared to be the most suspicious of all.

8

Edith Morrell

As a widow in possession of a good fortune, Edith Morrell was naturally one of Dr Adams's favourite patients. She was, in fact, one of the wealthiest people in Eastbourne, having married into the meat-packing Morrells, a Liverpool family whose business was massive in North America. In 1942 Morrell plants at Sioux Falls, South Dakota and Topeka, Kansas had packed three million hogs, and slaughtered more than three hundred thousand head of cattle. By 1950 Edith had been a widow for more than two decades and, bolstered by her meat-packing fortune, she had grown into the role of dowager – imperious and all powerful within her domain, and suitably heavy and imposing in appearance. She had a retinue of servants – a cook, a parlourmaid, a gardener, a chauffeur, and more – to whom she was a difficult and domineering employer, and she had a bevy of professional men – notably her bank manager, her solicitor and her doctor – to attend to her instructions about her business affairs, her wills, and her well-being.

People who knew Edith Morrell described her as 'trying', 'irritable', 'rude' or, in one instance, 'a wicked piece of work'. Occasionally, though, someone would find her very charming, and there is no doubt that she was a loving mother to her son Claude, who ran the British end of the Morrell business, and to her daughter, Doris. In Eastbourne, she had a group of friends, but her main interests were her garden – which was filled with prize dahlias – and her ten-bedroom house, Marden Ash, which was in the desirable Meads end of town, near Beachy Head, and the Hulletts' modern mansion, Holywell Mount.

Surviving letters give a sense of Mrs Morrell's character. During the war, she left East Sussex and decamped to the Pump House Hotel in Llandrindod Wells – a palatial Victorian performance of a building with pretensions to rival the Grand in Eastbourne. From there, she wrote to Dr Adams's solicitor, Herbert James, who at that time was handling her will: 'It is quite pleasant here with light and bracing air – but there is no need to say that I much prefer Eastbourne and miss it very much indeed – and I am only kept away by threat of "evacuees" – an absurd scheme really, because when the German "bombers" do come – <u>no</u> place in the United Kingdom will be safer than any other . . .' (She was proved right – it was not long before people were being evacuated *out* of Eastbourne.) Her other complaint about Eastbourne was that all her friends are 'all too deep in War work to have any time for me'. In another letter she writes: 'I feel April 1940 will go down in history with 1805 and 1815 – I do wish they would intern all the "spies". This country is riddled with them . . .'

She begins one of her letters to Herbert James, 'I am afraid you will think I have a tiresome propensity for making new wills . . .' When she dies, she says, the majority of her estate is to go to Doris – that is, Marden Ash and her motor cars. Earlier wills had contained bequests to charities, but in 1940 Mrs Morrell reconsidered, and thought she would not leave much money to charity after all as 'I have done so much in my life-time'.

Later in 1940 she left war-torn Britain altogether, and sailed the Atlantic to Canada. Writing from the splendid Ritz Carlton Hotel in Montreal, she says she has motored several times into the mountains to see the maple trees, and she is enjoying the company of her friends and relations there. 'The people here are loyal and friendly and all out to help win the war – into which they are putting every effort and I appreciate being able to come over here – but after all – there is no place like home.' While these might have seemed like the darkest of hours back in the United Kingdom, Mrs Morrell was optimistic. 'I feel full of hope about the future – as a country that can stand Dunkirk and France in the same year can stand anything!'

But the following year brought personal tragedy. In the spring of 1941 she wrote to Herbert James: 'This is the saddest day of my life – and I have hardly yet realised such overwhelming sorrow.' Her daughter, Doris, had died in England after an operation. 'I shall have to re-make my will or add a codicil to it . . .' she writes. 'I had left Marden Ash and many other things to Doris and I was thinking now it might be a good plan to leave the house to the Princess Alice Hospital as a convalescent home.' Shortly afterwards, she wrote again to say that she had decided to leave Marden Ash to her son, Claude, 'and only hope he survives to take it, but these are <u>terrible days</u> – and seem to get worse all the time'. She also told Herbert James that 'I desire to be cremated and that my ashes should be scattered over the sea and it is my particular wish that no relatives or friends of mine shall go into mourning for me and that my Executors will employ a doctor to ensure by all means that my life is extinct.' She had a particular fear of being buried or burned while still alive – and this desire to be properly certified as dead when the time came, reappeared in later wills.

By July 1945 Edith Morrell was back in Eastbourne, and the new will she made that month included in it her doctor, John Bodkin Adams, who was to receive £1,000. At this time she thought Marden Ash should go to the Friends of the Poor, or a similar charity, or be used as a convalescent home, or as a Home for Ladies in reduced circumstances. Dr Adams also benefited in a will she made the following month – again by £1,000.

In October 1946 she wrote to Herbert James in a shaky hand, saying that she had had a wretched summer. In July she had fallen and hurt her knee, and Dr Adams had told her to visit a specialist in Harley Street. But on the day that she went to London, she picked up a germ that gave her 'ptomaine poisoning' – an old-fashioned term for a condition that was probably a stomach bug. 'I nearly died,' she wrote, 'and I am still in my room or I should have been down to see you as there are several things I want to consult you about . . . I <u>would</u> like to <u>cancel</u> the £1,000 legacy I left to Dr Adams and rule it out. <u>If</u> this can be <u>done</u> simply and <u>separately</u> I would like to do it <u>but</u> if it means re-writing and re-making the whole will – we will just leave things as they <u>are</u>.' Somehow, she blamed Dr Adams for her germ and the fact that she 'nearly died'. Whether, in fact, he was dropped from the will at this point is unclear – but, if so, the situation was temporary, since Mrs Morrell was endlessly making new wills.

Then, early in 1949, her health took a bad turn. She had gone to Cheshire to see her son Claude and, during her visit, suffered a stroke. Claude contacted Dr Adams who dashed to Cheshire and brought Mrs Morrell home to Eastbourne by train ambulance. The following weeks were spent in various nursing homes – but she hated all of them and was relieved when she was able to return to Marden Ash. The stroke had caused her left arm, and much of the left side of her body, to be paralysed, and she had difficulty in walking. Several nurses now joined the household at Marden Ash, and in May 1949 Mrs Morrell also employed a live-in companion called Rosaleen Spray 'to attend to her comforts generally'.

Miss Spray, who was a nurse, was in a perfect position to observe the goings-on at Marden Ash. Her employer's health at that time, she told Detective Inspector Pugh, was 'very good' apart from the partial paralysis, and she was certainly well enough to go out for afternoon drives in her Rolls-Royce – a 1939 Silver Ghost. Sometimes the chauffeur, Thomas Price, would take Miss Spray along too, as well as Dr Adams who was visiting Mrs Morrell daily and sometimes several times a day. 'He would fuss over his patient and appeared to give Mrs Morrell the impression that she was the only patient he thought anything of,' said Miss Spray. One morning she watched as Dr Adams entered Mrs Morrell's bedroom, rubbing his hands together as he spoke. 'Good morning my dear,' he said, 'There is one thing I envy of you – it's your beautiful Rolls. It is like sitting in an armchair.' His behaviour, and this comment, 'brought a feeling of utter contempt for him', Miss Spray told the police.

But she felt 'reasonably sure' that Mrs Morrell liked his attentions. On one occasion she told Miss Spray that the doctor collected silver, so she would leave him an antique chest containing a large quantity of silver, and would also give him a pair of silver candlesticks as a Christmas present. One of Mrs Morrell's nurses remembered that, when assisting Mrs Morrell in walking around the house, Dr Adams would 'conduct her to the old silver chest, stop and admire it and its pieces'. Superintendent Hannam took a dim view of these guided walks to the silver chest. 'We comment that this is either covetousness or a technique to get Mrs Morrell to give it to him,' he wrote.

The chauffeur, Thomas Price, remembered that as well as the silver and the candlesticks, Dr Adams also took a keen interest in Mrs Morrell's fine dinner set of around 120 pieces. In the autumn of 1950, he said, 'I went into the lounge at Marden Ash and saw Dr Adams with what I could make out as a few plates of the dinner service which he was wrapping in paper on a chair. The doctor looked a bit sheepish on seeing me come into the room and when he had gone with the plates I looked into the cupboard where I had previously put the dinner service and there was nothing left – all the service had gone.'

Mrs Morrell's nurses commented on the doctor's manner. 'When Dr Adams entered Mrs Morrell's bedroom he always gave me the impression that he wished to be alone with her and sit by her bedside. I do not know what passed between them,' said Nurse Agnes White. She had encountered Dr Adams before, when she was nursing another patient – a Mrs Meyer who had 'plenty of money being the widow of a Ceylon Tea Planter'. Mrs Meyer, said Nurse White, was not really ill, but Dr Adams had visited her daily and it was always 'quite clear to me that he wanted to be left alone with the patient'. Mrs Meyer always looked forward to the doctor's visits, and wanted to look her best before he arrived. 'My opinion of Dr Adams is that he is a creeper,' she told Detective Inspector Pugh, 'particularly where there is plenty of money. He wouldn't visit a poor person three times a day and every day as he did when he had a rich patient.' Some of the other nurses at Marden Ash were less critical – instead commenting on the doctor's 'attractive bedside manner', and saying that he was 'very kind and attentive'.

During the doctor's visits, the conversation sometimes turned to wills and legacies. In April 1949, shortly after the stroke, Dr Adams telephoned Mrs Morrell's solicitor – no longer Herbert James, but now a Mr Hubert Sogno – and said that it was 'extremely urgent' that Mr Sogno should visit Mrs Morrell that day to talk to her about her will. The solicitor went to Marden Ash, and Edith Morrell told him that she had decided that the bulk of her estate should go to Dr Adams. Mr Sogno strongly advised his client against doing any such thing on a whim, and told her to give it more thought.

A year later, on 8 March 1950, Dr Adams called in at Mr Sogno's office and requested a 'very urgent appointment' with him. The doctor saw the solicitor that day and told him that Mrs Morrell had promised to leave him her Rolls-Royce, but she had just realised she had forgotten to put it in her will. He reassured Mr Sogno that Mrs Morrell's mind was very clear, and she was in a fit state to make a codicil to the will. He added that she also wished him to have some valuable jewellery that was held at the bank.

Mr Sogno advised against making hasty changes to the will. 'Dr Adams replied that Mrs Morrell was very uneasy and wished to get the matter dealt with at once,' wrote Herbert Hannam.

'He further said that Mrs Morrell seriously wished him to enjoy the gifts of the motor car and the jewellery and he suggested that Mr Sogno should prepare a codicil accordingly.' Mr Sogno was appalled, and told Dr Adams that his behaviour was quite improper. He would, he said, take his instructions from Mrs Morrell in person.

By early 1950 Mrs Morrell was, for much of the time, heavily drugged. Browne's the Chemist was sending its driver to Marden Ash at least four times a week with packages of medicines. In addition, Thomas Price, the chauffeur, regularly collected medicine for her, and it was observed that when Dr Adams gave his patient injections, they were generally of drugs that he had in his bag. The nurses said that Mrs Morrell was having regular morphia injections, and several people hinted that morphine was given because 'at times she played up a good deal and was a very trying patient'.

The Marden Ash cook, Bessie Woodward, was concerned about Mrs Morrell. 'Sometimes I thought she was a lonely woman – she gave me that impression,' she said. 'We understood each other as servant and mistress and neither of us abused the privilege.' On one occasion, said the cook, Mrs Morrell had had a row with one of her nurses. Afterwards, the nurse tried to bar Bessie from Mrs Morrell's room, but she pushed her way in anyway, she told the police, 'and was most disturbed to find Mrs Morrell lying in bed and she appeared unconscious'. Bessie asked the nurse: 'Is Mrs Morrell in great pain because she has to be drugged?' She received the reply: 'She is so tensed up, she must be kept quiet.' According to Bessie, after this Mrs Morrell's health gradually deteriorated.

One day, she saw one of the nurses in the kitchen washing a hypodermic syringe, and she had two white pellets in her hand. 'I [Bessie] said, "what, more drugs?" And the nurse said: "You and I would be dead if we had the same. This old lady is tough."' The reasons for the heavy drugs were far from clear, since Mrs

Morrell was in no pain. One clue to her treatment, though, was the diagnosis of 'cerebral irritation' that Dr Adams made – although, in truth, the term had no medical meaning. 'Cerebral irritation', it seemed, accounted for the fact that Mrs Morrell 'was a very difficult patient with a violent temper'.

There was also talk of 'brainstorms' – another non-medical concept. Sister Caroline Randall, who was a senior member of the nursing team, told Superintendent Hannam: 'She was a very difficult patient and she had brainstorms. I think there was no improvement in the cerebral irritation and she would go into a temper very quickly for no apparent cause. All the time on the doctor's instructions I gave injections of morphia and the quantity was slowly increased and oftener.' In addition, 'she had different tablets to take to induce sleep and sometimes had phenobarbitone in the day time. I believe sometimes she had heroin. Quite often in the night time she became ill and clammy and from my experience I attributed this to the effect of the heroin. Dr Adams did not agree with me and he thought the condition was not resultant from the drug. I think it right to say that Dr Adams did not like the unsolicited advice of the nurse on those matters.' Two other witnesses, a nurse and the chauffeur, Thomas Price, mentioned 'brainstorms' – and it is likely that they heard the term from Dr Adams.

On 12 September 1950 Dr Adams took a vacation. He left Eastbourne and went to Scotland to shoot grouse. While he was away, Dr Adams's partner, Dr Vincent Harris, was summoned, and he gave Mrs Morrell the morphia she was used to. But she was highly indignant about Dr Adams's holiday, so much so that she summoned her solicitor, Hubert Sogno, and on 15 September she told him to draw up a codicil cutting the doctor out of her will. She also sent a message to Scotland, informing Dr Adams that he must return to Eastbourne immediately, and he did catch a flight home, and attended her for one day – 16 September – before flying back to Scotland. He returned to Eastbourne on 24

September, and it was from this point that Mrs Morrell went into a devastating decline – although at some stage she rallied a little, and decided that she would, after all, like to include Dr Adams in her will. She tore up the codicil.

The short remainder of Mrs Morrell's life was spent confined to bed in a mental state that, for much of the time, was vague and confused. Sister Randall said: 'For the last month of her life, in my view, she was doped. I mean by this that she was always dopey because of drugs which were given to quieten her restless condition.' When Dr Adams visited at night, she added, he would often give her further injections, with drugs that he took from his bag. She was having morphine, heroin, various tablets and sometimes a powerful sedative called paraldehyde, said Sister Randall. She thought the drugs 'rather excessive', especially as Mrs Morrell was never in any pain.

About two weeks before Mrs Morrell died, Nurse Brenda Hughes told Dr Adams that she thought Mrs Morrell seemed very pale and lethargic. 'The doctor went into her room on his own and when he came out he said, "I have given her an injection to settle her. Good morning Sister." He then left the house. I was having coffee in the dining room and he did not obtain any drug for this injection from the dining room drawer. After about ten minutes I went into the patient. I found her very difficult to rouse, in fact I could not wake her. I went for Bessie the cook and she came with me and saw Mrs Morrell. I asked Bessie to stay with Mrs Morrell whilst I telephoned the doctor. I spoke to Dr Adams and explained the situation because I was very worried and he told me that we must expect these collapses because she was a very ill woman, but if I was unduly worried to ring him again.'

By the second week of November 1950, said the nurses, Mrs Morrell was comatose for much of the time because of the drugs she was receiving. It was now that she also had 'jerky spasms'. Then, on 12 November, the spasms became worse. Dr Adams visited Mrs Morrell at about 10 p.m. and left late that night. After attending to the patient, said the Marden Ash nightwatchman, James Dean, the doctor went to the garage to have a look at the Rolls-Royce. 'That's a beautiful car,' he told Mr Dean.

Sister Randall said that during his visit he gave directions that Mrs Morrell 'was not to come round' because of the spasms. 'Dr Adams prepared a hypodermic syringe containing an unusually large quantity for an injection,' she added. 'I did not know what it was. I gave the injection while Dr Adams was in the dining room. He filled another syringe with approximately the same quantity . . . After the first injection the jerky spasms appeared to increase, and acting on the doctor's instructions I gave the second injection. I telephoned him at his home before doing so, but could not contact him. Both these injections were given between 10 p.m. and 2 a.m., when she died. After the second injection she quietened down and in half or three quarters of an hour she died.'

Nurse Hughes said that Dr Adams came to the house at eleven o'clock the following morning. He went into Mrs Morrell's room, and cut her right radial artery (a rather intrusive way to confirm death). On the death certificate, he wrote that the cause of death was cerebral thrombosis, adding that she was in a coma for two hours before she died (although the nurses said her coma had lasted two or three days). Nurse Hughes remembered one of the other nurses telling her that Dr Adams took away with him Mrs Morrell's infra-red lamp.

After her death, Mrs Morrell's body was cremated, as she had requested, and her ashes were scattered in the English Channel. The cremation form was signed by Dr Adams, who answered the question: 'Have you, so far as you are aware, any pecuniary interest in the death of the deceased?' with the one word 'No'. When her final will was read, it turned out that £500 and her collection of prize dahlias went to the gardener, John Carter, and £1,000 went to her chauffeur, Thomas Price. The majority of the estate went to her son Claude. The position of Dr Adams was unclear. The codicil cutting him out of the will had been torn up – but that did not, in law, make it invalid. So technically, he was entitled to nothing. But Claude ignored the codicil. Without it, Dr Adams was to receive Mrs Morrell's oak chest full of silver, worth £246. In the body of the will, she did not leave him the Rolls-Royce (or at least, he would get it only if she were predeceased by Claude). None the less, Claude gave Dr Adams the car, along with a Jacobean cupboard. The Rolls-Royce was worth £1,500 and the cupboard £80. In addition, Dr Adams submitted to the executors a medical bill for £1,750 – enough to buy another Rolls-Royce, had he wanted to.

There was a lot in the Morrell case for Hannam to think about. His next step was to ask Detective Sergeant Leslie Sellors to visit Eastbourne's chemists to inspect records of prescriptions written by Dr Adams. The search proved fruitful, and in early September 1956 Hannam was able to send prescriptions written out for Edith Morrell and Clara Neil-Miller to L. C. Nickolls at Scotland Yard's forensic laboratory. On 11 September he received a response. There is no doubt, thought Nickolls, that in the last week of her life Edith Morrell was 'dispensed sufficient morphine sulphate and heroin to be lethal to anyone but a confirmed drug addict'. A further opinion should be sought from a physician, he added. In the case of Clara Neil-Miller, he wrote that 'again the prescribing is extremely heavy and is, in places, almost incomprehensible'. He could see that 'a fresh supply of hypnotic is being administered before previous supplies have been exhausted. One gets the impression that the general idea is to saturate the patient with barbiturates and then leave them in possession of a fatal supply and hope for the best.' However, the case for murder, or other unlawful death, was far from straightforward. The 'big trouble' with both cases was that, because both women were so old, it would be a good defence to say that it was not the drugs that killed them, but old age: 'Nevertheless, a report from a competent physician may elicit some phraseology "that no qualified doctor could possibly prescribe drugs in the amount shown without some peculiar intent".'

The difficulty at the heart of the case was the nature of Dr Adams's profession. Because he was a doctor, the means of killing was readily available. Because he was a doctor, his actions were rarely questioned or challenged. Because he was a doctor, he could be alone with a patient in her home, all other people banished from the room. If he was killing old ladies, as the police believed, then it was quite possible that nobody would ever be able to prove it.

9

Arrest

During August and September 1956 it seemed that half of Eastbourne was being interviewed by the police. Dr Adams's patients and their friends, relatives and nurses spoke to Hannam, Hewett and Pugh, and much of what they had to say was outright condemnation of the 'menace in their midst'. Lawyers and bankers were making statements, as were the few Eastbourne doctors who were defying the BMA ban. The press was hysterical about the whole thing – reporting that 300 patient deaths were under investigation. And through it all, the doctor was going about his business, apparently unruffled, seemingly unperturbed – holding surgeries for his NHS patients (many still showed up, despite everything), and sucking up to his remaining well-to-do widows. On the train to London, Percy Hoskins had been surprised by the extent to which Dr Adams seemed cut off from his predicament, unaware that the consequences might be fatal, not caring that he could end up facing the hangman. As the investigation against him intensified, he maintained this peculiar detachment, and it was hard to tell whether his attitude came from confidence that the fuss would blow over and he would be vindicated, or whether he was somehow psychologically disconnected, in a world of his own.

His close friend, Roland Gwynne, was a different matter. Gwynne was acutely sensitive to the gravity of the situation and on 7 September he telephoned Eastbourne Police headquarters and told Superintendent Hannam that he disliked all this rumour about Dr Adams, 'whom he said was the finest doctor in town and a great friend of his', and he asked Hannam to do all he could to dispel the gossip. Gwynne's situation was delicate. The old stories about a homosexual relationship between Dr Adams and Roland Gwynne were adding spice to the rumour mill (although the simple fact of the doctor's grotesque appearance and Gwynne's dashing good looks made a sexual liaison seem unlikely). And a perverse delight could be derived from the fact that Gwynne was chairman of the Eastbourne magistrates – and would have to step down from any future hearings involving Dr Adams. Then, in the midst of the furore, Roland Gwynne accompanied Dr Adams on a shooting holiday to Scotland. It seemed to all that Gwynne, whose elevated position in Eastbourne society was already precarious, had decided to stick by his friend. His loyalty seemed brave and bold, possibly reckless.

On 1 October, Dr Adams was back in Eastbourne when, by chance, he ran into Superintendent Hannam in the street. It was their first encounter since they had been introduced at the Bobbie Hullett inquest in August. 'It was a casual, unplanned meeting,' wrote Hannam. 'I said to him, "good evening doctor. Did you have a good holiday in Scotland?"' The simple enquiry elicited a long, gushing response – the doctor said he had been one of a party of ten who went shooting, and together they had had a very good bag. 'He then went on to tell me about his life,' continued Hannam, 'and I found him extremely loquacious.' He told the story of his father dying when he had been 14 years old, of his brother William dying so suddenly – 'like that – and he snapped his fingers', of the time that he had suffered a breakdown at Queen's University, of his return to his studies and achievement of his degree. He talked of going to work in Bristol, and of arriving in Eastbourne.

He told Hannam it was 'God's guidance and leading which brought him to Eastbourne'. As for the rumours about him, he said: 'those who know me know it is untrue and those who believe it, well, there is nothing I can do. I think it is all God's plan to teach me a new lesson.' Then he resumed his life story, telling Hannam about the death of his mother, Ellen, during the war, and of the death of his cousin, Sarah Henry, in 1952, explaining that she 'was a very sweet Christian soul' who 'died after six months of terrible agony. "I thank God," said Dr Adams, "for the sweet memory of such a dear woman. It is an inspiration to me even now."'

Eventually, he came to the matter in hand, and said to Hannam: 'You are finding all these rumours untrue, aren't you?' 'I am sorry to say that is not my experience, doctor,' Hannam replied. 'It is strange. I live for my work,' said the doctor. 'I gave a vow to God that I would look after my poor National patients . . . Day and night I will turn out for them and I never ask anybody else to do it for me. I think this makes people jealous of me. I get up at 6.30 each morning, listen to the 7 o'clock news, then visit a patient or go to Esperance [nursing home] . . . then I go to the hospital and get back here at 9 for private patients. Gwynne comes in then if he wants to.' He then launched into his afternoon and evening regime, concluding with the observation that he did more surgeries than his partners. 'If only others worked as hard as I do,' he said. 'What have you been told about me?'

Superintendent Hannam said he had found out that Dr Adams had forged prescriptions for some of his NHS patients, using the name of another doctor. 'That was very wrong,' he replied, '. . . I've had God's forgiveness for it. All of them were only to help the poor National patients. I love helping these National patients for I gave a vow to God that I would. The health people can afford it . . . You haven't found anything else?'

Hannam said he was anxious about some of the legacies that the doctor had received. 'A lot of those were instead of fees. I don't want money. What use is it? I paid £1,100 super tax last year,' Dr Adams replied. Hannam turned to Dr Adams's walks with Edith Morrell around her sitting room and to her valuable chest of silver. 'Mrs Morrell was a very dear patient,' said the doctor. 'She insisted a long time before she died that I should have that in her memory and I didn't want it. I'm a bachelor. I've never used it. I knew she was going to leave it to me and her Rolls-Royce car. She told me she had put it in her will. Oh, yes, and another cabinet.'

'Mr Hullett left you £500,' said Hannam. 'Now, now,' Dr Adams protested. 'He was a lifelong friend. He was a very ostentatious man about his wealth. He liked to talk about it. There is no mystery about him. He told me long before his death that he had left me money in his will. I even thought it would be more than it was . . . Every one of these dear patients I've done my best for. I've one thing in life, and God knows I've vowed to him I would, that is to relieve pain and try to let these dear people live as long as possible.'

Superintendent Hannam, unimpressed by the doctor's vows to God, now turned to his lies when filling in cremation forms. In the cases of Jack Hullett, Edith Morrell and others, he said, Dr Adams had written that he was unaware of being a beneficiary in their wills, when the opposite was true. Dr Adams objected: 'Oh, that wasn't done wickedly, God knows it wasn't. We always want the cremations to go off smoothly for the dear relatives. If I said I knew I was getting money under the will they might get suspicious, and I like cremations and burials to go smoothly. There was nothing suspicious really. It wasn't deceitful.'

'I hope I shall finish all these enquiries soon,' concluded Hannam, 'and we will probably have another talk.' Ominous mention of 'another talk' may have been designed to unsettle the doctor. But it did not. 'Don't hurry,' he replied. 'Please be thorough, it is in my interests. Good night, and thank you very much for your kindness.' The two men parted, and as soon as he was able, Herbert Hannam sat down to write up their conversation, and the doctor's voice is beautifully clear in those notes – the unctuous remarks about the 'the dear relatives', the sanctimonious references to 'God's will' and the jarring self-regard in comments like 'if only others worked as hard as I do'.

On the same day, the Home Office pathologist Francis Camps sent some comments on the Morrell case to Scotland Yard. If the drugs that Dr Adams had prescribed for Edith Morrell were actually administered, he wrote, they amounted to 'an enormous quantity of hypnotic and narcotic (morphine, heroin) drugs for one person' – and it was difficult to see why they were appropriate, unless she had inoperable cancer or some very painful disease – which she did not. He noted that the drugs were prescribed in increasing quantities, and would have resulted in addiction, and he pointed out that 'the cause of death given on the certificate would resemble clinical narcotic poisoning'.

Another expert, Dr William Thrower, had also been asked by Hannam for his opinion on the medical treatment of some of Dr Adams's patients. Dr Thrower thought the doctor's propensity for giving cerebral thrombosis as a cause of death 'a trifle unusual' and he was surprised that it had escaped the notice of the local Superintendent Registrar. He described the treatment of Edith Morrell in the final days of her life as 'almost unbelievable'.

Dr Thrower thought the chemists' prescriptions for Clara Neil-Miller were mostly harmless. And yet, towards the end of her life, he noted, she was given injections three times a day – of heaven knows what. The drugs for the injections did not appear in the prescriptions in her name found at Eastbourne chemists, and must have come from Dr Adams's bag. Once again, the cause of death was given as cerebral thrombosis. But 'patients with cerebral thrombosis particularly if near the end of their life hardly sit up in bed as is the evidence in this case'. Dr Thrower strongly recommended the exhumation of Clara Neil-Miller's body, so that a post-mortem could be performed.

Dr Thrower also had misgivings about the death of Jack Hullett, and the last injection administered by Dr Adams which was probably 'highly concentrated morphia'. 'Why the free use of morphia as the patient did not seem to suffer pain?' Also, given that Jack had colon cancer, why was cerebral haemorrhage given as the cause of death? 'The whole thing looks odd to me,' Dr Thrower concluded. Francis Camps agreed that Jack Hullett's death was 'extremely doubtful'.

Superintendent Hannam included these expert opinions in an almighty report that he sent to the Chief Superintendent at Scotland Yard on 16 October 1956. His investigations, he said, proved that 'there is substance' in many of the Eastbourne rumours. 'The doctor is an extremely greedy man who has exercised considerable influence upon aged and wealthy patients and . . . frequently with the aid of hypnotic drugs, has caused them to bestow gifts upon himself and to include him as a beneficiary under their wills.'

The report documented cases as far back as the 1930s. It told of the wealthy widow Matilda Whitton (died 11 May 1935) who had adored Dr Adams, and had photographs of him in her room at the Kenilworth Hotel, but who had been afraid of his injections. This was the first death to bear all the hallmarks that so concerned the police. It was too old to merit further investigation, but showed 'that the technique of Dr Adams that we are going to learn so much about in this report was well established over 20 years ago'.

From the 1940s, Hannam documented the drugging of Agnes Pike in the Lathom House hotel in 1941, telling of Dr Adams's sudden lunge at her with an injection of morphia 'because the patient might become violent'. He documented the case of Mary Mouat (died 31 January 1946) whose legs had been burned by an electric fire. On her deathbed, Dr Adams had tried to make her sign some mysterious document. 'We shall hear a good deal about similar attempts to get patients to sign Powers of Attorney or other documents when they are very ill,' wrote Hannam, adding that Mrs Mouat's death should have been brought to the notice of the Coroner.

He included the unseemly jostling for position among those who stood to gain from the will of Leslie Cockhead (died 15 December 1947) and the fact that Dr Adams took away a gold pen 'as a little reminder of the dear patient'. And he recorded his conversations with Edith Mawhood about her relationship with Dr Adams – the strange way he had of ordering things, the mackintosh, the boots, and charging them to her husband's account. Then, when her husband William died (8 March 1949), his attempt to get hold of William's fortune – and the way in which he had helped himself to a 22-carat gold pencil. 'We shall also see as we proceed,' wrote Hannam, 'that this taking of an article of value from the house of a deceased patient is not isolated to the Mawhood case.'

He mentioned the many wills made by Edith Morrell (died 13 November 1950), some including Dr Adams and others not. He described the heavy sedatives that she received, and wrote: 'That he had this woman under his complete influence there can be no doubt . . .' Her death was definitely not 'bona fide' and seemed very much like a case of manslaughter, 'and if it is we shall certainly show the clearest possible motive for desiring to see her life at an end'.

He reported the death of Annabella Kilgour (died 26 December 1950) who was given a strong injection by Dr Adams, and never came round from it. The nurse who attended Mrs Kilgour thought the injection had killed her – but she was not prepared to give a sworn statement saying so. 'Suspicion will always remain that Dr Adams disposed of Mrs Kilgour by his method of treatment, more quickly than might have been natural,' wrote Hannam, adding 'exhumation crossed our minds'. And he put particular emphasis on the case of Harriet Hughes (died 29 November 1951), the widow whose illness prompted Dr Adams to fuss around her bed with a new will, leaving a couple named Thurston £2,000. Immediately afterwards she had been given injections, and died of 'cerebral thrombosis'.

Superintendent Hannam thought this case, from a financial point of view, 'the most suspicious of the whole lot'.

He recorded his doubts about the death of Julia Bradnum (died 27 May 1952), who had died very suddenly after being given an injection by Dr Adams and 'it is by no means certain that the death of this lady was genuine'. Hannam suggested an exhumation, although 'her age is against us'. And he wrote of his worries about Clara Neil-Miller (died 22 February 1954) who, just eleven days before she died, gave Dr Adams £500 and Annie Sharpe £200. It was while 'Dr Adams had Miss Clara Neil-Miller completely under his domination and a victim of his hypnotic medication', that she made a will which left him £1,275. 'The whole circumstances surrounding her death are unsatisfactory,' said Hannam. He thought Mrs Sharpe had a lot more to say, and the potential to be a vital witness.

On Jack Hullett, he cited the expert view that this was 'an extremely doubtful death'. On Bobbie Hullett, he drew attention to the cheque for £1,000 that she had written for Dr Adams, shortly before she went into a coma. This, he said, was an 'extremely damning piece of evidence'. There was no doubt, wrote Hannam, that Dr Adams 'knew full well' that Bobbie's coma was due to barbiturate poisoning and 'gave no treatment whatsoever to counteract it'.

The main focus of his investigation had been on twenty-three patients who had, between 1946 and 1956, left Dr Adams money in their wills. Older cases had been given less attention, as had his treatment of those patients who had died in his care but had not left him any money. He had calculated that the doctor's total benefit from patient wills during the ten years was more than £36,000 and a Rolls-Royce, plus the second Rolls-Royce and the valuable chest of Georgian silver that came to him from Mrs Morrell. 'Surely,' concluded Hannam, 'Dr Adams must be prosecuted if only to expose his technique.' But this was the strongest wording he was prepared to muster when he submitted his report to the Chief Superintendent. He alluded to the strange circumstances of the deaths of many of Dr Adams's patients, but minced his words, and did not press for a murder prosecution.

At Scotland Yard the report was passed into the hands of those who had sent Percy Hoskins to Eastbourne to spy on Hannam, the men who were wary of him and thought him incapable of conducting a calmly forensic inquiry. Now that he saw Hannam's report, the Chief Superintendent was dismissive. He conceded that Dr Adams had 'feathered his nest in a manner frowned on in good circles', and may have induced his patients to alter their wills in his favour. But, he wrote, a criminal offence could 'never be proved'. Another senior officer, Commander 'C' at Scotland Yard, was similarly negative. The rumours and gossip that Dr Adams had 'quietly put some of his patients out of the way in order to inherit legacies', he wrote, 'have proved unsubstanti-ated'. But he acknowledged that Dr Adams's behaviour, private and professional, was 'rather shocking', and that there was scope for further investigation, if the Director of Public Prosecutions recommended it.

The top brass's analysis was dramatically at odds with Hannam's assessment of the situation. Although he had held back in his official report, he was forthright and opinionated when, after sending it off, he met journalists – including Rodney Hallworth of the *Daily Mail* – in the Beachy Head Hotel. 'It was a night tailor-made for murder talk,' wrote Hallworth, 'clouts of wind shook the building, rain spat on the windows and the heaving sea far below was a frightening mass of white water . . . Hannam took out a Henry Clay Havana from its case, struck a match and puffed the cigar alight ...[He] squared his shoulders, glanced around the near-deserted bar and said quietly and clearly: "I am quite confident Adams is a mass–murderer. He has certainly killed fourteen people. If we had arrived on the scene years ago, I think I could have said he killed more."'

Evidently, he would have to work harder if he was to persuade his superior officers that they were in danger of letting a murderer walk free. The time had come for Hannam to deploy his controversial 'cracking' approach – and he would start by cracking the key witness, the Neil-Millers' landlady Annie Sharpe, who, he believed, had been in cahoots with Dr Adams and was 'the key to the whole case'. It was decided that Hannam and Sergeant Charlie Hewett would revisit Mrs Sharpe. She had already been interviewed twice and was, they thought, 'very frightened'. As Hannam left her house after an earlier visit he had said: 'She's cracking, Charlie. We'll have it next time.'

But, before they managed to visit Mrs Sharpe, Hannam and Hewett were called to London to discuss the case with the Director of Public Prosecutions. And while they were away from Eastbourne, Mrs Sharpe died suddenly, and was cremated within the week. She had been 76 and it seemed that she had had cancer. Dr Adams had been looking after her. 'It was so coincidental that she died when she did – and was cremated so quickly,' said Charlie Hewett. 'I always had the feeling, and it was never stronger than that, that the good doctor speeded her on her way. And like so many of the cases, left us without a body.'

So the cracking strategy now focused solely on Dr Adams. Hannam decided to arrest him on minor charges – forging prescriptions and making false claims on cremation certificates – while simultaneously putting him under pressure on more serious matters, and searching his house. So, at 8.30 on the evening of 24 November 1956 he arrived at Kent Lodge with Charlie Hewett and Brynley Pugh. Dr Adams appeared on the stairs, done up to the nines in a dinner jacket. He was on his way out to dinner at the YMCA. Herbert Hannam asked if they could go into a private room, then he made his arrest. 'What a shock,' said the doctor, who asked if he might ring his solicitor Herbert James.

Hannam said he had a warrant to search for drugs under the

Dangerous Drugs Act. 'There are no dangerous drugs here,' replied Dr Adams.

While he was talking, he unlocked a compartment in a wooden cabinet, saying: 'I have quite a bit of barbiturates here, is that what you mean? . . . What do you mean by dangerous drugs, poisons?' Hannam replied: 'Morphine, heroin, pethidine and the like.' He answered: 'Oh, that group. You will find none here. I haven't any. I very seldom ever use them.'

Superintendent Hannam sent Brynley Pugh out of the room to close the curtains in the front of the house to stop journalists from looking in – so the account of what happened next came from Hannam's memory, and was corroborated by his loyal aide, Charlie Hewett. Pugh was not there to witness it.

Hannam recalled that he next asked to see the dangerous drugs register that Dr Adams was obliged, by law, to keep. But the doctor said he kept no records, and that he hadn't realised that he was supposed to. Hannam produced a list of morphine and heroin prescriptions for Edith Morrell. Dr Adams raised his hand and said: 'Now all those I left prescriptions for either at the chemists or at the house. She had nurses day and night.'

'Who administered the drugs?' asked Hannam.

'I did nearly all. Perhaps the nurses gave some, but mostly me.'

'Were there any left over when she died?' asked Hannam.

'No, none. All was given to the patient.'

'Doctor, you prescribed for her 75 $\frac{1}{6}$ grain heroin tablets the day before she died [a huge 4,870 mg].'

'Poor soul, she was in terrible agony. It was all used. I used them myself.'

'I have no medical training myself,' said Hannam, 'but surely the quantity of dangerous drugs obtained for Mrs Morrell during the last week of her life alone would be fatal? And is pain usual with a cerebral vascular accident?'

Dr Adams asked to look at the list. He pointed to two of the prescriptions, and said there might have been a couple of the final tablets left over, he could not remember. 'If there were I would take them and destroy them. I am not dishonest with drugs. Mrs Morrell had all those, because I gave the injections. Do you think it is too much?'

Hannam replied that this was not a matter for him, and asked whether the doctor had kept records of his prescriptions for Mrs Morrell. 'No,' he replied, 'I do not keep any records of what I prescribe for my patients.'

'Many of your patients' deaths, particularly those from whom you received some pecuniary advantage, appear suspicious,' said Hannam. 'Can you tell me what was the injection you gave to Mrs Bradnum?'

'She was a cerebral haemorrhage case, so it would have been a stimulant, quite likely caffeine. She was dying when I got there.'

'A few minutes before you arrived at her house, she got out of bed, walked across the room and unlocked her bedroom door to admit a member of the household, and got back into bed again.'

'I am not certain what it was I gave her, but it would be a stimulant.'

'What was the final injection you gave Mrs Kilgour?'

'Do you think I killed her too?' Dr Adams asked. 'This is terrible, I've got no dangerous drugs. I haven't bought any for years and years.'

Dr Adams's face at this moment was very flushed, said Charlie Hewett, and he wiped a tear from his eye.

'When Miss Hilda Neil-Miller died, what articles did you take from her room?' asked Hannam.

'I never took anything.'

'Mrs Sharpe was present and a nurse saw you.'

'What did they say I took?'

'I thought you didn't take anything!'

'I only take what the patient has wished me to have . . .'

'What about Miss Clara Neil-Miller? Eleven days before her death, when she was only semi-conscious from sedatives, you got her to sign a cheque for £500 in your favour and one for £200 for Mrs Sharpe, and you knew you were already to receive £500 when she died, under her will, and you were her sole residuary legatee.'

'A dear lady. She insisted I must have the £500 and said Mrs Sharpe must have a present and I arranged it to give her peace of mind only.'

'. . . Miss Clara was not in a condition to will you money, was she?'

'She would not have been happy if I had not taken it.'

'Why did she die?'

'She was very weak.'

Then, said Hannam, the doctor 'began to cry for a moment or two, and said: "wasn't her death natural?" I made no reply.'

At this moment, Brynley Pugh returned, and he agreed with the version of subsequent events that was recorded by Hannam and Hewett. As Pugh entered the room Dr Adams was flopped in a chair, and was holding his head in his hands. Hannam told Pugh to search the room and, as the search began, Dr Adams stood up and again opened the compartment in his medicines cabinet, saying 'there are a number of barbiturates there but no drugs'.

The cupboard, said Hannam, was extremely untidy. Bottles were piled up on the top of it, and more bottles were crammed inside, mixed up with boxes and slabs of chocolate, some packets of sugar, and pieces of margarine and butter. Some of the chocolate had actually stuck to the shelves. It was a horrible mess, a sharp contrast to the doctor's efforts to make a good impression externally – he liked his cars buffed and polished, his suits to be immaculate, and his accessories (gold pens, kidskin gloves) to be obviously expensive. Hannam reached into the cupboard, and found a bottle with twelve cachets inside, bearing the name 'Mrs Hullett', seven empty bottles with her name on them, another bottle with her name on, containing twenty-two tablets, as well as several containers which appeared to hold pheno-barbitone.

While Hannam was examining the bottles, Dr Adams walked to the other side of the surgery to another cupboard. 'I caught the eye of Inspector Pugh and we looked at Adams,' he wrote. Furtively, the doctor took a key that was on a chain attached to his trousers, and unlocked a compartment in the cabinet. Then he took out two objects, and slipped them into his pocket. Hannam pounced: 'What did you take from that cupboard, doctor?' He replied: 'Nothing. I only opened it for you.' So Hannam pointed out that he had hidden something in his pocket. 'No, I've got nothing,' he replied. Hannam moved towards him and said sternly: 'What was it, doctor?'

Dr Adams took from his pocket two cartons, each containing a bottle labelled morphine, and handed them to Superintendent Hannam who marked them up with an 'A' – to be used as evidence. 'Doctor, please do not do silly things like that, it is against your own interests,' he said.

'I know it was silly. I didn't want you to find it in there.'

'What is it and where did it come from?'

'One of those I got for Mr Soden who died at the Grand Hotel, and the other was for Mrs Sharpe, who died before I used it.' The doctor was told to sit in a chair in the centre of the room, and not to move without permission.

The solicitor Herbert James now arrived and watched as the search progressed and 'dangerous drugs' were removed from Dr Adams's bags and from an attaché case, and labelled. Superintendent Hannam opened a record cabinet that was beside the doctor's desk, and asked the doctor whether there were any records of any kind for Edith Morrell. No, he answered, there did not appear to be. The police search took nearly two hours, during which they came across the carved chest of silver mentioned in the Morrell case. In the basement, they found a jumble of unused china and silverware. In another room twenty new motor car tyres were piled up, still in their wrappings, and several new motor car leaf springs. Evidently, Dr Adams was a hoarder. He collected things that he never used.

A large store of wines and spirits was found, and on the second floor one room had been made into an armoury 'for in it we saw six guns in a glass-fronted display case, several automatic pistols and many cases full of 12-bore cartridges . . .' Another room on the same floor was filled with photographic equipment: 'a dozen very expensive cameras in leather cases were seen and large quantities of unused films of various types were set out in trays'. At 10.20 p.m. the police left, and escorted the doctor to Eastbourne police station, where they charged him officially with the forgery and cremation form offences. Afterwards, Dr Adams returned to Kent Lodge where Herbert James was busy. The solicitor was conducting his own search of the doctor's house for anything at all, diaries or prescriptions or records, which might be helpful to his client, or incriminating – anything that might have been missed by the police. And, as it turned out, he did find something – some ordinary-looking notebooks that would prove to be rather important.

Two days later, on Monday 26 November, Dr Adams visited Eastbourne police station for an official photograph. While there, he encountered Superintendent Hannam, and said: 'You told Mr James there might be other charges. I am very worried. What are they?'

'Hiding that morphine on Saturday night is a serious offence and I am still enquiring into the deaths of some of your rich patients, I do not think they were all natural.'

'Which?' asked Dr Adams.

'Mrs Morrell is certainly one.'

'Easing the passing of a dying person isn't all that wicked,' replied the doctor. 'She wanted to die. That can't be murder. It is impossible to accuse a doctor.'

This was the finest moment of the investigation. In Herbert

Hannam's opinion Dr Adams had cracked, had admitted that he had accelerated the death of Edith Morrell. After all the insinuations and vague suggestions, here was something concrete, something that would be useful in a court of law. On 5 December 1956 Hannam wrote a twenty-page report detailing 'the most amazing conduct and remarks by the prisoner during the search of his surgery'. The doctor had proved to be a most loquacious man: 'He commits himself even in the presence of a solicitor, and if ever we have to re-arrest him on a more serious charge, there appears every reason to believe that he will talk himself into a conviction.'

He could not fathom why Dr Adams had lied so much about dangerous drugs, why he had said he had bought none for years. It was so easy to prove that he had, in fact, bought huge amounts. The police had inspected the records of Eastbourne chemists and found that 'his acquisition of barbiturates seems almost incomprehensible. Just one example is on 3 January 1952, when he bought 5,000 pheno-barbitone tablets for use in his practice.' The number was astronomical and it was hard to think of an innocent explanation. Another peculiarity was the timing of certain prescriptions; for instance, Dr Adams had prescribed morphia for Jack Hullett on the day *after* he died, with directions that the drugs should be sent to Kent Lodge. In theory, the endless prescriptions might be explained by the doctor being a drug addict himself. In practice, there was no suggestion of that.

In October Superintendent Hannam's report to his bosses at Scotland Yard had been unclear on the murder point. By December, he was no longer prepared to hold back, and he stressed that the deaths of many of Dr Adams's patients were suspicious, and made the point that the Eastbourne GP Dr Estcourt 'is quite certain that Adams precipitated the death of some of his rich patients for his own pecuniary advantage', though he had to admit that Dr Estcourt 'has no direct evidence of any actual case'.

Overall, there seemed to be a mountain of vaguely sinister events, and a few promising hard nuggets of evidence – the prescriptions, the inexplicable injections, and the incriminating nature of the doctor's own words: 'Easing the passing of a dying person isn't all that wicked. She wanted to die. That can't be murder. It is impossible to accuse a doctor.'

On 18 December 1956 Superintendent Hannam and Sergeant Charlie Hewett returned to London for a meeting with the Attorney-General, Sir Reginald Manningham-Buller, in his elegant oak-panelled office in the House of Commons. Also present were the Director of Public Prosecutions, Sir Theobald Mathew, and the barrister Melford Stevenson, as well as the Home Office pathologist Francis Camps, and a Harley Street consultant, Arthur Douthwaite. Their purpose was to decide what to do next. Reginald Manningham-Buller asked Francis Camps and Arthur Douthwaite about the amount of heroin and morphia given to Edith Morrell. When the doctors assured the Attorney-General that Mrs Morrell's prescriptions showed doses that were definitely, unarguably fatal, he turned to Hannam and commanded him to 'go down to Eastbourne now and charge Adams with the murder of Mrs Morrell!'

According to Charlie Hewett, he and Hannam were far from happy. Edith Morrell was not their preferred case, as she had died a full six years earlier, and there was no body. They would have preferred to hold off the arrest, and investigate further a more recent death, with a body. There was some consolation to be had, however, in that permission was now obtained for the exhumation of the bodies of Julia Bradnum and Clara Neil-Miller. This, thought the police, might alter the trajectory of the investigation.

In the meantime, the arrest was to be made. At 8.30 in the morning of 19 December 1956 Superintendent Hannam met Detective Sergeant Hewett at Victoria Station, where they found three reporters – from the *Daily Mail*, the *Daily Express* and the

Daily Mirror. 'Each was unkempt,' wrote Hannam. It seemed that the journalists had been waiting for the police all night long, with a view to tailing them down to Eastbourne. Hannam was aware that his relationship with the press was arousing criticism at Scotland Yard, and he attempted to shake off the reporters by getting into his car as soon as he reached Eastbourne station, and driving around the town for a while. When he thought the coast was clear, he parked the police car some distance away from Kent Lodge and, with Hewett, walked to his destination.

They entered the house, but found that Dr Adams was busy with a patient. Six or seven more were in the waiting room, along with a press photographer and a reporter from the French magazine *Paris Match*. The journalists had been welcomed in by Dr Adams, who had posed for photographs in his surgery and given the reporter 'his own exemplary life history'.

'Our arrival at this opportune moment,' wrote Hannam, 'was an accidental piece of excellent fortune for the *Paris Match* reporters. I ordered them out of the house and we were engaged there for some twenty minutes.'

Dr Adams was arrested for the murder of Edith Morrell. His response was peculiar – 'Murder,' he said, 'murder. Can you prove it was murder?' adding, 'I didn't think you could prove murder, she was dying in any event.' As he was escorted out of the house, his receptionist came and gripped his hand. 'I will see you in heaven,' said Dr Adams. Then he was led by the police down the steps of Kent Lodge, watched and photographed by a band of reporters who were waiting in the front garden.

IO

All the World at Eastbourne

IN THE NEWSPAPERS, the arrest of Dr Adams was set against a background of tumultuous world events. By December 1956, armed intervention in Suez had proved disastrous and the most pertinent question, aired frequently in the papers, was how quickly the troops could be brought home. The conflict had caused a fuel crisis – shortages of petrol, rationing and a monstrous hike in prices at the pump to ten shillings a gallon. The prevailing mood echoed that of the Second World War, particularly when the Chancellor, Harold Macmillan, urged every British business to do its patriotic duty to keep prices down, cutting profits if necessary. Anthony Eden, the aristocratic Prime Minister, was hanging on by his fingernails, and in the middle of the calamity flew off to Jamaica on the grounds that the sunshine might do him good and restore his ailing health. He returned to Britain on 14 December, golden-brown and glowing, declaring that he was 'absolutely fit' – though, in truth he was not – and ignoring the reporters audacious enough to ask him about rumours that he was going to resign.

In Europe, the Hungarian Uprising had been quashed by the Soviet Union's 'Red Terror'. 'Hungary re-explodes' splashed the *Daily Express* on 10 December, reporting that martial law had been declared and 'purge courts' set up to order death sentences or imprisonment for anyone who dared to participate in armed resistance. 'Do or die battles blaze' was the headline on the *Daily Mirror* three days later. The advertisements in British papers tried to summon up a cheeriness that had a desperate edge when set against the backdrop of the international situation. 'OMO ADDS BRIGHTNESS, the brightness women want!' – a declaration with resonance that went beyond washing powder. Or 'THEY'RE GR...R...REAT! says Tony the Tiger of Kellogg's sugar frosted flakes, guaranteed to give you fast energy . . . that's why they're good for you'. Heinz's attempts to lift the spirits took the form of a front page advertisement in the *Daily Express* for a 'delicious savoury treat' that involved making a soufflé out of white breadcrumbs, milk and cheese, and tipping a tin of Heinz spaghetti on top.

Then, on 20 December, the weather made a dramatic contribution to the timbre of the news. 'KILLER SMOG BUILDS UP' reported the *Express* the following day: 'The fog covering forty counties of England and half Europe was threatening last night to become another killer. Weathermen forecast it could become the worst since 1952, when 4,000 people died in London alone.' Airliners could not land in the capital, and ships in the Thames were at a standstill, while troops returning from Suez were stuck in Southampton Water on board the stationary *Asciana*. Another story, further down the front page, was muted – this being Percy Hoskins's paper. That of two exhumations in Eastbourne.

Other papers were not so restrained. The *Daily Mirror* downplayed the smog and instead led with 'CID OPEN TWO GRAVES TODAY, WOMEN TO BE EXHUMED AT DAWN', the headline filling almost half the front page. The following day, it reported the exhumations of the bodies of Julia Bradnum and Clara Neil-Miller across a two-page spread, with pictures. 'In the grey light of dawn the bodies of two wealthy elderly women were exhumed at Eastbourne today,' wrote Harry Longmuir. 'There Dr Francis Camps, the Home Office pathologist, conducted preliminary post-mortem examinations lasting five hours . . . Just before dawn was breaking,

Superintendent Hannam of Scotland Yard arrived at Ocklynge Cemetery, wearing a bowler hat and gumboots . . .' A new stage of the Dr Adams story had begun.

While Hannam was attending grisly work in Eastbourne, the doctor became prisoner number 7889 at Brixton jail. 'When those iron gates clang behind you,' he said, 'you lose your whole feeling of contact with the world. You lose your individuality and become just another number.' He was made to strip naked while his clothes were examined – a particularly undignified experience for somebody whose blubbery flesh was usually concealed by expensive tailoring. But his spirit was far from broken. Instead, he viewed himself in a somewhat heroic light, enduring persecution and hardship without complaint, and depending on God. He drew strength from his clear conscience, he said, and faith in British justice, and he told Percy Hoskins of the *Daily Express* that he was determined to be stoical and 'to adapt myself to the prison routine without asking any special favours'. He was held in the prison hospital, which was normal for someone charged with a capital offence.

His legal representation was arranged by the Medical Defence Union, an organisation charged with helping doctors guard their professional reputations. For the MDU, the Adams brief was a call to arms, as to accuse a doctor of murdering a patient was so grave and so rare, and there was also a symbolism in the case. Many GPs were offended by the press portrayal of a monstrous rogue doctor, and saw Dr Adams as one of themselves, a beleaguered professional caring for patients who were elderly and frail. If such a person, at the unglamorous, arduous end of the business, could be accused of murder just because he gave powerful drugs to the dying, then most doctors were vulnerable to the charge. Well-meant actions might be misinterpreted, good faith called into question. It was alarming, and contributed to an already heightened sense of grievance over doctors' low pay under the NHS. 'FAMILY DOCTORS IN REVOLT, 40,000 FIX

WALK-OUT DETAILS' was the front page lead in the *Daily Express* on 28 December 1956. Chapman Pincher wrote: 'A mass walk-out of doctors from the Health Service if the government goes on refusing their claim for a 24 per cent pay rise was threatened last night.' The BMA was making plans for an unprecedented strike that threatened to be the last straw for Anthony Eden, and his tenuous hold on government. In the circumstances, the defence of Dr Adams was both personal and political.

The Medical Defence Union appointed Hempsons solicitors, and Hempsons' man Leigh Taylor paid a visit to Brixton jail to check on his client. Dr Adams 'seems, relatively speaking, quite comfortable,' wrote Taylor, '... he is at ease in his mind and assured me there was nothing that he lacked'. Dr Adams's close friend Herbert James organised the practical side of his life, paying the Kent Lodge gardener, the chauffeur and the house-keeper, Miss Chattey, who was assigned to go back and forth to Brixton with spare pairs of trousers. Herbert James paid Dr Adams's bills – the sundry amounts for the *Christian Herald* and the *Shooting Times*, the *Reader's Digest* and the *Daily Telegraph*, as well as larger sums for the regular deliveries of chocolates from Bond Street. Then, as time went on, the momentous decision was taken to cancel the chocolates, not only from Charbonnel et Walker – famous for their rose and violet creams – but also a supply of chocolate pineapples from Joseph Terry.

Herbert James and his colleagues also dealt with the press requests that were flooding in – for interviews, for photographs of Dr Adams, and for his story – should he be free to give it after the trial. Mr James told the doctor's chauffeur, Mr White, that he 'was not to give any interviews of any sort or kind to news-papers', and when the receptionist, Miss Lawrence, was offered a whopping £1,500 to write articles for the *Sunday Dispatch*, he firmly advised her against it – a blow for someone whose wages were a mere £4 a week. And it was Herbert James who dealt with the police when naughty schoolboys stole the metal name-plate on the gate-pillar in front of Kent Lodge. He advised that the boys should not be prosecuted, and also that it was not safe to reinstate the nameplate since, in the circumstances, it was likely that it would soon disappear again. 'I am most anxious to do anything I possibly can for Adams,' James wrote. 'I have known him for thirty years and it is completely inconceivable to me that he could have done any of the acts alleged against him.' He worked hard, and Dr Adams wrote to him, in praise of 'such a wonderful friend'.

The doctor's Christmas was spent in jail and, he said, 'my good friends and patients in Eastbourne wrote to me and sent me fruit'. On his 58th birthday, on 21 January 1957, the wealthy widow Lady Prendergast sent him a basket of fruit. 'Before my arrest I took tea with her every Tuesday. She never ceased to send me words of encouragement,' he told Percy Hoskins.

In the meantime, Herbert James made efforts to rally other types of support. He had already obtained from a Mrs Pearl Prince a letter defending Dr Adams from 'the prevalence of unfounded rumours'. Mrs Prince lived at Annie Sharpe's Barton guesthouse and Superintendent Hannam had thought her an obvious target for the doctor. More important by far, though, was an attempt to gain a supportive statement from Dr Adams's colleague Dr Vincent Harris – the doctor who had assisted in the treatment of Bobbie Hullett and had attended Edith Morrell when Dr Adams was away in Scotland on his shooting holiday. If anyone was in a position to state that Dr Adams was no mur-derer, that he was simply a GP doing his job in a reasonable way, it was Dr Harris since he had observed the doctor at the closest of quarters, and had the expertise to assess his treatments and behaviour. But, sometime in January 1957, it became apparent that Dr Harris was not inclined to save Dr Adams from the gal-lows. That month, he made it clear to Herbert James 'that he did not think he could be in any way helpful'.

Dr Adams's legal team were also keeping a close watch on the exhumations of the bodies of Julia Bradnum and Clara Neil-Miller. The post-mortems might send the case against the doctor in either direction. If Julia Bradnum had died of cerebral haemorrhage and Clara Neil-Miller of coronary thrombosis, as Dr Adams had stated on the death certificates, and if there was no sign of overdose of morphine, heroin or barbiturates, then the defence could proceed with some degree of confidence. Of course, the opposite result would be a disaster. The Medical Defence Union appointed the renowned forensic pathologist Keith Simpson, and asked him to observe the post-mortems which were carried out by Francis Camps. The two men had once been friends, but were now bitter rivals at the top of their profession. Keith Simpson later accused Francis Camps of bearing a grudge whenever Simpson was assigned an interesting autopsy, and also of being too eager to oppose Simpson in court. In 1953 the men had worked together, fractiously, on the Christie case. Now they were together again, on opposing sides.

Julia Bradnum's body had been in the ground since 1952, and was in a state of advanced decomposition. Francis Camps wrote a report on the post-mortem, recording no evidence of the brain haemorrhage that Dr Adams had diagnosed, though because the brain is very fatty, it decomposes quickly and not all of it was in a condition to be assessed. Generally, the liver endures better – and if Mrs Bradnum's last injection had been morphine, it would show in the liver even though the body had been in the ground for four and a half years. The same would be true of heroin or barbiturates. But Dr Camps writes of bodily material being so dehydrated that he cannot be sure that it is the liver – and toxicology tests were not made.

Clara Neil-Miller was the lady who had died after being made to lie naked by an open window in winter. She had died more recently, in 1954, but her grave was partly submerged in water and the lid of the coffin had caved in. None the less, Dr Camps did find some evidence consistent with coronary thrombosis, and also with pneumonia. The coronary evidence, however, was unremarkable, since most elderly people have coronary disease which is evident at post-mortem. In her case, some small amounts of morphine were found, and also barbiturates. But, overall, nothing useful could be said about drugs in either case.

It was a disappointing outcome, but was soon eclipsed as the story of Dr Adams entered a new phase – once again amid dramatic political events. On 9 January 1957 Anthony Eden at last resigned, and the following day Harold Macmillan became Prime Minister, telling the Queen that he could not guarantee that his government would last six weeks. Despite the turmoil, the Dr Adams story took precedence on the front pages of the popular papers when, on 14 January 1957, he appeared before Eastbourne magistrates for preliminary hearings in advance of his trial for murder (Roland Gwynne stepped aside, as was seemly). The event was puffed in the press as a dress rehearsal for the real trial – and the fuss was immense. 'Paris, Geneva, Berlin – all the world watches' ran a headline on the front of the *Daily Express*, describing the ranks of pressmen from all over the world who had descended on Eastbourne. And the public gallery was 'packed to the walls' with people, many of them elderly women, who been waiting outside since dawn. 'Spectators stood in a long queue outside the court in a raw cold wind,' wrote the *New York Times* correspondent, under the headline 'Eastbourne's whodunit'. 'Some put up umbrellas against the alternating snow flurries and misty drizzle', in the hope of a ringside seat to a case that, for the Americans and others, was already regarded as a classic murder trial – the most significant since that of John Christie. It was now that some of the principal actors in the forthcoming trial were seen for the first time.

The prosecution barrister was Aubrey Melford Steed Stevenson, who was already well-known to the British public as an indefatigable flog-them and hang-them type, consistently on the sterner side of the criminal law, and on the right wing of politics and anything else that might have a right wing. He lived in a house in Winchelsea, Sussex, that happened to be called Truncheons – a fitting name for the home of a blunt, heavy-handed barrister who, when directed at a target, could be lethal. Stevenson was among the last of the 'grand eccentrics' in the criminal courts and he 'had a biting wit, much enjoyed by most of the Bar and not so much by the litigants'.

In 1955 he had defended Ruth Ellis, who was charged with the murder of her lover, David Blakely. Stevenson did not handle the case with distinction, and Ellis became the last woman in England to be hanged. It was said that her lawyer had let her down by allowing prosecution witnesses to have an easy ride in the witness box and by opening his defence with the words: 'Let me make this abundantly plain: there is no question here but this woman shot this man [. . .] You will not hear one word from me – or from the lady herself – questioning that.' It was characteristic that his position was firmly stated, unambiguous and forthright – but unusual in seeming to be on the wrong side of the case.

In Eastbourne, Stevenson went at his subject with his usual bulldog determination and on the first day of the hearing he produced a sensation, stating that, in the case of Edith Morrell, the prosecution wished to present evidence of two further deaths at the hands of Dr Adams, both of which were murder. Jack Hullett, he said, had – like Mrs Morrell – died after an injection of morphine. Jack Hullett had, like Mrs Morrell, mentioned Dr Adams in his will. And, when Jack Hullett died, the doctor had lied when signing the cremation form, just as he had done in the case of Edith Morrell, stating he had no financial connection to the patient. Because of this the body was burned, and any evidence that it contained was destroyed. Jack Hullett, said Stevenson, had been given a huge dose of morphine. After the death, Dr Adams had written out a prescription for 5 grains (324 mg) of morphia in Jack's name, and asked for the drugs to be sent to Kent Lodge. If he was replacing the amount of morphia he had given Jack Hullett just before he died, then 'we say that was a fatal dose and a dose meant to kill'. The motive was money.

He turned to the death of Bobbie Hullett. The inquest had suggested no foul play – a simple suicide – and Herbert Hannam, during his massive investigation, had given her case barely any attention. But Stevenson thought the manner of her death entirely suspicious, and wholly relevant to the death of Mrs Morrell. Bobbie Hullett 'died in circumstances in which the Crown says amount to murder by Dr Adams,' Stevenson told the magistrates, 'whether she herself administered the fatal dose or not'. 'From 1 May 1956,' he said, 'the doctor had prescribed for her quantities of barbitone, and from that date he embarked on a course of drugging which led to her death'. It was no coincidence that she was a very wealthy woman, and he referred to the £1,000 cheque that Bobbie had given Dr Adams two days before she overdosed, and which had been ignored by the Coroner at her inquest. 'Dr Adams gave instructions to his bank that that cheque was to be specially cleared,' said Stevenson. 'Why? We say it was because Dr Adams knew quite well that Mrs Hullett was going to die that weekend.'

The Hullett cases were relevant to that of Mrs Morrell, he continued, because they involved 'similar facts'. Generally in English law, evidence from one case of alleged murder cannot be used in the trial for an entirely separate murder, but an exception can be made when the facts of the cases are very alike. A famous precedent for the introduction of similar fact evidence, or 'system', was the Brides in the Bath murder trial of 1915, in which George Joseph Smith was accused of murdering a young lady named Bessie Mundy in her bath, and the judge, Thomas Scrutton, allowed evidence to be heard relating to the deaths in baths of two other women. Stevenson argued that the Adams case was of the same type – featuring the repetition of a distinctive, unusual modus operandi. As the lawyer spoke, the doctor listened intently, and took notes in green ink. For most of the day, 'the public saw only the back of his florid neck and bald head'.

It was now that the world glimpsed for the first time the barrister who was to conduct Dr Adams's defence. He was Frederick Geoffrey Lawrence, and he was the opposite of Melford Stevenson – low key, no particular liking for the limelight, and certainly no element of bluster to his delivery in court. In appearance, he was as fine-featured, neat and small as Stevenson was bold and rough-hewn, and his approach was forensic and clever. *Time Magazine* described him as a 'puckish, mousy little man with a mind as orderly as a calculating machine'. His oratory style was considered 'magnetic', and it was observed that he could make 'polysyllables such as "cerebral" and "respiratory" sound like something out of Keats'. In private, he was an accomplished musician who played the piano and violin, and he was often out of doors, yachting, swimming or playing cricket. At work, he was assiduous and, until the Dr Adams case, had toiled mainly out of the public gaze, on matters of planning and parliamentary law, and divorce cases.

Nine days of preliminary hearings at Eastbourne drew towards their close with a two-hour speech by Geoffrey Lawrence. There was, he stated, a 'patent absurdity' at the heart of the prosecution's case. If Dr Adams's motive had been money, as Stevenson had claimed, then the possible inheritance of a Georgian chest of silver from Edith Morrell was a paltry thing – hardly worth murdering for. She was a wealthy woman, worth £157,000, and she was far more valuable to Dr Adams alive than dead, because of the medical fees that she was paying him. And Lawrence thought the cases regarding Jack and Bobbie Hullett so thin that, rather than contribute as evidence in the Morrell case, they served the opposite purpose. *Common sense* was against the charge of murder. His point was forcefully made but, at the same time, there was an air about Lawrence that suggested that he was keeping his powder dry, that he had more to say – not here, but at a trial. And, sure enough, the Eastbourne magistrates took just twenty-seven minutes to decide that Dr Adams would be tried at the Old Bailey for the murder of Edith Morrell.

After the hearings, Dr Adams's partner, Dr Vincent Harris, at last made his view of his colleague clear. He gave a statement to Superintendent Hannam, in which he distanced himself from Dr Adams and criticised his behaviour at the bedside of Bobbie Hullett. Dr Harris said he had supported his senior partner at the Bobbie Hullett inquest 'as far as was honestly possible'. But, now that he looked back, he could see that 'if Dr Adams did not intentionally mislead me in connection with Mrs Gertrude Hullett, he most certainly kept back material facts which I should have known about'. Dr Harris had had no idea that barbiturates were being delivered to Holywell Mount, and Dr Adams did not ever suggest that Bobbie might be suicidal. 'Had I known that Mrs Hullett had suggested suicide or that she had access to excessive quantities of barbiturates, I should certainly have insisted that she was removed to hospital.

'Throughout the course of Mrs Hullett's illness, Dr Adams was absolutely dogmatic that she was suffering from a cerebral haemorrhage and I did not feel that I was in a position to disagree with the diagnosis, with his superior knowledge as an anaesthetist of barbiturates and I felt that the treatment was entirely his responsibility.' As for Mrs Morrell, Dr Harris admitted that while Dr Adams was on his shooting holiday in Scotland, he had given her prescriptions for omnopon – a morphine-based drug – but he could not now remember why he had done so. Dr Harris had covered his own back with a statement that was helpful to the prosecution.

At the same time Dr Adams's great friend, Roland Gwynne, who until now had stood by him, phoning the police on his behalf, accompanying him to Scotland, changed his mind and endeavoured to shake off all connection. He told people that he thought he had been lucky to escape the doctor's friendship alive, and that he had decided that, when the time came, he would not be cremated, but would be buried in a sealed lead coffin – the implication being that he took a dim view of cremations because of the way they sent evidence of murder up in flames. On 1 February 1957, Herbert Hannam paid Gwynne a visit, and afterwards made a note of their conversation. 'He regarded Adams as a greedy man,' wrote Hannam, 'and said that all he had really done for him was to allow him the complete use for shooting purposes of some 2,000 acres of his various estates.' Gwynne said that Dr Adams had been his GP for the past eight years, and admitted telling friends that since the doctor had been in custody, and no longer prescribing medicines for him, he had felt much better. However, he now told Hannam, his recent sense of well-being 'might be due to his elation at the honour of a knighthood conferred upon him by Her Majesty last month'. Colonel Gwynne said Dr Adams had given him mild sleeping tablets, but never any injections. His comment about escaping with his life had, in fact, been a joke – and his wish to be buried in a lead coffin had been made long ago. However, he now thought he 'might be fortunate to have been relieved of Dr Adams', and, added Hannam, 'he told me finally that under no circumstances would he ever see Dr Adams again'.

Others among the patriarchs of Eastbourne were inclined to believe the worst, and to make jokes about Dr Adams. At a meeting of the Eastbourne Hoteliers Association held at the Burlington Hotel on 13 February 1957 the chairman, Edward Johnson, read out to the hundred or so members five 'scurrilous verses' that were said to have been written by a local doctor who had 'never been friendly to Dr Adams'. The verses had been printed, and circulated widely in the town, under the title 'Adams and Eves', and began:

In Eastbourne it is healthy
And the residents are wealthy –
It's a miracle that anybody dies;
Yet this pearl of English Lidos,
Is a slaughterhouse for widows –
If their bankrolls are above the normal size.

Herbert James learnt of the verses, and telephoned Mr Johnson to warn him that they were libellous and that he should consult his solicitor as he could expect to receive a writ. He also considered an action for contempt of court.

The flurry of legal activity that precedes a major criminal trial was now in full flow. Patrick Devlin was appointed as the judge who would take the case and the Attorney-General himself, Reginald Manningham-Buller, was to lead the prosecution, with Melford Stevenson as his second. They made a formidable pair – being alike in their politics and strident attitudes. Had they been born on the wrong side of the tracks, they would have had the stomping look of dockhands or East End gangsters (in common with the other main player for the Crown – Herbert Hannam). But Reginald Manningham-Buller had been educated at Eton and Magdalen College Oxford, had been a Tory MP since 1943, and was politically ambitious. It was widely known that he had his eye on the job of Lord Chief Justice, and that he might be keen to perform in a spectacular criminal trial in order to impress both the Bar and his political masters. As it happened, the judge, Patrick Devlin, was also in the running for the job which, in legal circles, lent a certain frisson to the dynamics of the courtroom.

Later, Patrick Devlin wrote an account of the trial of Dr Adams, in which he portrayed Reginald Manningham-Buller unfavourably, some would say unkindly. While everyone else was referred to by their surnames, Manningham-Buller was called 'Reggie' throughout – on the grounds that he was, in life, Reggie to friend and foe alike, and because he was the sort of person who obviously ought to be called Reggie. 'What was almost unique about him and makes his career so fascinating is that what the ordinary careerist achieves by making himself agreeable, falsely or otherwise, Reggie achieved by making himself disagreeable,' wrote Devlin. 'Sections of the press, which he permanently antagonised, liked to parody his name by calling him Sir Bullying Manner. This was wrong. He was a bully without a bullying manner. His bludgeoning was quiet.' His disagreeableness was 'pervasive', his persistence 'interminable', the obstructions he put in your way were 'far flung', and all in the name of objectives that were 'apparently so insignificant that sooner or later you would be tempted to ask yourself whether the game was worth the candle: if you asked yourself that, you were finished'.

In practice, many people found Reggie perfectly agreeable, and Patrick Devlin conceded that he was responsible for many small kindnesses and courtesies. But, his overall position on Reggie was, if not damning, then demeaning. It was also so eloquent, entertaining and recognisable that it became inevitable that Reggie was stuck with the Devlin view in perpetuity. 'His zeal for the conversion of souls,' Devlin wrote, 'was equal to that of any of the great mediaeval bulldozers of religious orthodoxy. He was neither a saint nor a villain. But since most of his convictions were wrong-headed, he was ineluctably a do-badder.' Reggie was an inspiration for the character of Kenneth Widmerpool in Anthony Powell's novels *A Dance to the Music of Time*, and Patrick Devlin writes that he did, indeed, seem very much like Widmerpool: 'The reappearance of Widmerpool, each time surprisingly on a higher rung of the ladder, are glimpses of how Reggie's climb in real life appeared to his contemporaries.'

On 21 February 1957 Reggie visited Patrick Devlin and told him that he had decided to ditch the line taken by Melford Stevenson at the Eastbourne hearings. At the Old Bailey trial, he said, he would not ask for the evidence relating to the deaths of Jack and Bobbie Hullett to be admitted. He would not, after all, be arguing that Dr Adams had a 'system' at work, that the doctor had killed others in a very similar manner. As Patrick Devlin put it: 'Exeunt the Brides in the Bath'. Instead, said Reggie, he would apply to the Lord Chief Justice to file a separate indictment for the murder of Bobbie Hullett. If the jury were to acquit Dr Adams on the case of Edith Morrell, then he would immediately proceed with the Bobbie Hullett case. If Dr Adams were found guilty of the murder of Edith Morrell, said Reggie, then the Crown might, or might not, go ahead with the Bobbie Hullett indictment. The decision would be of the keenest consequence for the doctor. The Homicide Bill was going through Parliament, which restricted the use of capital punishment, and would have the effect of saving Dr Adams's life should he be convicted for one murder only. A conviction for two or more murders, and he would hang.

When Geoffrey Lawrence heard of Reggie's about-turn he was incensed. He had argued, unsuccessfully, that the Hullett evidence should not be heard in public at Eastbourne. Now the world, and any Old Bailey jury, was well-acquainted with all the juicy details of the deaths of Jack and Bobbie Hullett as described by Melford Stevenson. He believed that a fair trial was impossible. 'I was taken aback by Lawrence's vigour,' wrote Devlin, 'which in any other man I should have thought to be slightly paranoiac . . . he was obviously and deeply disturbed.'

II

Trial

NEWS OF THE impending trial had reached Hollywood. One morning in late February 1957 the film director Alfred Hitchcock was in his garden pruning roses and allowing himself to daydream, when a neighbour called out: 'Well, I see you've got another juicy murder case on your hands over there!' Hitch glanced around to see if he had overlooked a corpse in the undergrowth, but quickly realised that by 'over there' his neighbour meant England. And the juicy murder case was one that had been all over the American newspapers, and in Hitchcock's mind had become 'The Unfortunate Occurrences at Eastbourne'. 'What do you mean "another"?' he asked, defensively. 'It was my impression there were occasional homicides in the United States too.' 'Oh sure,' the neighbour agreed. 'But *you* know – they aren't like those cases of *yours*.' Hitchcock, in fact, agreed; as he put it, 'crime in England does seem to have a specially fascinating aura'.

Alfred Hitchcock had always been curious about murder. As a boy, growing up in east London, he had often made the short journey to the Old Bailey, and sat in the public gallery at murder trials. He liked the fine detail of murder and had visited Scotland Yard's Black Museum to inspect the artefacts of notorious crimes. 'They've got all the shoes of prostitutes from the gaslight era,' he recalled. 'Did you know that the colour of every scarlet woman's shoes determined what her speciality was? If a man saw a prostitute walking along Waterloo Bridge at night he knew she did one thing in red heels, another thing in blue heels. I find that a fascinating bit of information.'

Now, decades later, he was a Hollywood great, with fifty movies and a popular television series to his name. He had directed such classics as *The Lady Vanishes*, *Shadow of a Doubt* (his personal favourite), *Strangers on a Train*, *Dial M for Murder* and *Rear Window*. In early 1957, while Dr Adams was in Brixton jail awaiting his trial, Hitchcock was taking a break from work because of a hernia operation, but he was contemplating the screenplay for the film he was about to make, the one that would become *Vertigo* – starring James Stewart and Kim Novak. He was a world-famous expert on 'the lamentable practice of murder' in general, and the state of the English murder in particular.

In March 1957 he shared his thoughts on the subject with the readers of the *New York Times*, and ruminated on the case of the doctor who was charged with orchestrating the 'rather phenomenal succession of demises of elderly, moneyed patients'. 'Murder – with English on it', by Alfred Hitchcock, posed the question: 'What makes high crime as practiced on the tight little island so special?' There were more murders in America than England, around twenty times more, Hitchcock observed. And yet, it was the English murder that 'managed to contribute so spectacularly to the literature of crime which occupies (without chauvinistic distinction) a half-dozen shelves of my library'. English crimes were intrinsically more dramatic, he thought, partly because the English had 'an ingrained racial sense of drama which, despite its concealment behind impassive visages, has appeared intermittently in history all the way from Shakespeare to Shaw'.

Drama, particularly crime drama, requires contrast. In films, Hitchcock liked to achieve this by juxtaposing a lurid situation with the understatement of ordinary life: 'A man is carrying a bomb in a satchel – a checkroom clerk refuses it – not because it has a bomb in it but because it is all greasy.' Hitchcock did not know it, but the Dr Adams investigation was shot through with just that sort of contrast and understatement – the perfect pitch of the doctor's observation that 'we always want cremations to go off smoothly for the dear relatives'; his explanation to a patient that 'she would probably want to go to sleep' after the injection that he gave her – an injection that the police believed had been fatal.

Geography also played a part. 'If one commits a murder in Hollywood . . . he has within a couple of hours' drive an expanse of desert bigger than the whole United Kingdom in which to dispose tastefully of the remains,' wrote Hitchcock. The English murderer, by contrast, had to look for cellars and trunks in which to hide the body. And if he chose the trunk, then inevitably he would check it in at a railway station. 'Right away you have "The Waterloo Station Trunk Murder," pregnant with drama.' And, because people lived so close together in England, there was an inflated sense of personal privacy to escalate the dramatic tension: 'In the Eastbourne affair, it apparently was years before anyone had the temerity to suggest that the doctor's therapeutic batting average seemed to be slipping badly.'

The national character was also inclined to make murder more interesting. England was not racially diverse, and had a distinct homogeneous population, known for its reserve: 'emotions and urges to which other peoples give ready vent are, by tradition and habit, bottled up. When they emerge, the manifestation is likely to be accordingly bizarre.' And the British judicial system seemed to be timed 'almost with an eye for dramatic pace'. By ancient tradition, if someone were sentenced to hang, then the execution should take place 'within three clear Sundays'. The possibility of 'a swift doom' added wonderfully to the tension in any capital trial.

Eleven years earlier George Orwell had written his celebrated essay 'Decline of the English Murder', in which he imagined a golden era for murder that ran roughly from 1850 to 1925. In the perfect murder, the sort that 'gave the greatest amount of pleasure to the British public', the means of death would be poisoning, and the criminal would be middle class, ideally 'a little man of the professional class – a dentist or a solicitor say – living an intensely respectable life somewhere in the suburbs ... he should be either chairman of the local Conservative Party branch, or a leading Nonconformist and strong Temperance advocate'.

Sex might be a motive, or respectability, or money in the form of a legacy. More often than not, the murder would come to light slowly 'as the result of careful investigations which started off with the suspicions of neighbours or relatives'. The prime examples included Dr Crippen, the poisoner Frederick Seddon, and the Brides in the Bath murderer George Joseph Smith. George Orwell argued that this sort of murder, middle class and domestic, was giving way to a less absorbing type of killing – unfocused and brutish. He cited the 'cleft chin murder' of 1944, in which a young couple, he an American soldier, she an aspiring striptease artist, had killed two people at random in order to show off to each other and establish their credentials as tough gangster types. 'The whole meaningless story, with its atmosphere of dance-halls, movie-palaces, cheap perfume, false names and stolen cars, belongs essentially to a war period,' he wrote. This was the iconography of public spaces and a bleak alienated society – far removed from the images of life in the drawing rooms of English towns and suburbs. It was Americanised and hard-boiled and, in literature, was more suited to the city streets of Raymond Chandler than the domesticated atmosphere of the vicarage and the village in Agatha Christie novels.

And yet, in 1957, the occurrences at Eastbourne were still entirely recognisable as an English story, and Alfred Hitchcock's article did not suggest that Dr Adams's world might be a disappearing one – perhaps because he had been living in America for many years. In Britain itself it was clear that society was less homogeneous than Hitchcock assumed, that the Dr Adams story belonged to a particular vision of England that, while familiar, was rooted in the past. It was a class-based story, of mistresses and servants, of the respectability of the professional middle-class man – the bank manager, the solicitor, the doctor – and it was furnished with the trappings of class, in particular the Rolls-Royces, jewels and furs of the newly rich whose money was made, not inherited. At its heart was deference – the deference, by now rather shaky, of the gardeners, cooks and parlourmaids at work in Eastbourne, and the deference that female patients showed a male doctor who insisted that, as well as attending to their health, he would manage their money. It was 'a damnable technique', said Herbert Hannam, in the language of old England. And, as a story, its potency came from nostalgia for a seemingly ordered, hierarchical past, and from the shocking suspicion that beneath the surface, something evil was happening.

Dr Adams fitted perfectly into the story. The prickly doctor who was an outsider, marked out by his Irish accent, who was constantly making heavy work of securing his social position, sucking up to Edith Morrell, Roland Gwynne, Lady Prendergast and the rest, while being rude and dismissive to the lower orders: the nurses and servants around him. Patrick Devlin was as hooked as the next man: 'The affair was so convincing dramatically,' he wrote, 'the casting so good . . . Dr Adams was a family doctor. True, he was a bachelor. But he was one of those bachelors with amplitudes which seemed to strain his waistcoat and with features so comforting as to make him the equal of any family man . . . He was in partnership with three other doctors with the reassuring names of Snowball, Harris and Barkworth. The fear that such a man with access to so many patients was a poisoner sent shivers down the spine. No one now supposed that the two or three patients whose cases were being exhibited by the police were the only victims. For most of the public the gap of six and a half years presented no difficulty. It was easily filled with any or all of the patients who during that time had died.'

All the talk, all the imaginings, were now to be distilled into something that amounted to evidence, and the Old Bailey was packed with spectators impatient to hear the testimonies, and observe the witnesses who would, at last, get to the heart of the story of Dr Adams. The author Sybille Bedford attended the trial, and described his first appearance in court, 'standing in front of the dock, spherical, adipose, upholstered in blue serge, red-faced, bald, facing the Judge, facing this day'. She watched as he was called by the clerk of the court to confirm his name, and as the words rang out:

> You are charged that on the 13th day of November 1950 you murdered Edith Alice Morrell. Are you guilty or not guilty?

'There is the kind of pause that comes before a clock strikes,' wrote Bedford. Then Dr Adams replied: 'I am not guilty, my lord.' It came out, she thought, with 'a certain dignity and also possibly with a certain stubbornness'. And it was said using the greatest number of words that anyone could manage to put into a plea of Not Guilty. 'A loquacious man, then,' she observed, correctly.

The trial began with the Attorney-General's opening speech. Reggie was not a natural orator, thought Patrick Devlin, 'but his manner was earnest and either, as some might say, impressive, or as others, ponderous'. A 'somewhat massive figure' in the court-room, he began, in full voice, with an instruction to the jury to put out of their minds anything they may have heard about the case, all the rumours, anything they had heard or read about Dr Adams. Instead they must listen only to the evidence before them, and he presented the submission of the Crown:

> that Dr Adams by the administration of drugs to Mrs Morrell, drugs given by him and given upon his instructions, killed her, and our submission is that those drugs were given to her with the intention of killing her.

He set out the doctor's credentials, emphasising that, since he was trained as an anaesthetist, 'he would know a lot about dangerous drugs', then promptly turned to the wealthy widow in the case. After Mrs Morrell's stroke in 1948, said Reggie, and her return to Eastbourne from Cheshire, she was given her first dose of morphia by Dr Adams. This was on 9 July 1948. Then, on 21 July, she was given the first prescription for heroin. Both were derivatives of opium and were very powerful drugs – heroin being the stronger – and throughout his speech Reggie endeavoured to make clear the exact nature and quantities of the drugs prescribed by Dr Adams, and their effects. Throughout the police investigation, the emphasis had been on a softer kind of evidence – the oddness of Dr Adams's behaviour, his grasping nature, the injections that he gave patients 'from his bag' – so it was a relief to hear some hard facts, clear and graspable.

Reggie said that during the ten and a half months of 1950, until she died on 13 November 1950, Dr Adams had prescribed for Mrs Morrell a whopping 165 grains (10,692 mg) of morphia and 139½ grains (9,039 mg) of heroin. The maximum daily dose, he said, was about ½ a grain (32.4 mg) of morphia and ¼ a grain (16.2 mg) of heroin. 'This enabled us to calculate,' wrote Patrick Devlin, 'that the doctor had kept near to the maximum in morphia but exceeded it in heroin by about 75 per cent.' Eventually, Reggie turned to 'the murder period' – and the amounts that were prescribed for Mrs Morrell in the last two weeks of her life.

Some 8 grains of heroin on 8 November, he said, and: 'Another 6 grains of heroin on the 9th. There was no point in prescribing them unless they were intended to be used. Another 6 grains on the 10th, another 6 grains on the 11th, 12 grains of heroin on the 12th.' As for morphia: '10 grains prescribed on the 8th, 12½ on the 9th and 18 grains on the 11th.' So, in those final days, Dr Adams was prescribing up to forty-eight times the maximum dose of heroin, and about twenty times the maximum dose of morphia. One of the expert witnesses, Dr Michael Ashby,

would tell the jury 'that in his view Mrs Morrell could not possibly have survived the administration of the whole of the drugs
prescribed in the last five days or any major portion of them . . .'

Why were the drugs prescribed in such large quantities?
Turning to the jury, Reggie said: 'Perhaps you may think that
the answer lies in the changes made by Mrs Morrell in her will
after she had been taking these drugs.' And he described Dr
Adams's visit to Mrs Morrell's solicitor Hubert Sogno, and the
doctor's insistence that she wished him to have not just her chest
of silver, but also her Rolls-Royce – a visit made when Edith
Morrell was heavily under the influence of heroin and morphia.

An expert witness for the Crown, Dr Arthur Douthwaite,
would testify that the only legitimate reason for giving massive
doses of heroin and morphia would be to relieve pain. But Mrs
Morrell had no pain. 'Why did he prescribe these large quantities
for which there was no medical justification?' asked Reggie.
'The submission of the Crown, members of the Jury, was that he
did so because he had decided that the time had come for Mrs
Morrell to die.'

He now raised the question of 'the last syringe' given on 12
November 1950, the evening before Mrs Morrell's death, when
she was lying unconscious or semi-conscious and was having
'jerky spasms'. That evening, Dr Adams visited and prepared a 5
cc syringe. 'A large one,' said Reggie, 'like *that*.' And, with some
drama, he held up a big syringe. 'You will hear that normally for
these injections of morphia or heroin, a syringe of 1 or 2 cc
capacity is used.' And he presented the jury with a normal-
looking syringe. He went through the events of Mrs Morrell's
last night – Dr Adams's instructions to Sister Randall to administer the huge injection, and his order that she should give a
second, similar, injection if Mrs Morrell's jerky spasms did not
die down. The nurse gave the second injection, said Reggie, and
'Mrs Morrell gradually became quiet, and about two o'clock in
the morning, about an hour after this second injection, Mrs

Morrell died.' The prosecution submit, he continued, 'that these injections, coming on top of the heavy dosage which she had already had, killed her'.

Then Reggie complicated matters. Even if these final injections had nothing to do with Mrs Morrell's death, he said, it was still his submission that Dr Adams had murdered her, because of the prescriptions for morphine and heroin in the period 8 to 12 November. And he emphasised that Dr Adams had said that he, personally, had administered *all* of Mrs Morrell's prescriptions, and there had been no drugs left over. He reminded the jury that 'doctors are not entitled to kill people even if they say they want to die'.

He told the court of the extraordinary conversation with Superintendent Hannam, when Dr Adams had said of Mrs Morrell: 'Easing the passing of a dying person is not all that wicked. She wanted to die – that cannot be murder. It is impossible to accuse a doctor.' At this point, half the court turned to look at Dr Adams, while Reggie continued: '"Easing the passing". That must refer, must it not, to something that Dr Adams did shortly before her death? It clearly refers, does it not, to the two injections that he had given to her, not himself but which he had given to Sister Randall to give to Mrs Morrell the evening before she died. Was it really easing the passing of a dying woman, or was it accelerating her death? What need, Members of the Jury, was there to ease the passing of an unconscious woman?' And, once again, he stressed that Mrs Morrell had not been in pain, no terrible agony that might justify heavy doses of drugs.

He came to Dr Adams's reaction to being charged with murder: 'Murder. Murder. Can you prove it was murder?' and then 'I did not think you could prove murder. She was dying in any event.' 'Is that what you would expect an innocent man to say when he is charged with murder? Or is it what a man might say if he had committed a murder but thought he had done it so cleverly that his guilt could not be proved?' And finally: 'I submit to you that the evidence which I and my learned friends will call before you, proves, and proves conclusively, that this old lady was murdered by Dr Adams.' The Attorney-General sat down. His speech had lasted nearly two hours. He had 'opened high' with a presumption that everything prescribed for Mrs Morrell was actually injected. How this was to be proved remained to be seen. But it was evident that Dr Adams's own words were to be significant – his assertion that he had, personally, administered nearly all the drugs.

A parade of Eastbourne chemists now stepped into the witness box – the men who had made up Mrs Morrell's prescriptions. At this point, Devlin put a question – asking how many grains a 5 cc syringe would hold. 'It is the first time we hear him speak,' wrote Sybille Bedford, 'and at once he reveals both grasp and charm.' The witness's reply was worthy of some drama – 12½ grains, he said. Given that the court had heard that Mrs Morrell's treatment relied overwhelmingly on two drugs – morphia and heroin – and that the maximum dose of morphia was ½ a grain, and of heroin ¼ a grain, the amount looked suitably and decisively lethal.

The trial was in need of some indisputable facts on the matter, so it was fortunate that the time had come for the testimony of the nurses who had attended Edith Morrell in her last illness, and who had observed Dr Adams at the closest of quarters.

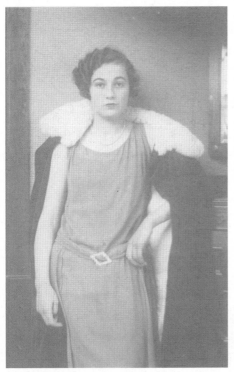

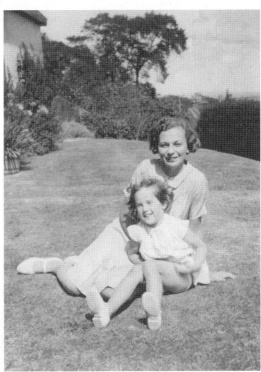

Bobbie: young, sultry and ready for love

Wishanger days. Bobbie with her daughter Patricia

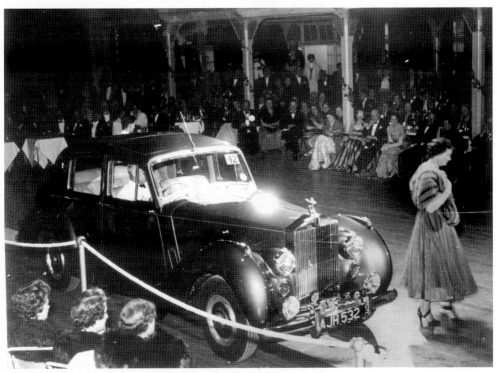

Bobbie, now a Hullett, in her mink and jewels. She is walking in front of the Rolls-Royce she left to Dr Adams. He sits among the spectators and takes photographs

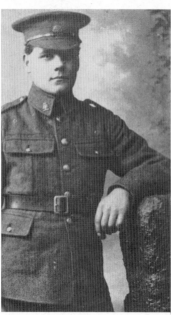

John Bodkin Adams as a young man.
He is in uniform, but did not fight

Dr Adams, now a family
doctor whose specialism
was the treatment of
wealthy widows

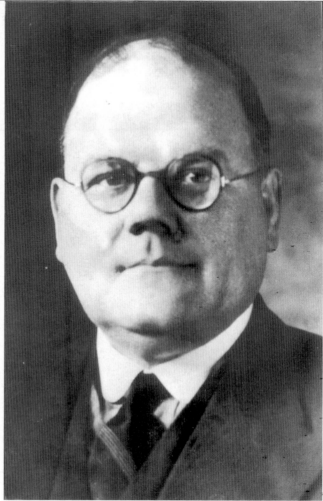

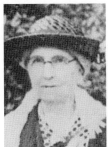

Julia Bradnum. Loves, Potters and
Onions wanted her house

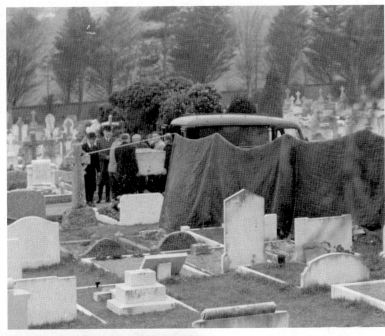

Ocklynge Cemetery.
The exhumation of the
body of Mrs Bradnum in
December 1956

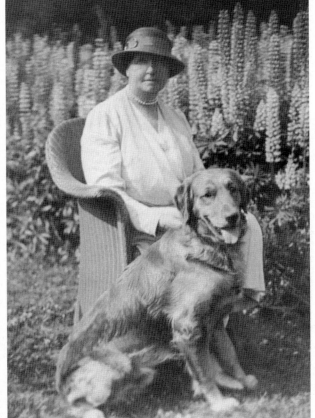

The redoubtable Edith
Morrell with prize blooms
and dog. Her bad moods
were treated with heroin
and morphine

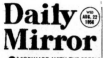

Daily Mirror

WED AUG. 22 1956

2D FORWARD WITH THE PEOPLE No. 16,390

SUEZ

● 17 NATIONS LAST NIGHT BACKED THE WEST'S PLAN FOR WORLD CONTROL OF THE SUEZ CANAL— See Back Page

RICH WIDOW DRAMA

Suicide verdict—CID to probe 12 other deaths

By HARRY LONGMUIR

DR. BODKIN ADAMS "I did my best."

DETECTIVE Superintendent Herbert Hannam, of Scotland Yard's murder squad, was called as a surprise witness yesterday at an inquest on a wealthy widow.

A crowded court at Eastbourne was silent as Superintendent Hannam was asked by the coroner, Dr. A. C. Sommerville: "Has the Chief Constable of Eastbourne asked Scotland Yard to help in investigating certain deaths in this neighbourhood?"

Superintendent Hannam replied: "Yes, sir."

Asked if he wished to apply for an adjournment of the inquest — on Mrs. Gertrude Joyce Hullett, 50 — he replied: "No."

The jury then returned a verdict that Mrs. Hullett committed suicide by an overdose of barbiturate drugs.

They had heard her doctor, Dr. John Bodkin Adams, say she was depressed. She had talked of suicide.

After the inquest Superintendent Hannam conferred with the Eastbourne police.

Tomorrow he will begin inquiries into the deaths of more than twelve elderly wealthy women.

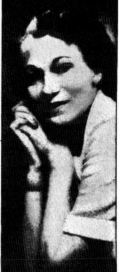

Mrs. GERTRUDE JOYCE HULLETT "Unhappy since the death of her second husband"

'SHE HAD IMPLICIT FAITH IN DOCTOR'

SUPERINTENDENT Hannam was in court throughout the five-hour inquest on Mrs. Hullett, who inherited £94,000 when her second husband died in March.

The coroner said that Mrs. Hullett complained of a headache on July 19 and went to bed at 10 p.m. at her home, Holywell Mount, Eastbourne.

Next morning she was found, apparently asleep, and later that day she was found unconscious. She stayed unconscious until she died on July 23.

A police scientist, Mr. Michael Stephen Moss, said he found 172 grains of barbiturate in Mrs. Hullett's body.

'Wise After Event'

Dr. F. E. Camps, pathologist, said 113 grains — or twenty tablets — would be a fatal dose. Most of it was taken after July 19.

Asked if he thought Mrs. Hullett might have been saved if barbiturate poisoning had been considered when she was taken ill, Dr. Camps replied:

"I think one must say — and naturally it's a case of being wise after the event — that specific treatment might have led to recovery."

Miss Evelyn Patricia Tomlinson, Mrs. Hullett's daughter by her first marriage, said her mother had been unhappy since the death of her second husband last March. She had said she did not want to live.

Mrs. Hullett had been taking sleeping tablets, which had been left for her by her physician, Dr. John Bodkin Adams.

A Lloyd's underwriter, Mr. Percy Robert Handscomb, said he was a great friend of Mrs. Hullett.

She was very depressed after the death of her second husband, but his mental health suffered.

Mrs. Hullett had implicit faith in Dr. Adams and he (Mr. Handscomb) did not think it necessary to advise her to ask for a second medical opinion.

The coroner: Here we have a fit woman, well off, with a daughter to look after. She is having tablets every night and is obviously under the influence of tablets part of the day and you still say you did not think it necessary to have another opinion to try and get her better?

Mr. Handscomb: I am afraid it never entered my head.

Have you ever heard her say she would take her own life? — Not in so many words.

Mr. Handscomb said he was an executor of Mrs. Hullett's will, which was drawn up on July 19.

Continued on Back Page

The press reports on the Bobbie Hullett inquest hinted that the real story involved any number of suspicious deaths. Some papers reported a dozen, others 300

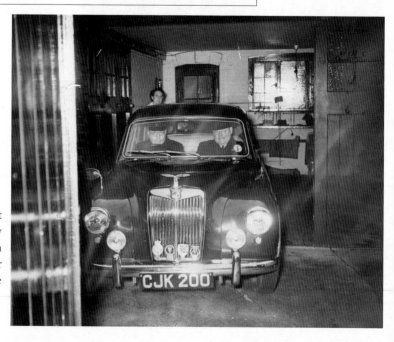

Dr Adams rides out in his customary Rolls-Royce, driven by his chauffeur James White

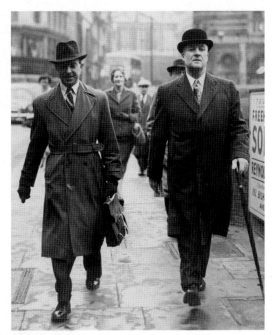

'The Count': Herbert Hannam of Scotland Yard, a man with a wardrobe full of elegant suits and smart bowler hats. His loyal sidekick Charlie Hewett is at his side

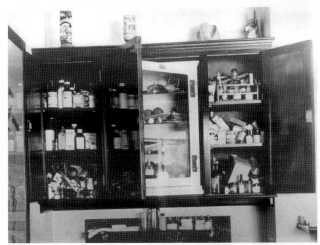

The messy medicine cabinet of Dr Adams. It contained assorted drugs as well as packets of sugar, melted chocolate, butter and margarine

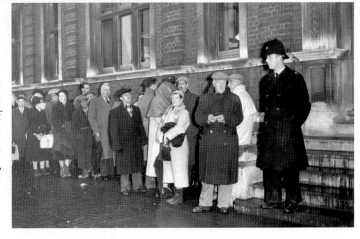

Spectators brave Eastbourne's 'cold raw wind' in the hope of seeing Dr Adams at the preliminary hearings of a murder charge, 14 January 1957

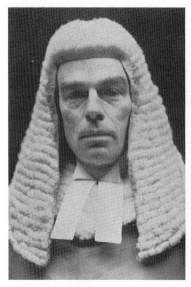

The judge, Patrick Devlin. His was the coolest head at the trial of Dr Adams; his vision was clear, his analysis sharp

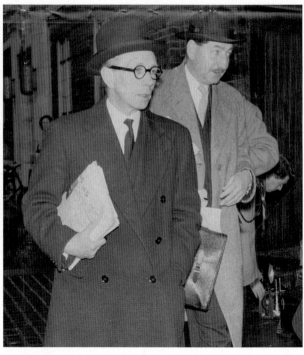

Geoffrey Lawrence QC, who performed brilliantly at Dr Adams's trial for murder. His style was quiet and forensic, and utterly mesmerising

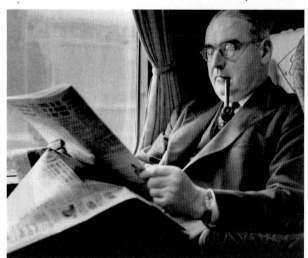

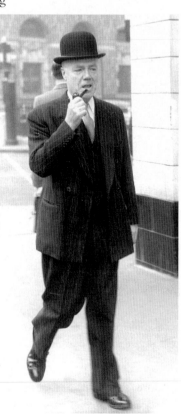

Sir Reginald Manningham-Buller in 1957, when he was Attorney-General. In cross-examination, Reggie was 'all thunder and disapproval'

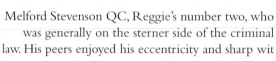

Melford Stevenson QC, Reggie's number two, who was generally on the sterner side of the criminal law. His peers enjoyed his eccentricity and sharp wit

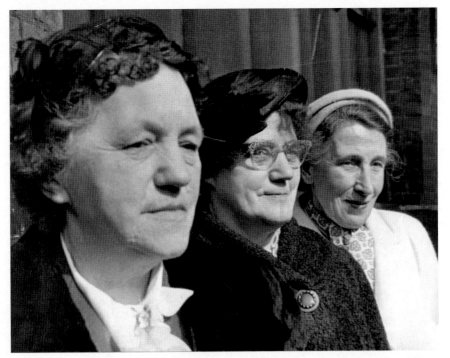

The infamous nurses: Caroline Randall, Helen Stronach and Annie Mason-Ellis. Strong characters but shambolic witnesses

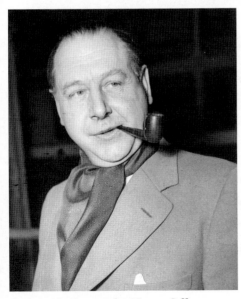

Dr Francis Camps, the Home Office pathologist whose name was synonymous with murder. He identified 163 suspicious cases in the police files on Dr Adams

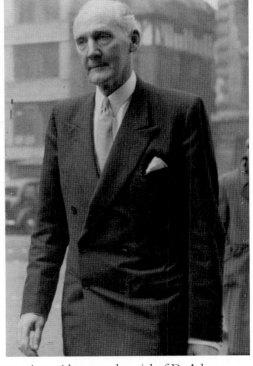

The urbane Dr Arthur Douthwaite on his way to give evidence at the trial of Dr Adams. His style was lofty and commanding, but his theories were sometimes implausible

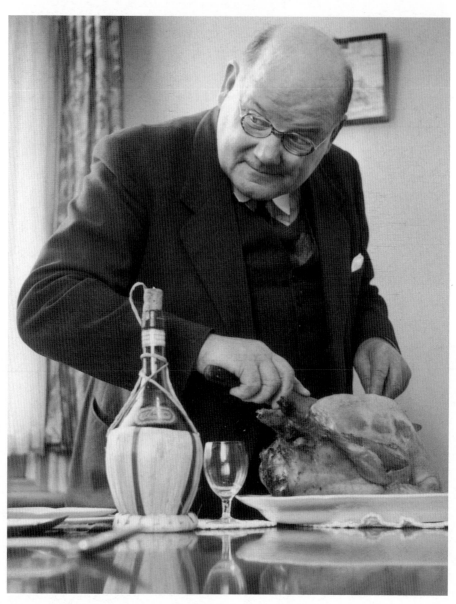

Dr John Bodkin Adams in his element – carving a fat chicken

12

Nurses

THE FOUR NURSES at the trial of Dr Adams were to achieve celebrity. Two of them, Nurses Randall and Stronach, had the appearance of tough old boots, middle-aged ladies decked out in shapeless woolly coats, sensible shoes, and ugly little hats. The 1950s suited rich women like Bobbie Hullett, with her jewels and furs, her minxy make-up and come-hither eyes. But for poorer working women over 50, like these two, the decade was unkind. Their hair was permed into a helmet of unforgiving grey curls, their faces were weather-beaten, complexions pallid, and their mouths pinched. They seemed like women whose lives were taken up with manual tasks, the scrubbing of clothes on wash day, the forcing of bed sheets through the mangle, the making up of the fire at dawn, and the clearing out of the grate. And they were spinsters, at a time when 'spinster' was a term of rejection, meaning unsexual and unappealing. Bobbie Hullett looked like she might be taken up any minute by Hollywood, but these nurses, thanks to their rougher lives, resembled an Ealing comedy battleaxe.

The third nurse, Sister Mason-Ellis, was of a similar age and background, but had something a little willowy and delicate about her. She was better dressed than the other two, and finer boned. And she wore lipstick. It is evident from the statements of Nurses Stronach and Randall that they thought Sister Mason-Ellis gave herself airs – they referred to her several times as 'calling herself Mason-Ellis' because, on marrying, she had chosen a double-barrelled surname.

The fourth nurse was younger and different. Sister Brenda Bartlett was, in Patrick Devlin's words, 'girlish and zestful'. She was now married and was Mrs Hughes, but throughout the trial was known to everyone by her 'stage name'. Photographs show her to be pretty, a little of the coquette about her. And, unlike the older women, she is clever with make-up.

It was one of the battleaxes, Nurse Randall, who was scheduled to appear first. But the Crown had miscalculated its timings, so it was the other battleaxe, Nurse Stronach, who appeared in the witness box.

'Stocky, a face of blurred features except for a narrow mouth and strong jaw,' wrote Sybille Bedford of 62-year-old Helen Stronach. For the Crown, it was Melford Stevenson who examined her, asking about the injections that she had, on Dr Adams's instructions, given each night, during her period of duty at the end of October 1950. The content, she said, was ¼ a grain of morphia. Dr Adams would come each night and give another injection.

'Did you see Dr Adams prepare the syringe ever?' asked Melford Stevenson.

'Yes. But I could not tell you what it was.'

'Do you know what the injections which Dr Adams gave her were?'

'No, sir. I have no idea.'

At this point, before the examination had established any sort of rhythm or identity, the day's proceedings drew to a close. The second day of the trial began with Nurse Stronach back in the witness box, still on the subject of Dr Adams's nightly visits, and the injections he gave Mrs Morrell.

'Where did he get the injections from?' asked Stevenson.

'From his bag.'

'How many injections did you see him give on each night? One or more than one?'

'One.'

This, said Nurse Stronach, took place after she had given Mrs Morrell the ¼ grain of morphia injection, at about eleven o'clock at night.

'When the doctor came on these visits late at night, was Mrs Morrell awake or asleep, or how was she?'

'Well, she would be very dopey. She would be half asleep . . . because I had already given her an injection.'

Nurse Stronach said that on her very last day with Mrs Morrell, 2 November 1950, 'she was in an almost semi-conscious condition and rambling'.

'Did you ever see any signs that she was suffering pain?' asked Stevenson.

'I cannot say I saw any real signs, although she did tell me that she had pain, but I considered it to be neurotic.'

As Melford Stevenson drew to the end of his examination, Patrick Devlin spoke. He wished to know what happened to Mrs Morrell's drugs once they had been delivered to Marden Ash by the chemist, 'where they were put, whether they were kept under lock and key and who had access to them'. Melford Stevenson put the question to Nurse Stronach.

'They were kept in a drawer, to the best of my knowledge,' she answered.

'Do you know whether it was locked or not?'

'I think so.'

Early in the second day, Geoffrey Lawrence rose for the cross-examination. He established that Nurse Stronach was a busy woman, who had been nursing patients constantly during the past six or seven years. He ascertained that, when she arrived at Marden Ash, Nurse Stronach had been aware of Mrs Morrell's stroke, of her paralysis down the left side, and knew that she was a 'very old lady' of 81.

'She had great variations in her condition, did she not?' asked Lawrence.

'She had.'

'Sometimes up and sometimes down?'

'That applies to every patient.'

'But all the time, whether there were these ups and downs, all the time she was going downhill, was she not?'

'Steadily.'

'Generally deteriorating?'

'Oh yes.'

'And at the end she was, as you have said, very very weak?'

'Extremely weak.'

'And frail?'

'Yes.'

'And from time to time she had attacks of great irritability, did she not?' asked Lawrence.

'Due to her condition,' answered Nurse Stronach.

'When you say "due to her condition" you mean due to the injury to the arteries of the brain?'

'Not only that.'

'. . . What else?'

'I should say that it was due a great deal to the amount of drugs she was having.'

'Yes, I thought you were going to say that . . .'

Geoffrey Lawrence changed his line, and referred back to the injections of ¼ of a grain of morphia that Nurse Stronach had given the patient. But, he established, no other drugs:

'No heroin?'

'No.'

'No omnopon?'

'No, not with me.'

'And then Dr Adams came and gave a further injection?'

'That is so.'

'And that is what you still say?' asked Lawrence.

'I do.'

'There is now a definite sense that counsel is building something,' wrote Sybille Bedford, recognising that the question 'and

that is what you *still* say?', delivered in Geoffrey Lawrence's controlled, understated manner, contained in it the promise of a
revelation of some sort. 'He goes on,' wrote Bedford, 'treading
very lightly':

'I am reminded of something that Sister Mason-Ellis said. I just
want to ask you about it. When she gave her evidence at
Eastbourne: "I knew what I was injecting but I cannot accurately
remember now, but whatever I gave was booked in a book and
passed on to the next nurse"?'

'Yes, that was quite correct.'

'That is quite correct?'

'We wrote down every injection we gave . . . We kept a
report of every injection we gave, which is a usual thing when
you are nursing, to keep a report of the injections you give.'

'It is a usual thing?'

'Yes, it is the proper thing to do.'

'Well, all experienced and trained nurses do it, do they not?'

'Yes, they do.'

'And that is what you did?'

'Yes, indeed we did.'

'So far as you know, all of you?'

'Yes.'

'. . . And whatever you wrote in that book would be accurate,
would it not?'

Lawrence asked this gravely, with weight on every word. And
if Nurse Stronach felt that she was being led into a trap she did
not show it. Instead, she went with the flow – accepting the flat-
tering implications of Lawrence's line – that she was, indeed, a
highly professional nurse who would, because of her profession-
alism, always keep notes in a book.

'Oh yes,' she replied.

'Accurate, because it was done right at that very moment?'

'Yes.'

Everything of any significance would go into such a book, she confirmed, not only injections, but medicines and 'that sort of thing'.

'And doctors' visits?'

'Well, we would just put down that the doctor visited and the time, usually.'

'And, as distinct from memory, six years later, of course these reports would be absolutely accurate, would they not? I mean yours would, at any rate?'

'Oh yes, they would be accurate for each one of us.'

'So that if only we had got those reports now we could see the truth of exactly what happened night by night and day by day that you were there, could we not?'

'Yes, but you have our word for it.'

Geoffrey Lawrence now delivered his bombshell. He took into his hand an ordinary-looking exercise book with an orange cover and handed it to Nurse Stronach. 'I want you to look at that book please,' he said. 'Would you look at the day report for the 4 June 1950?'

Patrick Devlin intervened. 'Is this one of the Exhibits, Mr Lawrence?'

Geoffrey Lawrence replied that it would be an exhibit, in due course – and that it was one of the books in which the nurses made their day and night reports about Mrs Morrell. There was immediate discombobulation in the Crown team, which until this moment had no idea that the defence had in its possession any of the nurses' notebooks relating to Mrs Morrell. The members of the press at once realised that the existence of the notebooks was explosive. They might contain the proof needed to convict the doctor. But the fact that they had been produced by the defence suggested the opposite – that they would throw the Crown's case completely off course. The journalists rushed for the door to telephone their editors. 'Mr Lawrence hangs fire,' wrote Sybille Bedford, 'and Nurse Stronach is reading.'

'There is no doubt about it, is there, Miss Stronach,' continued Geoffrey Lawrence in his composed, superior tone, 'that is the very book of daily and nightly records kept by nurses when you started your first spell of duty in June 1950?'

'Yes, that is so.'

'. . . Of course one cannot remember things after six years, I am not suggesting you can. In view of what you said, if we look at this book we can see what happened as recorded by you . . .'

As he spoke, Nurse Stronach looked intensely at the book. It seemed she was aching to see whether the comments inside bore any resemblance to the accounts she had given police in her statements. But Geoffrey Lawrence did not allow her to gather her thoughts.

'Are you listening to me or are you reading that book?' he asked.

'I am listening.'

'Please listen to me.'

He ascertained that the book was authentic. Nurse Stronach recognised it, and the handwriting inside. He presented two further books. These too were genuine. Geoffrey Lawrence addressed Patrick Devlin:

'My Lord, at this stage I desire to say we have the whole of the nursing reports on this case from June 1949, 21 June 1949, until 13 November 1950 when Mrs Morrell died. There are eight of these books.'

Thus, he indicated, he had a day-by-day, hour-by-hour record of the activities of Dr Adams, the very activities that the Crown alleged were murderous. And with great daring, he was presenting the record as evidence for the defence. 'Normally while the prosecution's proof is being unfolded the defence tactic is to harry it by sniping,' wrote Patrick Devlin. 'Sometimes a raid may be mounted into prosecution territory so as to reduce the opposing forces to the point where the reasonable doubt can enter. But here was the defence marching into the heartland of the prosecution and taking command of it.' Sybille Bedford put it succinctly: 'Mr Lawrence must get full marks for audacity.'

Lawrence proceeded to put Nurse Stronach through a sort of torture:

'Miss Stronach, I want your help now, if I may have it, on your own record of what happened when you were nursing Mrs Morrell. In fact, we all want your help. So will you please be good enough to help us?'

'Certainly.'

'Will you look now at the first entry [in the notebook] . . . for 4 June. Have you found it?'

'Yes.'

'Do not try to read them in advance.'

'I was not reading them in advance. I was finding the page.'

Nurse Stronach agreed that when she came on duty for the first time at Marden Ash, at 9 p.m. on 4 June 1950, it was recorded that an injection had already been given to Mrs Morrell. An injection of a ¼ grain of morphia with ⅓ of a grain of heroin. Nurse Stronach, according to the book, had given Mrs Morrell a sedormid sleeping tablet, some milk and brandy and 'one special tablet (yellow)'. Thereafter Edith Morrell had 'quite a good night'.

'You did not give any injection, nor did the doctor visit. That is right, is it not?'

On Nurse Stronach's second day at Marden Ash, 5 June 1950, she had written in the book that she had once more given Mrs Morrell a sedormid tablet and a milk and brandy at bedtime: '6.15 a.m. patient woke up in a temper, said she had rung her bell and I had not answered it. Also that I had left her bed all untidy and that I was a nasty common woman.' In the morning, she recorded another milk and brandy and at 7.40 a.m: '1 yellow tablet, given with water. Depressed this morning and weeping. Taken breakfast. Seems brighter.' The yellow tablet, suggested Lawrence, was dexadrine (an amphetamine, given to produce wakefulness). It was strange that Mrs Morrell had been given dexadrine before bed, but Geoffrey Lawrence was not concerned about that:

'There is no indication there, for all the detail that you give, of any injection of morphia or that the doctor visited, is there?'

'No.'

'You see, the injection, as you would have seen it, is given by the day nurse at 8.40 p.m., is it not, and not by you? That is right, is it not?'

'Yes.'

And so it went on, Geoffrey Lawrence taking Nurse Stronach through her daily routine, as recorded in the notebook, with much mention of harmless milk and brandies, single sedormid tablets, yellow tablets and aspirin, but nothing sinister – no doping with morphia. Looking at 8 June 1950, Lawrence said:

'Again, no record of an injection and again no record of a doctor's visit, is there?'

'No,' replied Nurse Stronach. 'But it does not say that he did not call though.'

'It does not say that he did not call?'

'It is no proof that he did not call that night because I did not put it down here.'

'You realise this is a serious case, don't you?'

'Yes, indeed I do.'

'You realise that before you saw this book you told me that everything of importance, including the doctor's visit if there was one, would have been put down by you, as a trained nurse, in your contemporary record made at the time, didn't you?'

'Yes.'

Having put Nurse Stronach firmly back on his straight and narrow path, and fearful of leaving it, Geoffrey Lawrence continued with his litany of Mrs Morrell's treatments, the most common being brandy – warm water and brandy in the morning, milk and brandy in the evening, brandy and soda at bedtime, and more milk and brandy during the night. And so it went on until he reached the last date of Nurse Stronach's night duty – 25 June 1950. The regime during the summer of 1950, as recorded in the notebooks, was sharply at odds with the expected drugging scenario, the anticipated rivers of morphine and torrents of heroin. But Lawrence was still to address the key months of October and November 1950 when, according to the prescriptions, the drugging increased dramatically.

First, though, he wished to rub salt in the wounds of Nurse Stronach:

'It is quite clear, isn't it, that in that first spell of night duty, when you were there from nine o'clock onwards, you never recorded yourself as having given any injection at all of any kind?'

'No.'

'And you never recorded a visit of the doctor in the evening when you were on duty, did you?'

'No, I did not record it.'

Her tone suggested room for manoeuvre, and Geoffrey Lawrence pounced:

'You are not saying this, are you, that as a trained nurse of experience, recording every dram of brandy, for instance, that you would not have recorded a visit from the doctor and an injection by him if in fact it had occurred?'

'I cannot answer that quite.'

'Do not mutter please. We cannot hear what you are saying. The question I put was clear. If you do not understand it you will tell me and I will try again.'

'Well, we usually report it.'

'As such a trained nurse, you would not have omitted to record the visit by the doctor and an injection given by him if in fact it had taken place while you were on duty, would you?'

'No, I do not think I would have done.'

Lawrence judged this answer good enough, and moved on.

He now guided Nurse Stronach to the third of the notebooks –
the records for her period of day duty at Marden Ash, which
began on 12 October 1950.

'Now, here you are not on night duty but on day duty and this
is only a month before Mrs Morrell died, is it not? . . . Is it not?'

'Yes.'

'Now just take your eyes off that book and please do not go
on turning the pages in advance. When you went back in
October there was a very big difference in Mrs Morrell's
condition, was there not?'

'Yes.'

'She had deteriorated very much, had she not?'

'Oh yes.'

He drew her attention to the first injection she gave to Mrs
Morrell, according to the notebooks. It was given on 12 October
1950.

'Is this in your writing: omnopon ⅔ rd given at 4.30 p.m.?'

'That means that you gave that injection, does it not?'

'It does.'

'And it is an injection of omnopon?'

'Yes.'

'Now, Miss Stronach, do not think that I am blaming you in
any way or criticising you for this . . . But you do remember telling me earlier this morning, before you saw the contemporary
records, that you had never given Mrs Morrell any injection
except morphia?'

'Well, I believed that to be true.' (She did not point out that
omnopon contained morphine.)'

'Well, this entry shows that your memory was playing you a
trick, does it not?'

'Apparently so.'

'Well, it is obviously so, is it not?'

'Yes.'

'Obviously so. Miss Stronach, may I ask you to face this

squarely. Obviously your memory played you a trick, did it not, when you said you had never injected anything but morphia?'

'Yes. Of course, you have got to remember it is a long time ago for us to remember these things.'

Geoffrey Lawrence was delighted. 'That is exactly what I was suggesting to you,' he said, 'that it was a long time ago, and that mistakes of memory can be made.' He then pointed out that in the early evening of 12 October, Dr Adams had come to Marden Ash, and Nurse Stronach had recorded the visit.

'"7.30 p.m. Visited by Dr Adams. Hypodermic injection morphia gr ¼, heroin gr ⅓, omnopon gr ⅓." Is it there, in your writing?'

'It is.'

'You have there recorded the exact nature and the exact quantities of the injection which was given to Mrs Morrell when the doctor visited, have you not?'

'Yes I have.'

'So that it is quite clear that on that occasion at any rate, you knew what the injection was, is it not?'

'Yes, it certainly is.'

Earlier, she had said she did *not* know the contents of Dr Adams's injections. The spectacle of Geoffrey Lawrence skewering Nurse Stronach, and pinning down the notion that the notebooks, and not distant memories, were the core of the case, was mesmerising. The press thought it so, as did commentators like Sybille Bedford, and the judge, Patrick Devlin – who underlined this passage in red pencil in his copy of the transcript of the day's events. On 14 October, according to the notebooks, Nurse Stronach was once more on night duty – and not day duty, as she had said in her statement. Once again, she recorded that Dr Adams visited – this time at 10.20 p.m., and gave Mrs Morrell an injection. And, once again, she detailed the precise contents of that injection – morphia ¼ grain, heroin ⅓ and omnopon ⅓ – exactly the same as before.

'Let us see how the night goes on,' said Lawrence. '"Various drinks given and jelly. Position changed. 6.45 a.m. warm milk, soda water and brandy . . . Mrs Morrell has been very restless even when asleep. Brain is very muddled, does not know where she is. During sleep breathing was Cheyne Stokes." That means periods of heavy breathing alternating with quiet, shallow breathing, doesn't it?'

'Yes.'

'Typical with elderly people with strokes in the last stages of senile deterioration?'

'Yes.'

'You have seen it before I expect?'

'Many times.'

According to the notebook, the next night Mrs Morrell was restless again, and Nurse Stronach gave her an injection to calm her down – morphia ¼ grain, heroin ⅓ grain and omnopon ⅔. The following morning she was 'more herself', and had some toast, marmalade and tea. And so it continued. On 21 October, she got up in the night and started stripping the bed which, Nurse Stronach confirmed, was 'the sort of thing which happens to those senile patients towards the end'. 'She was obviously going very rapidly downhill at this stage?' suggested Lawrence. 'Yes,' replied Nurse Stronach, 'she was deteriorating very much.' On 25 October, she became worse still, refusing milk or tea, and pushing away a glass when it was offered – 'a sign of the final stages of this type of case'. She received no injection, and had no visit from the doctor.

On 28 October Nurse Stronach returned to day duty. That day, Dr Adams did visit and give an injection – but this was in the morning, not the evening. Mrs Morrell had some appetite back: 'For lunch took a little chicken broth, refused pudding. During afternoon ate a whole pear and had jelly and cream. For supper, mushroom soup and croutons and asked for another jelly.' That evening, Nurse Stronach recorded in the book:

'To have big hypo injection each night just after 9 p.m.'
'Was that recorded as the result of some instruction you had
from the doctor?' asked Geoffrey Lawrence, dropping Reggie
Manningham-Buller and Melford Stevenson their first crumb of
hope since the notebooks had been produced. 'Yes, it must be,'
answered Nurse Stronach. However, as she was no longer on
night duty it was Nurse Randall, not Nurse Stronach, who was
responsible for administering the injection and, said Lawrence,
'we must find out from Nurse Randall whether that was done or
not'.

With Nurse Stronach's help, Lawrence made the case that
from 30 October 1950 onwards Mrs Morrell's health deteriorated
into 'general deterioration and break-up'. The instructions from
Dr Adams were now for injections of heroin, without morphia
or omnopon. Finally, he came to her last day of duty, 2
November 1950 – two weeks before Mrs Morrell died, when
according to Nurse Stronach, her patient had been dopey and
semi-conscious:

'Do you observe that . . . this semi-conscious woman ate for
lunch that day a small quantity of partridge, a small quantity of
celery, a small quantity of pudding and a small quantity of brandy
and soda? Do you see that?'

'Yes.'

'You have written it? You have recorded the lunch of the
partridge and celery and the pudding?'

'Yes.'

'Consumed by this semi-conscious woman?'

'Yes.'

'Miss Stronach, let us face this: it is another complete trick of
your memory to say that on the last day, when you left, Mrs
Morrell was either semi-conscious or rambling, isn't it, now you
see what you wrote at the time?' (A pause.) 'Isn't it? What?'

'I have nothing to say.'

'You have nothing to say?'

'No.'

The cross-examination was drawing to its close with Nurse Stronach wholly defeated by Lawrence's skill in turning her words into a trap. 'It has been beautifully done,' wrote Sybille Bedford, 'the sequence and control of details, the moods of tone.' At the same time, she observed an American journalist in the court write on his pad: 'The nurse being all mixed up doesn't mean the old lady didn't get plenty of dope from whoever it was.' He had a point. Geoffrey Lawrence had demonstrated that, after six years, the nurse's memory was faulty in the extreme – but the notebooks *did* show that Mrs Morrell was being injected with powerful drugs – with morphia and heroin, just not in the exact mixes and measures that Nurse Stronach had remembered, or at the exact times, or by the particular people she had identified.

The court's attention now turned to the prosecution team, to see what Reggie Manningham-Buller and Melford Stevenson could make of the revelation of the notebooks. It seemed entirely possible that a brilliant mind equal to Mr Lawrence's might turn the books around, might make them seem to support the Crown's case, but it was also far from obvious that the prosecution possessed such a brilliant mind. Over a frantic break for lunch, Reggie and Stevenson pored over the books, re-evaluating their approach, deciding on a new way forward. Afterwards, it was the Attorney-General who rose to re-examine Nurse Stronach.

Reggie kept his examination brief, ignoring the discrepancies and uncertainties raised by Lawrence and, instead, establishing that Dr Adams had given Mrs Morrell many mysterious 'special injections', and reaffirming that, in general, she was not in any pain. He did not attempt to use the notebooks in a forensic way, and seemed to be playing for time. At the end of the cross-examination, Patrick Devlin asked Nurse Stronach about the drugs that were kept in the house. These, she answered, were kept in a cupboard which was always locked. If Dr Adams wished to obtain drugs from the cupboard, he would have to ask a nurse for the key. Often, though, the drugs he administered came from his bag. Devlin told Nurse Stronach that, on no account, was she to discuss the case with anyone – and that instruction included the other nurses who were about to give evidence.

The second day of the trial ended with the entrance of Nurse Annie Mason-Ellis – the lipstick wearer who gave herself airs. She was 'a thin, rather pale, tallish, fairish woman, dressed in beige, apparently not strong', and quite unlike Nurse Stronach who had seemed edgy and affronted by her experience. In the witness box, Sister Mason-Ellis was timid, scared even. Reggie examined her first. When he produced the nurses' notebooks, she immediately took the line that, as a record, they were all but infallible. From Reggie's point of view, some of her answers were exasperating:

'Did you see Dr Adams at that time?' he asked.

'Only if it was mentioned in the book.'

'Did you yourself ever see Dr Adams give an injection to Mrs Morrell?'

'I cannot answer that.'

'Why not?'

'It is too long ago.'

'What was her condition throughout 12 November when you saw her?'

'I am sorry, I can't remember these things. It is much too long ago . . .'

'Was she conscious on 10 November?'

'Please don't ask me these questions. I can't tell you.'

She seemed distressed, and as a prosecution witness she was close to useless. But Sister Mason-Ellis confirmed that, like Nurse Stronach, she had given the injections of a mixture of morphia, heroin and omnopon that were recorded in the books.

And she had, on occasion, witnessed Dr Adams giving injections, though she could not say where he took the drugs from. On where the drugs were kept in Marden Ash, she contradicted Nurse Stronach – making no mention of a locked cupboard, but insisting they were kept on a tray in the dining room.

Geoffrey Lawrence now had his chance with Sister Mason-Ellis. He established that Mrs Morrell's stroke had left her with 'signs of cerebral brain irritation' which manifested itself in 'quite unrational outbursts of temper, for no apparent reason' (a condition doctors would now call 'post-stroke lability of mood').

'You used to refer to that among yourselves as brainstorms, didn't you?'

'Yes, we did.'

'You could see as the weeks and months went on a steady deterioration in her condition, couldn't you?'

'Yes, that would be understood.'

'And in the latter months I suppose there was no question of her being able to get out of bed and being able to walk about even with assistance?'

'Not when she was having drugs to the extent she was.'

Geoffrey Lawrence now drove home that Mrs Morrell's cerebral irritation was the reason for her regular, routine sedation, rather than the result of it. Sister Mason-Ellis agreed. He had barely got into his stride, however, when Patrick Devlin interrupted to say that it was late, and the court would adjourn. All day, Dr Adams had sat calmly watching the testimonies, his arms folded across his chest, only occasionally moving to pick up a pen and make some notes. At the end of the proceedings, he tucked beneath his arm two copies of the nurses' notebooks, one blue, the other red, and hurried down the steps of the dock.

13

Inquisition

THE NEWSPAPER HEADLINES were suitably dramatic: 'QC AND NURSE IN DRAMA OF BEDSIDE NOTEBOOKS' in the *Daily Mirror*, which also blasted 'PARTRIDGE LUNCH FOR MRS MORRELL' across a double-page spread, and reported that, according to the notebooks, Mrs Morrell had been 'hysterical, wanting to die and weeping'. The *Daily Express* continued to be more restrained and was subtly on Dr Adams's side with the headline 'I COULD NOT TRUTHFULLY ANSWER QUESTIONS ABOUT MRS MORRELL SAYS NURSE No. 2', alongside a photograph of Geoffrey Lawrence with the comment 'he is astute in cross-examination and a suave advocate'.

Day three of the trial began with the suave advocate making a merciless attack on Sister Mason-Ellis. He turned to her:

'After you had left the witness box yesterday afternoon, you were talking to Nurse Stronach and Nurse Randall, weren't you?'

'That is quite right, sir. Yes.'

'And is this right; that the three of you travelled together last night from Victoria to Eastbourne on the 6.45 train from Victoria?'

'Yes, we did.'

'All three of you in the same carriage?'

'Yes.'

'Reading the reports together of this case. Is that right?'

'Yes, I think that is so.'

'And discussing it together?'

'Discussing what was in the newspapers, yes.'

'Is it right that all three of you travelled back to London this morning from Eastbourne to Victoria on the 8.04 train from Eastbourne?'

'Yes, it is, sir.'

Again, the nurses had all been in the same compartment of the train, with the newspapers in front of them. Again they had been discussing the case.

Everyone, including the judge, was wondering how on earth Geoffrey Lawrence knew. Patrick Devlin said he heard later that a civil servant, or possibly a city stockbroker, had happened to be travelling in the same railway carriage as the three nurses when they had returned to Eastbourne from London the night before. He had heard them discuss the case quite freely, and was so shocked at their brazen breaking of the rules that when he saw them boarding the train for London the following morning, he once again sat by them and listened to their conversation. Afterwards he had telephoned the Old Bailey and had demanded to be put through to the lawyers defending Dr Adams. By 10.30, when the court sat, 'Mr Lawrence was fully armed.' The barrister's tone to Sister Mason-Ellis was utterly scathing:

'At one point were you discussing the cupboard or cabinet in which the drugs were kept in the dining room at Mrs Morrell's house?'

'That was discussed, I think . . .'

'Did one or other of you . . . say this about that drug cabinet . . . "Don't you say that or you will get me into trouble"?'

'No, I cannot answer that one.'

'You cannot answer it?'

'No. No.'

'Perhaps I did not make my question clear to you. Let me try again . . . did one of you say something to this effect, either these words or something like it – now listen – "Don't you say that or you will get me into trouble"?'

'Yes, I think one of them did say that, but which one I am afraid I cannot tell you.'

'Was it you?'

'Oh no . . .'

'Then it was either Nurse Stronach, who has already given evidence, or it was Nurse Randall, who has not yet given evidence. That is right, is it? . . . Which one of those two was it?'

Sister Mason-Ellis was distressed. She looked anxiously about the court, and then turned to the judge: 'Must I answer that, sir?' He told her that she must.

'Then it was Miss Randall.'

And what was it that Sister Mason-Ellis was asked not to say? After a long pause, the nurse tried out decorum as a method of evasion:

'Really I cannot remember, because I was not terribly interested, if I may say so.'

Geoffrey Lawrence now brought down the full force of his scorn and directed it not just at the behaviour of Sister Mason-Ellis in particular or the misdemeanours of the nurses in general, but at the weakest point in the prosecution's case:

'I am not asking you to remember something which happened six years ago, like the Attorney-General did yesterday. I am asking you to remember something which happened in the train this morning! What was she talking about when she said "Don't you say that or you'll get me into trouble"?'

'About the drugs.'

'About the drugs. And what was it that you were not to say?'

'There has been a little confusion about it, I think, sir. You see the drugs were kept in a drawer, not in a cupboard, and there was no key attached to them.'

Sister Mason-Ellis now revealed that the nurses had discussed the newspaper reports of Nurse Stronach's evidence, in which she had said that the drugs were kept in a locked cupboard, and had agreed that, in fact, there had been no cupboard and therefore no lock and no key. It was all untrue.

In a sense, the fact that the drugs were easily accessible favoured the prosecution. They instantly became a source for all those 'special injections' that Dr Adams had given Mrs Morrell. But, in practice, that was not the effect of the incident. Instead it made the nurses seem like shambolic second-rate witnesses, and undermined any evidence they might give that was at variance with the notebooks.

Geoffrey Lawrence now returned to his expedition through the notebooks, dragging a wounded Sister Mason-Ellis through the minutiae of the daily reports. Her spirit was broken:

'Outside the contents of these books and your entries in them you would not pledge your recollection to anything, would you?'

'No.'

'And you do not want to?'

'No, I don't, because I couldn't speak truthfully.'

So Lawrence trudged onwards, with more talk of Mrs Morrell's brandy and milk, her jellies and baked apples, her injections of morphia and heroin. He referred to her moods and outbursts – pausing for effect over a note that she 'wished she was dead and that she knew a doctor who would put her to sleep forever'. She wished a doctor would 'put her to sleep', repeated Lawrence, and yet she was still carrying on, day after day, in the apparent absence of such a doctor. He came back, repeatedly, to the idea that Mrs Morrell was 'going downhill', entirely from natural causes, from August until her death in November 1950. He noted that, on 24 September, Mrs Morrell's breathing had been very fast.

'When people are under the influence of morphia and heroin their breathing tends to get slow, does not it?'

'Yes.'

'This was just the opposite?'

'Yes.'

'And quite typical of the closing stages of a cerebral thrombosis case with poor circulation, and so forth?'

'Yes.'

When he came to Mrs Morrell's final day, Geoffrey Lawrence observed that according to 'the fountain of truth' – the notebooks – she had taken her last ever glass of milk and brandy, and so could not have been in a coma as the prosecution had stated. Sister Mason-Ellis agreed:

'Not according to my report, which was correct at the time of writing, and her condition was such at the time of writing.'

'More than once you have agreed with me that these reports are the place where truth is to be found?'

'Yes.'

'You don't want to go back on that now, do you?'

'Not at all.'

'As a trained and experienced nurse you would not enter anything in these reports which was not accurate, would you?'

'Certainly not . . .'

'When at 5.30 p.m. you write the word "awake" on the last afternoon before Mrs Morrell died, it means she was in fact awake, doesn't it?'

'She must have been.'

'And, therefore, could not possibly have been in a coma?'

'No, because it is the opposite condition.'

The battering of Sister Mason-Ellis had lasted four hours. Now the Attorney-General rose to re-examine her – a process that would take only twenty minutes. He started by emphasising that Mrs Morrell had never suffered any serious pain. Mirroring the style of Lawrence, he established that Sister Mason-Ellis would 'most certainly' have recorded any pain in the notebooks, had it occurred. 'And it was not there, was it? No pain at all.' Then he moved to the morphia and heroin injections. Sister Mason-Ellis confirmed that, in her experience, it was most unusual to give morphia and heroin routinely, day after day, to any patient. She could not remember any other doctor ever instructing her to do so. She stuck to her earlier statement that Dr Adams often gave Mrs Morrell injections with drugs from his bag. These final observations felt significant, but fell far short of indicating murder – and that was the state of things when her evidence came to an end. That night she made sure she travelled alone back to Eastbourne, taking the No. 11 bus from the Old Bailey to Victoria, and then finding an empty compartment on the 4.45 train – at least, empty of anyone other than the photographer whose picture of her gazing sadly at her newspaper filled half a page of the *Express* the following day.

It was now the turn of Nurse Randall to face the court. Of the four nurses, she was the most important witness since, on Dr Adams's instructions, she had administered the final injections to Mrs Morrell, the injections that had come in the large 5 cc syringes. She was a strong-looking woman, who entered the witness box like a boxer, buzzing with 'compressed energy'. She looked like she might be a feisty performer.

First the Attorney-General examined her. On 6 November 1950, the week before Mrs Morrell's death, Nurse Randall had recorded three heroin injections during the day – of ½ a grain each – well above the supposed maximum daily dose. The jerky spasms started, and the injections of morphia and heroin were intensified. The notebooks showed that on the night of 11 November there were several injections, and Dr Adams visited at 10.45 and gave 'a hypodermic injection of morphia ½ a grain and heroin ½ a grain', a dose that was repeated at 2.10, this time given by a nurse. At 3 a.m. that night Mrs Morrell was 'more wakeful and jerky' and a full grain of heroin was given.

Reggie turned to the infamous final injections with the 5 cc syringe, administered on the night of 12 November and in the early hours of 13 November. Reggie had said in his opening speech that the prosecution could not know what was in that syringe. But in the nurses' report for 12 November, Mrs Morrell's last night, Nurse Randall had recorded an intra-muscular injection at 10.30 p.m. of 5 cc paraldehyde – a strong rapidly acting hypnotic and sedative drug. Mrs Morrell, at the time, 'certainly wasn't conscious. She might have been semi-conscious.' And she reflected that for her last two or three days 'she was in and out of that sort of heavy coma'.

After the 5 cc paraldehyde injection, said the nurse, Dr Adams refilled the syringe, and said that 'if she was restless to give it'. He left Marden Ash and soon afterwards the disturbing jerky spasms came back. Nurse Randall was unhappy about giving such an enormous injection so soon after the last one, and she tried to get hold of Dr Adams on the telephone. But she could not find him, and so she gave the last 5 cc injection at 1 a.m. Edith Morrell became very quiet, and at about 2 a.m. she died. Nurse Randall was absolutely certain about this last injection, even though there was no sign of it in the notebooks.

Geoffrey Lawrence rose for the cross-examination. Despite the skewering of Nurse Stronach and the battering of Sister Mason-Ellis, Nurse Randall seemed self-assured, braced for combat. But Lawrence judged the moment well – and was less confrontational than he had been before. There was a less acerbic tone to his questions, and a quiet assumption of his total command of the journey through the notebooks, and, under his influence, Nurse Randall's demeanour changed. She seemed to have no will to struggle, and instead surrendered herself to Lawrence's narrative and his flattery, accepting his pretend regard for her superior knowledge of medical matters, soaking up his feigned deference, as he peppered his questions with 'I do not understand these things because I am not a State Registered Nurse', or 'Am I right in thinking, as a layman?' In fact, Lawrence seemed no longer there to demand answers, but more – as Patrick Devlin put it – he simply 'sought the help of the conquered', and Nurse Randall, though 'supposedly under cross-examination' was 'really playing the part of the Greek chorus to Lawrence's rendering of the notebooks'.

As he bowed to her professional understanding of Dr Adams's intentions, Lawrence put it to her that, 'as a trained nurse' she appreciated that the doctor's object was simply to give his patient some rest and some sleep at night.

'Yes,' answered Nurse Randall.

'That is quite right?'

'Yes, sir, yes.'

The main points of contention between the prosecution and the defence were now crystallising. The drugging of Mrs Morrell could, according to the Crown, be justified only if she was in severe pain, which she was not. Otherwise, it was sinister because it was lethal. Nobody could have survived it. The defence position was that the sedation was justified by Mrs Morrell's 'restlessness', her 'nervy' outbursts and her 'brainstorms'. The Crown argued that the 'brainstorms' were caused by the drugs. Lawrence was firm that it was her stroke that caused them. Both sides agreed that the 'routine sedation' ended around the end of October, when a period of heavier, more heroin-based sedation began. The Crown saw this as the 'murder period' or the 'fatal fortnight'. The defence argued that this was simply the period in which a very old lady, who was seriously ill, went into a last decline. As for the final two injections, the Crown had it that with or without them, Mrs Morrell had been murdered – but they *may* have been significant. The defence argued that that paraldehyde was an appropriate treatment for Mrs Morrell's condition. It was hard to tell who was right, and by now the court was in sore need of expert witnesses to shed light on the matter.

In the meantime, the jury was treated to a startling attempt by Nurse Randall to change tack, to slip the leash and go off in a direction which did not please Geoffrey Lawrence. His response, wrote Patrick Devlin, was 'to throw in all his reserves and the thunder of them was like the charge of the Imperial Guard at Waterloo'. The subject under consideration was the extent of Mrs Morrell's last 'jerky spasms'.

'Let us turn to the last night,' said Lawrence. 'There is no mention, is there, from start to finish in your writing of any twitching or jerkiness at all?'

'No, sir, not here.'

'This is the situation, is it not, that although, as a trained nurse, on the night before you had used the word "jerky" twice . . . that that is the only record throughout the whole of these books of the word "jerky" by you on that patient.'

'Yes.'

'You simply put "very shaky" and underline it. That is right, is it not?'

'Yes, sir.'

'Are you standing there in face of this record made on the last night by you, are you standing there and saying, as a trained nurse with twenty-five or more years' experience, that when you wrote those words "very shaky" and underlined them on the last night report they were intended to mean something quite different from what they had meant when you had used those very words in your earlier reports?'

'Yes I do. They were more intense.'

'What was more intense?'

'The shakiness, or the jerkiness.'

'Ah! But you just told me that the shakiness recorded in your earlier notes had nothing whatever to do with twitchings or jerkiness, didn't you?'

'No because they are quite different.'

'What?'

'Shakiness and jerkiness.'

'Are quite different?'

'Yes, sir.'

'Well, that is what I thought. Then why, why, if you were

recording something quite different on the last night, in the peace and quiet of what was then the room in which Mrs Morrell had died – if you were recording something quite different, why did you use the same words?'

'I just don't know. I suppose I just wrote it down quickly.'

'You suppose you just wrote it! Let me suggest the reason why you use the same words and underlined them. The reason was that you then, six years ago, were describing the same condition of shakiness that you had described months before but that it was greater in degree but still the same kind of thing, was not it?'

'I can only remember now how very dreadful they were, the jerks.'

Patrick Devlin had a question: 'Have you got now, apart from what is written down in the book, a clear recollection in your mind of her being jerky an hour and a half before she died?'

'I have. I never want to see anything like it again.'

The vividness of Nurse Randall's recollection was striking. 'I never want to see anything like it again' suggested something extraordinary had happened, that the jerky spasms were alarming and unforgettable. It gave the impression that her memory was right and the notebooks wrong, that they were fallible after all. The nurse seemed pleased that she had stood her ground. Lawrence's persistence on the point alerted the court that the jerky spasms were important, and would come up again. For now he let them go, but another confrontation quickly developed. This time, it was over whether or not Mrs Morrell was, as Nurse Randall had testified, in a coma during the last days of her life. Geoffrey Lawrence said:

'It is quite obvious in these reports made by you during these last three or four nights that Mrs Morrell was not in a coma, isn't it?'

'She would be in a coma, or in a heavy sleep, after the injections, for a time. Almost like a coma.'

'A heavy sleep and a coma are not the same thing . . .'

'No.'

'Miss Randall, are you trying to be as accurate as you can be at this stage?'

'I am, sir, yes.'

'If a patient is properly described as awake she plainly is not in a coma, is she?'

'No, sir . . .'

'If you record a patient as being "not sleeping – seems more wakeful", that is not recording a coma, is it?'

'No, sir.'

'You told the Attorney-General when he was examining you in chief that she was in and out of a heavy coma, did you not?'

'I probably meant a heavy sleep.'

'Miss Randall, you and I are agreed, are we not, that there is all the difference in the world between a heavy sleep and a coma from a nursing or medical point of view?'

'Yes, sir . . . But having so many drugs she would be so heavily asleep it would be like a coma.'

'Did you think I had asked you any question to which that is an answer?'

'No, sir.'

'If you want to say you want to alter or withdraw that evidence, what is it you want to alter?'

'I know that she was heavily asleep, or whatever it was, and she would not respond to light or having her mouth cleaned at times, whereas if she was not in a coma she would have sucked on the swab.'

'But that is exactly what you record her as having done on the last night but one, is it not? Just look at the bottom of your report of 11/12 November, do you see that?'

'Yes, sir.'

'Now and again will suck a swab on forceps?'

The focal point of the trial had become the battle for supremacy between the truth in the notebooks, and the reliability of

memory. With the demolition of the coma, Lawrence ensured
that the notebooks were in the ascendant. He did not linger on
the point, but turned swiftly to Nurse Randall's recollections
about Mrs Morrell's final two injections. He asked her to turn to
the relevant pages in the notebooks. It was quite plain, he said,
that the first paraldehyde injection was given by Dr Adams, and
not by her. She had remembered giving it herself, but her
memory was wrong. As for the second large injection, there was
no record of it in the books.

Nurse Randall let it pass that the first paraldehyde injection
was, in fact, given by Dr Adams – but she would not let Geoffrey
Lawrence triumph on the point of the second injection.
Although there was no record of it in the notebooks, she insisted
she *had* given the injection. She was quite certain about it. As for
it actually being paraldehyde, as Dr Adams had said it was, she
was uncertain.

Geoffrey Lawrence responded with a brilliant attack on the
reliability of Nurse Randall's memory. According to the notebooks she had been wrong about who gave the first of the two
5 cc injections. When she had been asked about the nurses'
conversations on the train the previous day she, like Sister
Mason-Ellis, had claimed she could not remember what was said.
So, Lawrence asked, if she could not remember what had happened the day before, why should her memory of that last
injection six years ago be relied upon? Having tied her up in
knots, he put it to her that 'your memory is not trustworthy, is
it, on details?' At last, Nurse Randall capitulated. 'It appears not
to be,' she answered.

Reggie Manningham-Buller rose to re-examine Nurse
Randall. He had a lot of work to do if he was going to redress the
damage, and he began by taking up the 'coma' question, and
boldly putting it in the context of the drugs, asking if she could
describe the last stages of life in someone whose life was ending
'as a result of excessive injections of morphia and heroin'. 'Well,

they just get more heavy,' answered the nurse, 'and have to have more injections and just get more heavier sleep and get excited if they do not have it.'

Did Nurse Randall know that paraldehyde has a distinctive and powerful smell? 'Yes,' she replied, she did know that. And it was strange that, although Dr Adams had told her he was injecting paraldehyde, there was no smell. None at all. Nurse Randall still insisted that she *had* given the second 5 cc injection that had been prepared by Dr Adams. Afterwards she had washed the syringe, and again she did not notice the tell-tale, unmissable smell of paraldehyde. The judge pressed the point harder than the Attorney-General had done, asking whether she had thought something else might have been in the injection, such as morphia or heroin. But Nurse Randall said she could not remember.

Then, while speaking of the final injection, she threatened to open up a new line of thinking which was wanted by neither the prosecution nor the defence. Referring to the final syringe, she said:

'It was given to me to give to her if she did not get quiet . . . and as she was so very restless, the spasms were so intense, I gave it. Mrs Morrell told me that Dr Adams had promised her he wouldn't let her suffer at the end.'

Reggie cut her short as quickly as he could with the comment: 'I did not ask you that last bit, Miss Randall.' None the less, it was out there – the idea of Dr Adams, not as a legacy-hunting killer, but a compassionate doctor prepared to 'ease the passing' of a dying patient.

Nurse Randall represented the high point of the nurses' evidence – but there was one more nurse to come. This was Sister Brenda Bartlett (who was now Mrs Hughes). She stood out because she was young and pretty, and turned up in court with her hair tucked up into a knitted green skiing cap. Hers was the shortest time in the witness box of all four – and was memorable for her recollection that, in her final two or three days, Mrs

Morrell was 'sort of semi-comatosed. I cannot explain it in any other way' – thus reviving the idea of an old lady, close to coma if not actually in one, not in any pain and being pumped full of drugs. On this note, the first week of the trial drew to a close.

The extravagant rhetoric of Reggie's opening speech seemed a distant memory. Long gone was the picture of a murderer implementing a dastardly plan to kill an old lady in order to inherit her Rolls-Royce, or her chest of silver. Thanks to the notebooks, the plot had changed, and the spotlight was not on some evil master plan, but on the day-to-day ministrations at Marden Ash – the injections of morphia and heroin, the upping of the doses in the fatal fortnight, and the significance of the 'last injections'. There was a pressing need for the evidence of the expert witnesses who were waiting in the wings.

14

Murder, Can You Prove It?

PATRICK DEVLIN SPENT the weekend at his elegant house in the Wiltshire countryside where, with a small glass of brandy and a large cigar, he went through the transcripts. It was obvious, he thought, that everything depended on the medical experts, but he was not sure that the case would last long enough to hear them. In his opinion, the trial had gone so badly for Reggie that on Monday morning he would probably 'throw in his hand'.

The decision would rest on a careful analysis of the contents of the nurses' notebooks. Before the discovery of the books, the prosecution was confident that the 78¾ grains (5,103 mg) of opiates prescribed for Mrs Morrell in her last six days was so excessive that it could only mean murder. Now, the Attorney-General's team would be spending the weekend adding up the amounts that, according to the notebooks, were actually injected. So far nobody had come up with a total, but, wrote Devlin, 'I think it must have been the general guess – it was certainly mine – that it would be substantially less.' What would be the expert opinion on this lesser amount? Could it possibly be high enough to eliminate all reasonable doubt that Dr Adams intended to kill Mrs Morrell?

Much would depend on the willingness of the expert witnesses for the prosecution to be firm in their opinion, and unswayable in the face of a skilful cross-examination. Patrick Devlin was keenly aware of the power in the courtroom of an impressive expert. In 1930, as a junior lawyer, he had observed the legendary Home Office pathologist Sir Bernard Spilsbury give controversial but decisive evidence at the trial of a young man named Sidney Harry Fox charged with the murder of his mother, Rosaline. Rosaline's body had been dragged from a fire in a hotel room in Margate on the Kent coast, and at first it looked as though a terrible accident had occurred. But Sidney made a claim on her life insurance, and suspicions were raised.

Spilsbury was called in to examine the body, and when the case came to court he testified that a bruise at the back of the larynx had been caused by 'some mechanical violence' – in other words, Rosaline had been strangled. The defence pathologists in the case had also examined the body, but they found no bruise and saw no other signs of violence. In court, Spilsbury could not be moved from his position. He 'never admitted to a doubt' and spoke 'with the voice of doom'. Thanks to his evidence, Sidney Fox was found guilty and hanged at Maidstone Prison. Spilsbury was a professional witness who was able to convince a jury that his was the only possible view. Any admission that a different view might also be reasonably held would open the way for 'reasonable doubt' and an acquittal. But the expert witnesses for the Crown in the case of Dr Adams were no Spilsburys. They were not accustomed to appearing in murder trials, or to facing barristers of the calibre of Geoffrey Lawrence.

When the trial resumed on Monday morning, there were other matters to be addressed before the expert witnesses were called – and one of these was the question of motive. The Crown wished to revive the idea that Dr Adams had murdered Edith Morrell because he was desperate to get his hands on a legacy, and the chief witness to his attempts was Mrs Morrell's solicitor, Hubert Sogno.

Mr Sogno told the story of Dr Adams's visit to his office to insist that Mrs Morrell wished to leave him her Rolls-Royce and some jewellery. Despite Mr Sogno's disapproval, the visit had resulted in a codicil to Mrs Morrell's will dated 19 July 1950. A fresh will followed on 5 August 1950 and yet another on 24 August 1950. This was her final will – and in it she left Dr Adams the 'oak chest containing silver in my drawing room at Marden Ash together with all the silver articles usually kept in it'. Her Rolls-Royce and Jacobean cupboard, she said, should go to her son Claude, unless he predeceased her, in which case they were to go to Dr Adams.

Geoffrey Lawrence rose for the cross-examination – and turned to Dr Adams's shooting holiday in Scotland in September 1950. Mr Sogno said that Mrs Morrell had been 'very angry' with Dr Adams when he went away, and had asked him to draw up a codicil cutting the doctor out of her will – the final will of 24 August. This had been done. He told of Mrs Morrell later tearing the codicil into little pieces, believing that her action would make it invalid, and would return Dr Adams to the will. Lawrence asked the solicitor whether, in his view, the codicil remained in force. Yes, he said, he believed it did. Lawrence said:

'So that when she died on 13 November he was not, in your view, a beneficiary under her will?'

'That is correct.'

'For anything?'

'For anything at all.'

So the court learned that if Hubert Sogno was right, all that Dr Adams had received after Mrs Morrell died – that is, the Rolls-Royce he so desired, and the chest of silver – came to him as a gift from her son Claude. He had been entitled to nothing.

Lawrence was set on making the motive of inheritance look flimsy, and now asked Mr Sogno about the actual beneficiaries under Mrs Morrell's last will. A number of people, including two executors and her chauffeur, Thomas Price, received £1,000 each. The gardener received £500 and her prize collection of dahlias. Nurse Randall had received £300. The oak chest and the silver that she believed she had left to Dr Adams looked piffling by comparison to most of the legacies – its value being £276. 5s., and a tiny proportion of her total estate, valued at £157,000.

Patrick Devlin thought that Mr Sogno's evidence 'dissipated the Crown's theory of a doctor who bartered for legacies prescriptions of heroin. So abject a failure after two years of prescribing was too much to swallow.' It had left a picture of a grasping, bungling idiot rather than a criminal mastermind. None the less, the motive question was not entirely destroyed. What counted now was not the position in law relating to Dr Adams's legacy from Mrs Morrell, but what he *believed* he would get. And there was evidence still to come on that – from the policemen who had interviewed him.

Superintendent Herbert Hannam's appearance was familiar from the newspapers. 'He strides into the box,' wrote Sybille Bedford, 'chest out, chin in, as a tenor might go forward for his aria.' Questioned by Reggie, he told the court of the doctor's professed belief that he would get her Rolls-Royce, as Mrs Morrell had told him so. Also that he would receive another cabinet, and that she 'insisted' he should have the chest of silver. 'I didn't want it,' Dr Adams had said, 'I am a bachelor. I never use it.'

Dr Adams had admitted, quite readily, said Hannam, that he lied about his financial interest in Mrs Morrell's will when filling in the cremation form, and he repeated Dr Adams's words: 'Oh that was not done wickedly. God knows it was not. We always want cremations to go off smoothly for the dear relatives. If I said I knew I was getting money under the will, they might get suspicious, and I like cremations and burials to go smoothly.'

Reggie asked about the quantities of morphine and heroin that had been given to Mrs Morrell. Superintendent Hannam explained that he had shown Dr Adams the full list of prescriptions for Mrs Morrell. 'I said: "Who administered the drugs?"' said Hannam.

'What did he say?'

'He said: "I did, nearly all. Perhaps the nurses gave some, but mostly me."'

'What did you say?'

'I said: "Were any left over when she died?" He said: "No, none. All was given to the patient."'

So, there it was. The jury heard that Dr Adams had said he had personally administered *everything* that was prescribed for Mrs Morrell – the full and fatal 78¾ grains of opiates. Of all the evidence against him, that which came out of Adams's own mouth was the most damning. What was this to mean? That the notebooks were flawed? Or that the doctor, and not the notebooks, was an unreliable source of information? It seemed obvious that Geoffrey Lawrence would put Dr Adams in the witness box, and have him tell the court that the notebooks were a far more accurate record than his memory. That, after all, was what each of the nurses had said of their own evidence. Such a claim would be strengthened by the fact that the doctor, by his own admission, did not keep written records.

The seventh day of the trial started with Superintendent Hannam once more in the witness box, again telling of the doctor's volubility and his willingness to talk himself into trouble. This time, it was his reaction to learning that the police were suspicious about the death of Mrs Morrell. Hannam stated:

'He said: "Easing the passing of a dying person is not all that wicked. She wanted to die. That cannot be murder. It is impossible to accuse a doctor."'

And he repeated the other quote that had such resonance – the response to being cautioned for murder: '"Murder, can you prove it was murder?" and then: "I did not think you could prove murder. She was dying in any event."'

Geoffrey Lawrence rose for the cross-examination. He might have been merciless with the nurses, but with Herbert Hannam he went further. The nurses, he had intimated, had faulty memories and were flawed witnesses. But Hannam, he implied, was far worse – a police officer who was prepared to lie to secure a conviction. Lawrence spoke with passion, fuelled by apparent belief that his client was a persecuted man. Hannam's first interview with Dr Adams, he suggested, had happened not because of a chance meeting in the street near Kent Lodge, but because Hannam had planned it. 'The truth of the matter is that you were waylaying him, weren't you?' he said. 'Indeed I was not,' Hannam answered.

As for motive, Dr Adams's comment 'I knew she was going to leave me her Rolls-Royce car. She told me she had put it in her will. Oh, yes, and another cabinet,' was never, in fact, made, Lawrence stated. 'Let me put this quite squarely to you,' he said, 'that in fact he made no reference on that occasion to the Rolls-Royce car or the cabinet at all.' Hannam was robust. 'Oh yes, sir, indeed he did,' he replied. These 'are not things that Dr Adams said at all,' continued Lawrence, 'but they are the reflection of things that you were saying and putting to him and to which he was making no reply.' 'That is quite untrue,' Hannam insisted. 'These were his actual words and I recorded them accurately.'

Geoffrey Lawrence turned to 24 November 1956, when the police came to Kent Lodge with a search warrant. He intimated that Hannam's record of Dr Adams's words during the search was another pack of lies. On the question of dangerous drugs kept at Kent Lodge, said Lawrence, 'I put it to you that he did not say "I haven't any".' 'Oh he did,' Hannam snapped back. 'I was very amazed at the time.'

Hannam stood his ground, as he had done three years earlier when at the receiving end of a similar grilling, not by Lawrence, but by Peter Rawlinson at the trial of the Towpath Murderer, Alfred Whiteway. The insinuations were the same – that he was a dishonest officer. The courtroom attack was just as fierce, and at one point Lawrence began a fresh assault with an oblique reference to the Whiteway trial. 'This is not the first time you have given evidence in a criminal trial, is it?' he asked. Then he observed darkly that some of Dr Adams's supposed incriminating comments had been made to Hannam while Inspector Pugh was out of the room, ordered out by Hannam.

'When Pugh left the room, did you go over to Dr Adams's desk?' asked Lawrence.

'Yes, I was standing by the desk.'

'. . . when you got to his desk you opened a brief case that you had got with you and produced a handful of papers from it?'

'. . . I certainly opened my brief case and took one small quantity of papers, Exhibit 25.'

'Did you say this: "This is a list of drugs you prescribed for Mrs Morrell"?'

'Yes.'

'. . . I suggest that at that time Dr Adams was . . . across the room, and he just said, quite casually, "Oh yes"?'

'He was standing right beside me and I had that list in my hand.'

'You see, I have to put the best of Dr Adams's recollection?'

'Yes, I agree.'

'And that you said something to the effect of a question: "Were they all given to her?" and that he said, "I can't remember about that", or words to that effect?'

'No, sir, that is quite untrue. He was most emphatic about it.'

'And that you persisted in the question and that he still maintained that he could not possibly remember the details and he would not discuss it with you?'

'That is quite untrue, the whole thing. He was most loquacious, and always has been since I have known him.'

It was evident that Lawrence wished to demolish the Crown's assertion that *all* the prescriptions were administered, and the line of questioning suggested that Dr Adams would appear and assert that he had never incriminated himself, had never spoken the words – and that Hannam had fabricated them.

Lawrence turned to Dr Adams's other moment of self-destruction. On 19 December Hannam had arrested the doctor for murder, and cautioned him. And the doctor had responded: 'Murder. Murder. Can you prove it was murder?' and then 'I did not think you could prove murder. She was dying in any event.' In his opening speech, Reggie had said these sounded like the words of a guilty man. A man who thought he had murdered, but could get away with it. Now Lawrence asked:

'The inflexion of the voice on that word "murder" was interrogative, wasn't it?'

'Now sir,' answered Hannam, 'I think it is only fair to say this: Dr Adams was a very, very shaken man indeed, and I am not going to suggest there was any inflexion of any kind. I think he was very distressed.'

'I think we can leave it that way. It was quite obvious your announcement of your arrest for murder was a shock?'

'It certainly was. He was very shaken.'

Patrick Devlin underlined this exchange in red pencil in his transcript, and later commended Superintendent Hannam. For all the insinuations that he was dishonest, or had handled the investigation badly, when it came to this vivid piece of evidence, Hannam seemed at pains to be fair to Dr Adams, not to misrepresent him. The effect was to underline his credibility as a witness and, in fact, to help the prosecution. The 'murder, murder' comment may not have been a 'cracking' moment, an admission of guilt. But the 'easing the passing' comment was brought into sharp relief. And the assertion that Dr Adams had administered 'nearly all' the prescribed drugs for Mrs Morrell appeared genuine, and had escaped Geoffrey Lawrence's attack. In the papers, the clash between Lawrence and Hannam was reported as 'DRAMA OF A DUEL AT THE OLD BAILEY'.

After Hannam, Brynley Pugh and Charlie Hewett appeared briefly to agree with his evidence. Then Dr Vincent Harris came to the witness box – and testified that he had made twenty-eight visits to Mrs Morrell during the time that she was under Dr Adams's care, at least eight of which were not mentioned in the nurses' notebooks. He said that he had continued with Dr Adams's treatments, and while his partner was in Scotland in September 1950, when Mrs Morrell was very angry, Dr Harris had actually given her an *increased* dose of morphia. Sybille Bedford thought Dr Harris 'blossomed' under the questioning of Geoffrey Lawrence, and never more so than when he agreed that Mrs Morrell had done extremely well to survive for two years and four months after her stroke. Dr Harris had flipped back again. His evidence was useful to Dr Adams – and the court was left with the impression that Dr Harris had never, in all his twenty-eight visits to Mrs Morrell, found anything shocking or improper about her regimen of morphine and heroin.

15

Dr Douthwaite

THE FIRST EXPERT witness was Arthur Douthwaite of 49 Harley Street, a tall and languid man, accustomed to the comfortable ways of the medical elite. In an age of deference, he was at the apex of the deference hierarchy, being a senior physician at Guy's Hospital, the respected editor of a medical textbook, a Fellow of the Medical Society of London, and an expert on opiates. He lived elegantly. It was his custom to arrive by limousine at Guy's, and step out in full morning suit and bowler hat. Legend had it that he once walked into the hospital and informed the casualty officer, 'I am Arthur Henry Douthwaite and I have just perforated my duodenal ulcer, please arrange my admission.'

'He is a most handsome man,' wrote Sybille Bedford, '. . . Greying hair, handsome in the way of the good-looking soldier who has reached, perhaps, the rank of Lieutenant-General. Such appearance is not unobtrusive, and the most striking thing about it is his height . . . Dr Douthwaite stoops slightly and even so gives the impression that his head touches the canopy.' Patrick Devlin also thought him 'very handsome' and 'very commanding but very courteous, always frank, never evasive. Also very decisive; things either were or they were not.'

As Dr Douthwaite made his entrance, there was a sense of relief. At last, a top man who could speak with the authority conferred by medical science. The journeys through the notebooks with the nurses had been dramatic, entertaining even; but the medical story that emerged had been on the chaotic side, a tangle of events that needed to be unpicked – the morphia injections, the heroin, the paraldehyde, the jerky spasms, the last days, the cerebral thrombosis – Dr Adams's favourite diagnosis at death. Dr Douthwaite seemed the very opposite of Nurses Stronach, Mason-Ellis, Randall and Bartlett, who had proved to be flotsam and jetsam, wreckage moved this way and that by the talented Mr Lawrence. In contrast, Dr Douthwaite had the bearing of someone in command of the scene.

Reggie began by asking his witness to consider Mrs Morrell's stroke in 1948. In all probability, said the doctor, this *had* been a cerebral thrombosis: a clot in an artery in the brain which cut off the blood supply to that part of the brain – in other words, a stroke. Afterwards a patient might improve over several months, but could become 'depressed and irritable, lachrymose'. The correct treatment was to mobilise her as soon as possible, since this might prevent another clot. Reggie asked whether there was any justification for injecting morphia and heroin after a stroke caused by cerebral thrombosis. 'No, there is no justification.' It would be 'wrong in all circumstances'. 'This has a ring of such absolute, such towering, such *natural* certainty that the court sits stunned,' wrote Sybille Bedford. Except for Dr Adams, who appeared not stunned but incensed, outraged. 'The doctor is actually bouncing on his chair in anger, pinching his lips and shaking his head, an expression of obstinate mortification on his face . . .'

Giving morphia and heroin to Mrs Morrell, Douthwaite continued, would 'greatly interfere' with her rehabilitation, causing her to be still when she should be moving about, and ensuring 'severe addiction' to both drugs. Dr Adams's insistence that Mrs Morrell be 'kept quiet' during the day was the opposite of the correct treatment because it increased the risk of another stroke. As for his suggestion that the morphia and heroin would help calm her when she was irritable, Dr Douthwaite stated with great certainty that the injections would make the irritability worse, and within a few weeks they would turn her into an addict.

'Morphia,' asked Reggie, 'produces generally a feeling of pleasure in the person to whom it is administered?'

'Yes,' answered the doctor.

'And that feeling of pleasure would lead to dependence on the doctor who was supplying the drug?'

'He, naturally . . . obtains a complete ascendancy over that patient.'

The only legitimate purpose for injections of morphia over a long period was severe pain. If the pain was agonising, then the dose could be given once an hour. The normal dose was ¼ of a grain, and the British Pharmacopoeia gave the maximum as ⅓ of a grain. Morphia, he said, was dangerous, but heroin was worse. Like morphia, it was highly addictive, but it carried the additional risk of being a powerful depressant on respiration. The maximum dosage of heroin was ⅙ of a grain. 'We seldom give heroin more than once in six hours,' he said, although 'one might be prepared to give it more frequently in the face of terrible pain'. The contrast with Dr Adams's instructions was stark – in her final days Mrs Morrell's treatment had been a full grain of heroin every hour 'if needed'. If given very often, added Dr Douthwaite, heroin did not have a sedative effect – flying in the face of Dr Adams's reasoning.

A tolerance of both morphia and heroin could quickly develop, requiring ever greater doses to secure the initial effect. Until her final weeks, Mrs Morrell was receiving a level dose, which would have left her 'in a state of almost constant craving for more drugs and . . . excitable, bad-tempered, impossible to live with'. Reggie asked whether the 'twitchings', or 'jerky spasms', could be produced by heroin. 'Oh, yes,' replied Dr Douthwaite. It could 'give rise to jerky movements, twitchings, convulsions'.

On the paraldehyde, Dr Douthwaite confirmed that its

distinguishing feature was its revolting smell. The drug, he said, acted as a depressant on the whole of the central nervous system, and could be used to stop twitchings. By itself it was not danger- ous, but if someone were in a coma, it would deepen the coma, and if paraldehyde were superimposed on the use of heroin by itself, or heroin and morphia together, then 'that would be likely to produce death'. So the paraldehyde was not neutral – it was lethal. For now, the mystery of the missing smell was ignored.

Looking at the nurses' notebooks, Dr Douthwaite said that sometimes when Mrs Morrell became 'shouting and hysterical' it was the natural consequence of a temporary lowering of the amount of drugs she received. She was experiencing withdrawal symptoms. Conversely, when the dosage was increased rapidly then 'one would expect the individual to go into a deep sleep or coma'. And in the case of a sudden increase in heroin, 'it would be very likely to produce jerky movements'. On 9 October 1950, for instance, he could see that after her morning injection, Mrs Morrell became semi-comatose, her lower lip was blue, and she could not be roused – even by brandy. This, said Douthwaite, was consistent with the effects of a large injection of morphia or a mix of morphia and heroin.

He was of the firm view that when Mrs Morrell had experi- enced Cheyne Stokes breathing, it was caused by drugs, and not by the senile deterioration suggested by Geoffrey Lawrence. He could tell, because it happened after a huge dose, and did not recur. As for the injections given during the 'murder period', Dr Douthwaite was shocked. He said that the two-hour intervals between high heroin doses were 'dangerously short'. And when, on 9 November, Dr Adams told the nurses to give 1 grain of heroin hourly 'if necessary', this was 'an astonishing instruction' to give six times the maximum dose, and unbelievably often. The amount of heroin Mrs Morrell was given between 8 November and her death on 13 November, he said, 'would have produced jerking spasms or convulsions, and ultimately death'.

And, this was just the heroin. On top of this she also had the morphia.

Reggie asked the vital question:

'On the nurses' notebooks alone, not the prescriptions, what conclusion did Dr Douthwaite draw from the dosages given in the last few days before Mrs Morrell's death?'

'The only conclusion I can come to,' replied Douthwaite, 'was that the intention was to terminate her life.'

'I want to ask you about one other matter,' said Reggie. 'On the cremation form Dr Adams, we know, has recorded as the immediate cause of death, cerebral thrombosis. Are there any signs in the nurses' reports in your opinion which justify that conclusion?'

'No,' replied Dr Douthwaite.

The doctor had been everything the prosecuting counsel wanted him to be – clear, authoritative, convincing. And the impression in the press gallery was that the case had swung around dramatically in the Crown's favour. When the journalists now said, 'it's a walkover', they meant Dr Adams would certainly be found guilty. The revelation of the notebooks had been neutralised by Dr Douthwaite's observation that they, without a shadow of a doubt, pointed to murder. And Geoffrey Lawrence's masterful cross-examinations of the earlier prosecution witnesses seemed diminished. The expert had arrived, and taken the trial to a new plane.

Geoffrey Lawrence rose for the cross-examination, and the question was hanging in the air. Would his remarkable skills be matched by the eloquence of Dr Douthwaite? Lawrence began by saying he wished to be quite sure that he had understood Dr Douthwaite properly. Was he saying that Dr Adams had formed the intention to terminate Mrs Morrell's life on 8 November 1950, and 'carried that intention into effect over the next five days'? Dr Douthwaite confirmed that, yes, this was his expert opinion.

'I think it follows . . . that that murderous intent in your view was present in his mind from and including 8 November onwards to the end?'

'Yes.'

'I hardly suppose that you have often given a graver or more fateful opinion on a matter of medicine than that, have you?'

'No.'

'Before going into the witness box and expressing that view upon oath in this court, have you satisfied yourself that you have had every piece of relevant evidence before you on which to judge?'

'Yes.'

'You gave evidence in this case before the magistrates at Eastbourne, didn't you?'

'I did.'

'For the prosecution?'

'Yes.'

'Supporting the charge of murder?'

'Yes.'

'At that stage of the matter your knowledge of the medication, the treatment of Mrs Morrell, began at the beginning of January 1950, didn't it?'

'Yes.'

'When you gave evidence at that stage you were entirely in ignorance of what her treatment by Dr Adams had been before January 1950, weren't you?'

'Yes.'

'And you gave that evidence at least partly upon the hypothesis that for the last three or four days of her life this lady had been in a continuous coma, didn't you?'

'Yes.'

'That has turned out on the facts now to be quite wrong?'

'Yes, not a continuous coma.'

From time to time during the trial of Dr Adams a mood of

great expectation filled the Old Bailey, an atmosphere created by the realisation that Geoffrey Lawrence was, in his quiet, stealthy way, building something.

Lawrence continued:

'It would be most interesting to know, wouldn't it, before damning Dr Adams's treatment from the start, as you did yesterday, to know what happened in Cheshire [where Mrs Morrell had her stroke]?'

'It would be interesting to know what happened in Cheshire, yes.'

'And it would be most interesting because – just follow this, Dr Douthwaite – because it might throw a great light upon the treatment that he adopted at the Eastbourne nursing home in July of 1948, when she got to Eastbourne from Cheshire?'

'Yes, I agree.'

'And so far you do not know what that information is, do you?'

'I do not. No.'

Then, in a flourish that was reminiscent of the moment of the production of the nurses' notebooks, Geoffrey Lawrence produced another contemporary record out of thin air. Somehow, he had found the original nurses' notes for Mrs Morrell's stay in the Neston Cottage Hospital in Cheshire, and he drew Dr Douthwaite's attention to a course of events that began in June 1948, immediately after her stroke. At first she had had little sleep and was restless at night. She was given sleeping tablets, but they had 'very little effect'. On 27 June, the report read, 'patient very distressed and complaining of severe pain'.

'There,' Lawrence continued, 'is the very phrase "severe pain" that you were using rather freely yesterday. According to the report, Mrs Morrell was given pills for the pain, but was unable to swallow them. Then: "Morphia gr ¼ given at 11.30 a.m. Has slept since." So there it was. Mrs Morrell had been started on morphia, not by Dr Adams, but by the doctors in the Neston

Cottage Hospital. We will go through the whole of this, Dr Douthwaite, before I ask questions about it,' said Lawrence.

At this point, Dr Douthwaite asked the judge if he might sit down. 'Yes, please do,' said Patrick Devlin.

Then, as Geoffrey Lawrence went through the reports day by day, it emerged that on eight nights during Mrs Morrell's ten days at the hospital, she received a morphia injection authorised by a Dr Turner.

Lawrence asked: 'Does the field of condemnation that you are spreading from that witness box extend to include Dr Turner for having given this patient morphia after this stroke?'

'If that was the treatment for the stroke, yes.'

'It does?'

Geoffrey Lawrence threw up his hands. 'Good gracious me! . . . We are left with this, are we not, that three doctors, two other doctors [Dr Turner and Dr Harris] who are not in the dock on a charge of murder at all, two doctors in addition to Dr Adams, gave – and deliberately gave – this particular patient, who had had a stroke, injections of morphia, not a single injection but night after night?'

'Yes. The first being given when pain was reported.'

'But you cannot shelter behind that, can you?'

'I am not trying to shelter behind anything.'

'Because the morphia goes on night after night, but as you pointed out just now, there was only one complaint of severe pain?'

'Yes.'

'. . . This at least is clear, isn't it, of the three doctors, Dr Turner, Dr Adams and Dr Harris, in whose practice of giving morphia you disapprove, every one of those three saw the patient themselves in the condition she was in at the time, didn't they?'

Dr Douthwaite admitted it.

'They had actually seen Mrs Morrell, and he had never set eyes on her. And he agreed that it was only "the man on the spot" who could really judge the full picture.' Lawrence continued: 'And in all the multitude of varieties of human illness that the general practitioner, the man on the spot, has got to exercise the best judgement he can?'

'Yes, most certainly.'

'He has not got to be the perfect physician?'

'No.'

Geoffrey Lawrence had reached the crux of his argument. Dr Adams, he asserted, was no murderer, just a less than perfect physician, and that was not a crime. He now turned to Mrs Morrell's general state of health, and put it to Dr Douthwaite that, given that she was in her late seventies when she had her stroke, she might have been expected to live for another six to twelve months after it. The doctor agreed. Lawrence drew his attention to the treatment she had received at the Esperance Nursing Home, when she returned to Eastbourne. He had, on hand, a list of all her prescriptions there. Once again, she had received morphia. Equally interesting, there were several prescriptions for the painkilling tablet Veramon, with the instruction that they were to be given 'when pain is severe'. Dr Douthwaite agreed that it seemed that, at some point, she had suffered some pain.

When Mrs Morrell had returned to Eastbourne, heroin had been added to her morphia – a drug that leaves the patient 'with a sense of well-being'. This, Lawrence suggested, was added to make the remainder of Mrs Morrell's life 'as bearable as it could be'. Dr Douthwaite went along with the scenario, agreeing that this may have been the objective. During Mrs Morrell's first months back in Eastbourne, the heroin and morphia were given at night time, and she was helped by nurses to get some exercise during the day. Somehow, under the guidance of Geoffrey Lawrence, the treatment plan seemed perfectly reasonable.

He now produced a blue notebook for Dr Douthwaite to look at.

'Would you look first of all – I am so sorry, doctor, you are not hearing me sometimes, are you?'

'I think I have heard you clearly.'

'My learned friends said that you were exhibiting signs of distress and straining to catch what I am saying.'

'It may be just a manner. I have not had any difficulty in hearing you. If I do not, I will tell you, certainly.'

'Please do . . .'

Then Lawrence directed Dr Douthwaite's attention to the fact that, twelve months after Mrs Morrell's stroke, Dr Adams had attended to the fitting of a new pair of boots for her, so that she might be mobile during the day. Entries in the blue book included 'walked around bed alone three times' in the new boots in June 1949. And walking around the bed four times, recorded in the books two weeks later.

'It is quite obvious he was still doing his best to keep her mobile?'

'Oh yes.'

The following month she went out in the car, with Dr Adams, to watch the launching of a life-boat. Activity of some sort continued right into the summer of 1950, and Dr Douthwaite acknowledged that on 9 August she 'walked the length of the tennis lawn twice'. So, two years after her stroke, there was ample evidence that Dr Adams was 'keeping her up and about and interested'.

'And by September 1950 she has already exceeded the reasonable prognosis for the expectation of life by thirteen months, or thereabouts?'

'Yes.'

It seemed that Dr Douthwaite conceded that Mrs Morrell had done very well on the mix of gentle exercise in the day, and a dose of morphia and heroin at night.

Then, when Dr Adams went away on his shooting holiday in Scotland in September 1950, Mrs Morrell suffered 'a marked degree of cerebral irritation', and Dr Harris increased her dosage of morphia. From then on, the doses became bigger still.

'Of course,' said Lawrence, 'if a doctor is using morphine as a treatment, a time always comes when a level dosage will not be adequate, and a choice has to be made between increasing the dose or stopping the drug.'

Dr Douthwaite agreed.

'And stopping the drug causes suffering?'

'Yes.'

'And an old lady of 81 might very well collapse if the drug were stopped? With the risk of death?'

Dr Douthwaite continued to agree.

'So the choice would be – increase the dosage or risk death. And in Mrs Morrell's case,' asked Lawrence, 'she was, in any case, in the terminal stages of illness?'

'Yes.'

'And what to do in those circumstances is one of the most difficult problems that faces a doctor, a general practitioner, is it not?'

'Oh yes, very difficult.'

'Also,' said Lawrence, 'the notebooks showed that both Dr Harris and Dr Adams had experimented with reducing Mrs Morrell's heroin. Each time, she had had trouble sleeping, and the dose was increased again to give her a comfortable night.'

The ease with which Geoffrey Lawrence led Dr Douthwaite along the defence's chosen path was striking. The doctor was a changed man. The superior and commanding tone that he had adopted with Reggie was gone, and now he followed Lawrence obediently down each and every byway. If he took a moment to disagree on some small point, the moment quickly passed, and the doctor was once more brought to heel.

Patrick Devlin was unimpressed by Dr Douthwaite. The expert witness, he wrote, should be 'something more' than an ordinary witness, and must advance his theories in the witness box, when he gets the chance: 'There is an art in this. In the cross-examination of the expert the art of the examinee must match the art of the examiner . . . Lawrence was artful in giving the witness no opportunity to argue; Douthwaite was artless in not trying to make one.' As a result, Lawrence was able to construct a picture of a doctor managing the health of an elderly, sick patient, dealing with day-to-day challenges. It was a picture that did not deal with the prosecution's theory that Dr Adams was drugging Mrs Morrell in order to get her money. It simply ignored it, causing the motive question to disappear altogether.

Geoffrey Lawrence now asked Dr Douthwaite to direct his attention to the autumn of 1950, and the days immediately before the 'murder period'. Mrs Morrell, at the time, was suffering 'awful restlessness' and 'cerebral irritation' and the nurses had been instructed to give morphia and heroin injections whenever they felt they were needed. So, when the amounts Mrs Morrell received went up, it was because the *nurses*, and not the doctor, thought it necessary. Then, as she had more injections, her tolerance of morphia and heroin increased:

'So that the general practitioner in a case like Mrs Morrell's is fighting a battle that is growing more and more difficult for him?'

'Yes.'

'The disintegration of senility and the terminal stages of the patient are going on?'

'Yes.'

Dr Douthwaite attempted a qualification of his answer, pointing out that he had not said the terminal stages of Mrs Morrell's illness were due to senile degeneration. (In fact, he had said, quite clearly they were due to the drugs.) Lawrence was not going to let it lie:

'But all the symptoms are compatible with senile degeneration, aren't they?'

'They are certainly compatible with it, yes.'

'[The nurses] said over and over again that these symptoms

recorded in their notes as we went through them were typical, or characteristic, of senile degeneration?'

'Yes. By and large they were. I agree.'

There was no fight in Dr Douthwaite. Did he still believe the symptoms were, in fact, an inevitable consequence of the drugs? That, regardless of any senile degeneration, Mrs Morrell would have experienced them? The court was not told.

Lawrence continued into early November 1950, when the restlessness and night-time wakefulness of Mrs Morrell worsened, the morphia was stopped for five days, but the heroin injections increased. The fateful day approached – 8 November, the date on which, according to Dr Douthwaite, Dr Adams must have had a murderous intent. From then on, he thought, there was no other explanation for his actions. On the night of 6 November, Lawrence told the court, Mrs Morrell had been suffering from:

'. . . restlessness and lack of sleep and thumping the bed and trying to get out of bed and all the rest of it. If that had been allowed to go on without any sedation to get her to sleep, she would rapidly have reached exhaustion and collapsed, wouldn't she?'

'Yes.'

The following day Mrs Morrell was irritable, pushing things away and restless, and was given injections of ¼ a grain of morphia and ½ a grain of heroin by Dr Adams, who said the injections could then be repeated at two-hourly intervals through the night if Mrs Morrell did not sleep. On the night of 7 November, she was restless again, and the nurse gave three injections. Then, the following morning, Dr Adams:

'. . . visited her at 11.20 and I suppose, if you are right, formed the intention to murder her. Is that right?'

'On the 8th? . . . Yes.'

That morning, noted Lawrence, Adams had prescribed a cough medicine, containing heroin, for Mrs Morrell, since a cough had contributed to her sleeplessness. So, Lawrence remarked archly, on the very day he made up his mind to murder Mrs Morrell, he also prescribed a linctus to help her cough?'

'Maybe,' answered Dr Douthwaite.

'What do you mean, maybe? He is, is he not?'

'He is prescribing linctus, yes.'

Later that day, Dr Adams gave Mrs Morrell another injection – ½ a grain of heroin with ½ a grain of a different sort of morphia, this one being hyperduric, and slower-acting. However, that night was bad again, and the following morning Mrs Morrell got out of bed and for an hour sat in a chair in her fur hat and coat and demanded to go out. Eventually, she was persuaded to return to bed, but had another restless day. Lawrence made the point: 'this is the 9th. It is the second day of this murderous intention?' 'Yes,' confirmed Dr Douthwaite, 'it was.' 'Let us see,' continued Lawrence, 'this is the second day of the "murdering" period, let us see what this "murderous" doctor did.'

Lawrence told the court of Edith Morrell's poor state, having had only fifteen minutes sleep the night before, and twenty minutes that day. She had received two injections from the nurses during the night, and ½ a grain of heroin that day at 6 p.m. In the context of all that had been heard already, it seemed like a normal day for Mrs Morrell, not one on which she was being murdered.

Perhaps, suggested Lawrence, Dr Douthwaite had reached the conclusion of murder by the aggregated amounts of morphia and heroin received by Mrs Morrell, but without any reference to the circumstances in which they were given? Had he, perhaps, regarded Dr Adams's instruction to 'keep her under' as suspicious, but had not looked at it in the context of her terrible lack of sleep? If Mrs Morrell were in the last stages of her illness, continued Lawrence, and 'manifesting the last stages of cerebral irritation', it would be Dr Adams's duty, would it not, 'to prevent her from getting restless and excited'?

'Yes,' answered Dr Douthwaite, weakly.

'And . . . he would have to use drugs for that purpose, of some sort, wouldn't he?'

'Of some sort, yes.'

'He could not cut her off from what she had been having because that would have meant almost certain death, wouldn't it?'

'At this stage, yes.'

It was another triumphant moment for Geoffrey Lawrence. He had led Dr Douthwaite into putting Dr Adams in the position of saving Mrs Morrell from certain death, when he was supposed to be in the middle of murdering her. On the tenth day of the trial, Lawrence continued in the same vein. In Mrs Morrell's final days, her drugs had sometimes been increased, sometimes reduced – allowing Lawrence the satisfaction of depicting 'this murderous doctor' reducing the dose – an absurd act if he were trying to kill his patient. The barrister rode the wave of his mastery of the courtroom, hardly bothering to mention the paraldehyde, and arrived at a destination that had the appearance of having been in his sights all along. 'What I put to you,' he said to Dr Douthwaite, 'was that, given the history of Mrs Morrell's last days, there was no need, at any stage to postulate any intent to murder.'

The doctor stuck to his original proposition – he was, he said, forced to postulate intent to murder because of the huge quantities of drugs. Lawrence came back:

'Did Dr Douthwaite acknowledge that, whilst he thought there must be an intent to murder, it was quite possible that another doctor, looking at the same facts, might not reach the same conclusion?'

'I think that is clear, is it not?' answered Dr Douthwaite. 'There could always be a difference of opinion.'

For the prosecution, the answer was disastrous. If there could be a reasonably held, but opposite, opinion, then the way was open for 'reasonable doubt'.

Reggie rose for the re-examination of Dr Douthwaite, and did his best to force the pendulum back. When Mrs Morrell had left Cheshire, Dr Adams had doubled her morphia. This, said Dr Douthwaite, in no sense was 'continuing the treatment'. As for her pain, it could not have been very severe since she had been given only a mild painkiller. Her sleeping was not as bad as Lawrence had intimated, very often she had five or six hours' sleep. He repeated his core case: morphia and heroin were not a justifiable treatment for Mrs Morrell, and the doses she received were 'colossal'. As for 'keeping her under' during the day, there was no medical reason for this.

'Has anything been said in this court, any evidence you have heard, affected your opinion as to the cause of death of Mrs Morrell?'

'No.'

'To what do you attribute her death?'

'To drugs, morphia and heroin, possibly assisted by paraldehyde. In the absence of paraldehyde, in my opinion, morphia and heroin administered in the last few days would have killed her.'

Patrick Devlin now interjected to clear up some matters that were bothering him. He wished to clarify exactly which of Dr Adams's actions Dr Douthwaite considered to be the murderous ones. Did he think the dose given to Mrs Morrell on the night of 7 November was cause to 'postulate murder'? The doctor answered that it was not that dose alone, but taken together with the doses that came before and after. And then he added something astonishing, since it was a totally new idea. Dr Douthwaite now said that when Dr Adams had dropped the morphia, for the period 1 to 5 November, and given Mrs Morrell only heroin, this was part of his murder plan. The lack of morphia, he said, was plainly designed to lower Mrs Morrell's tolerance of it, so that when it was reintroduced in the evening of 5 November, the effect would be lethal. When pressed on the point, he became firm and unbudgeable. Devlin asked:

'You explore every other hypothesis and reject it before you come to the conclusion that it is murder?'

'Yes.'

'Is it your view that in dropping the morphine Dr Adams was merely changing the drugging, or is that an impossible view?'

'I think that it is an impossible view.'

He thought the 'lethal intent' absolutely certain. The judge asked again:

'The *only* possible medical explanation of the dropping of the morphia was that he intended to reintroduce it with lethal effect?'

'Yes, my lord,' answered Dr Douthwaite.

'And then and thereafter all the subsequent injections are given and any one of them could have been lethal?'

'Could have been lethal, yes.'

'And can only be explained on the basis that they were intended to be lethal?'

'Yes, my lord.'

'And that goes on until the morphia and heroin is dropped, and then he takes to paraldehyde . . . so as to bring about her death more quickly than the accumulation of morphia and heroin would have done?'

'Yes, my lord.'

Dr Douthwaite had made an about-turn. When questioned by Lawrence, he had agreed that in dropping the morphia Dr Adams might simply have been trying out different treatments. Now he thought that same action was definitely, unarguably murderous. And the 'murder period' had changed. Instead of starting on 8 November, as he had previously said, it now started on 1 November, when the morphia had been withdrawn. This was the state of things when the court adjourned.

There was much for Patrick Devlin to ponder that weekend. He thought Dr Douthwaite's evidence shambolic, and the changing of the 'murder period' was really the 'last straw'. He compared the doctor with the experienced Home Office experts who would not dream of trying out experimental theories for the first time in the courtroom. They would 'commit themselves to nothing that is not their last word,' he wrote. 'To imagine the great Sir Bernard Spilsbury making a substantial concession is extremely difficult: to imagine him voluntarily changing his mind in the course of his evidence is an exercise to bring the word "boggle" briefly into its own.'

Once again, Devlin thought the sensible course of action would be for Reggie to throw in the towel. But it was unlikely that he would do so, since 'this was not Reggie's style. He was the fighter who never gave in.' His problems went beyond the vacillations of Dr Douthwaite. The motive question was badly damaged – and he might think it an option to let it go, and argue instead that this was 'euthanasia with a taint of legacy hunting'. If so, Devlin would have to instruct the jury that 'if they were satisfied that there was an intent to kill, it was imma- terial whether the intent was merciful or diabolic'. And he would need to address Dr Adams's own idea of 'easing the pass- ing' of a patient. 'I felt that, whether or not it was in issue, the jury would want to know how far the law allowed the orthodox doctor to go in easing the passing. To ignore a natural curiosity may be to leave a puzzled jury and a puzzled jury may not be a good jury.'

Reggie did not bow out over the weekend, and on Monday morning, the eleventh day of the trial, Dr Douthwaite returned to the witness box so that Geoffrey Lawrence could re-question him, in the light of his changed mind about the murder period. Lawrence proceeded as though he could scarcely believe what Dr Douthwaite had done. Did Dr Douthwaite's theory have two limbs, he asked, the withdrawing of the morphia, then its reintroduction, followed by ever-increasing doses of morphia and heroin? Dr Douthwaite confirmed that this was now his firm position. Lawrence asked:

'Having started on this policy of reintroducing morphia, each single dose was given with the intention to terminate life?'

'Yes.'

'And because the earlier single injections had not succeeded in that, he went on with more single injections. Is that right?'

'Yes, he went on with more single injections.'

'Each one singly being intended to effect the purpose?'

'No. Each one was of lethal dosage, but I have never suggested that he expected any one of those immediately to produce death . . . within the next two or three hours. The whole thing was based on this mounting up of drugs in an individual who . . . was dying and, therefore, excreting or destroying the drugs in her body slowly.'

His answer being somewhat convoluted, Patrick Devlin intervened. Let us suppose, he suggested, that 3 grains of heroin was a fatal dose. Was it Dr Douthwaite's opinion that Dr Adams had refrained from giving one large lethal dose, 'perhaps because he thought: this is too large and may arouse suspicion'?

'Yes,' answered the doctor.

'And what he did was to give a series of doses over a period, the combined effect of which he knew would kill?'

'That is exactly what I meant, my lord,' said Dr Douthwaite.

Geoffrey Lawrence allowed himself a moment of abandonment, and described Dr Douthwaite's views as 'absolute rubbish'.

The judge intervened once more. He reminded Dr Douthwaite of the picture painted by the prosecution of Dr Adams as a legacy hunter, who had murdered Edith Morrell in order to gain from her will, who wanted her to die before she altered her will to cut him out of it. In the light of that portrayal, it was important to know how long Mrs Morrell could be expected to live anyway, without any murderous interference by her GP.

'I see your point, my lord,' said Dr Douthwaite, 'and I would say, as far as I can see from the medical picture, if I had seen her in October, I would have expected her to live only for a matter of a few weeks, probably not more than two months.'

So, as Dr Douthwaite stepped out of the witness box, the court was left with the implausible image of a GP who, according to the prosecution, had carried out a complicated and risky murder plan in order to speed up Mrs Morrell's death by a week or so. And all because he was worried that she might rally for a moment on her death-bed, and find the time to alter her will.

16

Other Opinions

THE SECOND EXPERT witness for the Crown was Dr Michael Ashby of 148 Harley Street, a consultant neurologist to five London hospitals. An eminent man, though – in every sense – not as elevated as Dr Douthwaite. In manner, he seemed 'serious . . . possibly both high-strung and controlled', a style that suited the drama of the trial, as it now fell to Dr Ashby to answer the question of the moment. Would he attempt to support the convoluted theories of Dr Douthwaite, or plough his own separate furrow? After the shambles of Dr Douthwaite, neither course seemed a particularly good option. The first path would commit the prosecution to an argument that was weak and open to attack; the second would mean division in the ranks.

Reggie rose for the examination, and began on an unexpected note. He intended questioning his witness, he said, with reference to some graphs that Dr Ashby had drawn, showing all the prescriptions written for Mrs Morrell during her last two weeks. The judge was astonished. He thought that the nurses' notebooks had rendered the prescriptions obsolete.

'I am not sure,' said Devlin, 'that I quite follow now what the prescriptions have to do with the case . . . are you suggesting, then, that all the quantities prescribed were given to Mrs Morrell?'

'Yes, my lord,' Reggie replied. He was relying on Dr Adams's statement to Superintendent Hannam that he had *used all* the drugs prescribed for Mrs Morrell, apart from a small amount left over when she died. The Attorney-General was not going to let this admission fade away – and he asked Dr Ashby to comment on his graphs.

The doctor told the court that, without a doubt, the levels of morphine and heroin prescribed for Mrs Morrell were enough to kill her. The fatal element, he said, was the very sudden increase in the doses in her final fortnight. A cancer patient might have been able to tolerate those amounts, if they had been built up gradually over a period of weeks – but with Mrs Morrell, the extraordinary doses came suddenly and that made them lethal.

He had no idea why she was on morphine in the first place, and was scornful of the proposition that Dr Adams was simply continuing the morphia treatment that Mrs Morrell had received in Cheshire. After Cheshire she had experienced no significant pain and 'just at the time when I should have thought the morphia should have been stopped or tailed off, it was instead doubled'. He had never, in all his experience, known a doctor to use heroin and morphia on a patient who was not suffering severe pain. And he was mystified by the later addition of ever greater amounts of heroin – 'the most dangerous drug of addiction known to man'.

The Attorney-General reminded Dr Ashby that Dr Adams had often visited Mrs Morrell, and been alone with her. On these occasions he had always asked Nurse Randall for a glass of hot water. What would that be for? 'To rinse out a syringe,' said Dr Ashby. 'I do not think it could be to rinse his thermometer, because hot water is dangerous to a thermometer.' Reggie's proposition was not declared, was not explicit, but was none the less obvious – Dr Adams's own injections accounted for the discrepancy between the prescriptions and the notebooks. After all, he could easily have helped himself to the drugs at Marden Ash since they were not kept under lock and key, but were in a drawer in the dining room.

For good measure, Reggie asked Dr Ashby his view on the

effect of the injections that were recorded in the notebooks, alone and without the extra amounts indicated in the prescriptions. The doctor replied that these would have been fatal because of the 'very sudden' increases in the doses, and the jerky spasms were significant because they were evidence of an excess of drugging. So far, all had gone reasonably well for the Crown. Dr Ashby had seen both the notebooks and the prescriptions as evidence of an intent to kill, though the jury was left with the peculiar notion of the notebooks recording a fatal dose, and the prescriptions being, somehow, more fatal.

Reggie now turned to the difficulty at the heart of the medical evidence – Dr Douthwaite's pronouncement that the temporary withdrawing of the morphia, and its subsequent reintroduction, could only be explained by an intent to kill. It quickly became clear that Dr Ashby was his own man, and was not prepared to follow Dr Douthwaite's lead. 'I must say that it had not crossed my mind that this was very sinister,' he said. And, once it was articulated, it seemed that disagreement was the best course. It disrupted the prosecution's line, but did not destroy it, since the two doctors agreed on the essential point – that the doses prescribed for, and received by, Mrs Morrell must have been designed to kill her.

Unlike Dr Douthwaite, Dr Ashby did not think that by 1 November 1950 Mrs Morrell was definitely dying. Even then, he thought, her prognosis may have been good, and it may have been possible to wean her off morphia and heroin. But, by her last five days, the point of no return had been reached. Her death, he thought, was largely the direct result of the drugs she received. But there was a second element at work – the fact that Mrs Morrell was constantly 'kept under' would accelerate her death. At this stage, it seemed that Dr Ashby had acquitted himself well, had been a credible and authoritative witness.

Geoffrey Lawrence rose for the cross-examination. Could Mrs Morrell's final deterioration, he asked, have been caused not by the drugs, but by a second stroke? Dr Ashby replied that this was possible. Lawrence asked whether the drugs given to Mrs Morrell in her final days might have been administered 'with the sole object of promoting her comfort', and Dr Ashby replied that this was 'one interpretation, certainly'. And, at the very end, the day of her death, said Lawrence, it was surely not possible to rule out that her death was due to natural causes.

Dr Ashby agreed: 'that cannot be ruled out'.

'And, if that were the case, the cause of death given by Dr Adams – cerebral thrombosis – may very well have been a quite honest entry by him?'

'Yes,' answered Dr Ashby, 'I think he could well have thought that that was the immediate cause of death, certainly. There is just no evidence at all as to what it was . . .'

When questioned by Patrick Devlin about the degree of doubt in his mind, he said it was impossible to rule out the possibility that Mrs Morrell had died a sudden death from natural causes – for example, she might have had a cerebral haemorrhage in the middle of the night. Such things happened with old ladies of 81.

The problem with Dr Douthwaite was that he had appeared to force the evidence to fit sinister theories. Along the way, he had grudgingly conceded that there could always be a 'difference of opinion'. As a prosecution witness, Dr Ashby was weak in a different way. He had his ideas and opinions, but undermined his own case with his startling eagerness to state that any number of alternative views were entirely possible. The judge was not impressed by either expert, and thought that 'barring accidents' the trial was all going Dr Adams's way.

The time had come for Geoffrey Lawrence to consolidate his advantage, to drive home the disarray in the prosecution's case, with the help of the witnesses for the defence. But, when he rose, instead of calling his first witness, he turned to address the judge, asking if he might make his point without the jury present. Devlin declined the request, so, in full view, Lawrence suggested that the Crown's evidence had not been sufficient to support a charge of murder, and he asked Patrick Devlin to stop the trial. In a speech that lasted nearly two hours he argued that, in effect, there was no case to answer. Devlin was not convinced. As he saw it, the prosecution's medical witnesses had been a disaster but they had both, at some point, said that Dr Adams had killed Mrs Morrell with the drugs he gave her, and must have intended to do so. The holes in their evidence should, he believed, be a matter not for him but for the jury – and he told Lawrence he would let the trial run its course.

Geoffrey Lawrence now informed Devlin that 'the defence have decided in the circumstances of this case *not* to call Dr Adams'. To the spectators, the decision seemed extraordinary. The medical evidence had left ample room for Dr Adams to argue that he was helping Mrs Morrell, not killing her. And, given that the prosecution case was crumbling, it seemed odd to choose an option that reflected so badly on the defendant. Although he had every right to remain silent, it gave the impression that he would damage his own case if questioned in court, that he had something to hide. The journalists who were watching were astounded, and Sybille Bedford wrote of 'the disturbance of a dozen and a half reporters stumbling over benches and each other to run the news to a telephone'. Patrick Devlin realised that Reggie, too, would have been surprised. Lawrence's decision 'to sacrifice his evidence', he wrote, 'was as disconcerting to an opponent as the unexpected sacrifice of the queen' in a game of chess.

It was Geoffrey Lawrence's weakest moment – suddenly his mastery of the courtroom had disappeared, and there was a gap where his star witness should be. After so much had gone his way, it was disconcerting to see him on the back foot. And it was disappointing that the jury and the press were deprived of the opportunity to hear Dr Adams account for himself. For two weeks, he had been such a massive presence in the court – his pink, bulky mass at the centre of things, his little eyes watching so attentively – and an inevitable curiosity had built. What would he sound like? The evidence had suggested so many options, maybe he would sound reasonable, compassionate even. Or, self-righteous and pompous, maybe downright evil. Or merely an idiot, a bungler.

The question would not be answered and in the absence of Dr Adams, attention now switched to a medical witness for the defence – Dr John Harman, another Harley Street man. Dr Harman was physician to three hospitals, the author of several scientific papers, and an expert on cerebral thrombosis in elderly people. 'Dr Harman is dark, well-built and fluent,' wrote Sybille Bedford, who thought him perfectly at home in the witness box, and considered his manner, by turns, airy, self-possessed and urbane. Lawrence began by securing from Dr Harman the assurance that he had a great deal of experience of patients like Mrs Morrell, who had suffered strokes:

'Does pain accompany or follow a stroke?' he asked.

'It does, but not usually . . . one does occasionally have to use morphine as a sedative in restless people who have had strokes.'

'Are you prepared, therefore, or not, to condemn the use of morphine in those circumstances?'

'I am certainly not prepared to condemn it.'

Sybille Bedford thought his answer came 'a shade too quickly'. Dr Harman said it had been perfectly normal for Dr Adams to continue the morphia treatment that Mrs Morrell had first received in Cheshire. The fact of him doubling the dose was not mentioned. As for the addition of heroin, Dr Harman admitted this was 'unusual'. Heroin, he told the court, was 'very calming', but did not send people to sleep.

'Do you see anything at all sinister in the introduction of heroin into this medication at that stage?'

'No, nothing at all sinister.'

'Or in its continued use at a level dosage as time went on?'

'None at all.'

Sybille Bedford found the doctor's style 'carefree rather than Olympian or dogmatic'. The witness, she wrote, 'has his own brand of certainty'.

Dr Harman raised his game. The increasing heroin doses, he thought, were a good thing. Without them, Mrs Morrell would have suffered unpleasant withdrawal symptoms. He had read the notebooks and thought it plain that the morphia and heroin mix was helping make the remainder of her life bearable, and were a suitable treatment for her bad temper and irritability.

'In practice,' asked Geoffrey Lawrence, 'have you known any doctor to prescribe heroin for a patient who was not in extreme pain?'

'Yes,' answered Dr Harman; he had done so himself.

Dr Harman thought it likely that Mrs Morrell's final deterioration was due to a second stroke, and not the drugs – though he could not be sure. On Dr Douthwaite's theory about the withdrawal and reintroduction of morphia, Dr Harman agreed with Dr Ashby, that it was 'of no particular significance'. And, on the increased doses of heroin and morphia in the final days, Dr Harman saw only 'that they were being given to stop her getting excited, to keep her peaceful', but in the end 'they were not working very effectively'.

As for the paraldehyde: 'it is agreed I think universally that it is quite the safest of the powerful hypnotics'. He was not alarmed by the large 5 cc syringes. This, he thought, was a moderate dose, and he added: 'I never give less than six.' According to the notebooks, death came quietly at two o'clock in the morning of 13 November 1950. Did Dr Harman think this was 'a morphine death'?

'No,' he replied, 'by far the commonest form of morphine death is death in a coma and from respiratory paralysis . . . and before respiration completely stops it is slowed, it becomes very slow. It may be only ten times or six times a minute.' This was at

odds with Mrs Morrell's respiratory rate, which was recorded as
50 – 'remarkably high'.

Dr Harman insisted that both Dr Douthwaite and Dr Ashby
had been wrong when they said that the morphia and heroin that
Mrs Morrell received in her last week would certainly kill her.
He had known other doctors give the drugs at these high doses,
he said, and it was almost impossible to pin down the concept of
a fatal dose because individuals varied so much in their tolerance
levels. Dr Douthwaite had said the doses given to Mrs Morrell at
the end were colossal and lethal. Dr Harman thought they were
not freak doses at all.

He told the court that he had used both heroin and morphia
for elderly patients with no severe pain, to treat restlessness and
'hopeless misery'. So, Dr Harman ended on a note of compassion. Doctors Douthwaite and Ashby had declared morphia and
heroin suitable only for physical pain, Dr Harman thought tor-
ment of the mind equally deserving of treatment with powerful
drugs. It was not hard to imagine that, had she been able to contribute to the debate, Edith Morrell would roll up her sleeve for
another injection, and give her vote to Dr Harman.

The Attorney-General rose for the cross-examination, all
thunder and disapproval, and began with a personal attack. Had
the witness ever actually been in general practice? Only for one
fortnight. Had he ever made any special study of heroin and
morphia? No, he had not.

'You are a recognised authority, are you not, on a disease
known as Q fever?' asked Reggie. (Q fever being obscure, and
irrelevant to the case.)

'I have described cases,' answered Dr Harman.

'And is Dr Douthwaite a recognised authority in relation to
heroin and morphia?'

'He is.'

Dr Harman's opinions, Reggie intimated, were of an inferior
quality to Dr Douthwaite's, and he suggested they had been

formulated on an incomplete source of information – the nurses' notebooks – with no regard for the prescriptions, and Dr Adams's admission to Herbert Hannam that he had used very nearly all the prescribed drugs on Mrs Morrell.

'Do doctors normally prescribe morphia and heroin for a patient without the intention of using them on the patient?' he asked.

'I should think not . . .'

Dr Harman had seen the prescriptions for Mrs Morrell's last five days, which made a total of some 39 grains (2,527 mg) of heroin and 41 (2,657 mg) of morphia, but he was 'very unwilling' to suggest what the effect might have been, had all the drugs been administered. Reggie pressed him. Dr Harman replied that it was certainly possible that Mrs Morrell would have survived the dosage. Reggie pressed further, and Dr Harman refined his position. Survival, he said, was possible, but not likely, in fact so unlikely that he would call it 'remarkable'.

'Would you,' asked Reggie, 'have expected the drugs to do Mrs Morrell any good?'

'They might have done,' replied Dr Harman.

Sybille Bedford thought his response 'rather cocky'.

'Do you think you would ever prescribe doses of that magnitude?' asked the Attorney-General.

'I don't think I would.'

'Did you hear Dr Douthwaite's evidence that in his opinion each one of those prescriptions, if administered . . . was a lethal dose?'

'I don't agree with that opinion.'

The Attorney-General now swooped on Dr Harman's lack of experience in treating drug addiction. He had, he admitted, only treated two cases – one morphia, one heroin.

Reggie was scathing: 'One heroin addict is not a very representative pattern, perhaps, on which to base a general opinion . . . How many years ago was that?'

Dr Harman said it was before the war, and he had not seen a case of heroin addiction since. However, he was very familiar with sedation of the elderly. Reggie reminded him that Mrs Morrell had been on a routine of morphia and heroin for two long years, and asked:

'What is the longest that you have kept anyone who has had a stroke under morphine and heroin?'

'I do not recall using morphine and heroin for a patient with a stroke.'

'Not one?'

Although he had treated hundreds of stroke patients over the years, it emerged that Dr Harman had never given any of them the cocktail of morphia and heroin that he deemed so appropriate for Mrs Morrell.

Reggie came to the paraldehyde, and Dr Harman stood fast, insisting that those last two injections had had no effect, and did not cause death. The Attorney-General hammered away at Dr Harman in pursuit of a different answer, but it did not come. On the high respiration rate, Reggie seemed at first to botch the questioning. The respiration rate of 50, he put it to Dr Harman, was consistent with Mrs Morrell's death being due to the injections of morphia and heroin.

'No,' answered Dr Harman, 'it is quite inconsistent.'

But, Reggie came back, the high respiration rate *was* consistent with Mrs Morrell's semi-comatose state. But, said Dr Harman, there was no semi-comatose state.

Reggie gathered himself:

'Never mind the notebooks, all the nurses had suggested a semi-comatose state. All had said that every time Mrs Morrell woke up she had been given another injection. And if the nurses were right about the semi-comatose state, then Dr Harman would surely not be surprised by the high respiration rate.

'No,' he conceded.

'Nor would you be surprised if that led to death, would you?'

'No, I would not.'

The acknowledgment was a small success for Reggie, but no more.

As Dr Harman stepped down from the witness box, the press-men and the jury waited to hear who else would be called for the defence. There were some obvious candidates. Mrs Morrell's son Claude, perhaps, would testify that Dr Adams had always shown great care when treating his mother. Dr Adams's partners, Doctors Snowball and Barkworth, might tell of his competence and conscientiousness as a GP. But, no. It soon became clear that Geoffrey Lawrence had no regiment of witnesses waiting in the wings. Dr Harman was the best he could offer.

17

Verdict

DURING THE THREE weeks of the trial, Geoffrey Lawrence had proved to be the better examiner – quick, clever and unsparing. He had given everything, and it was noticed that, by the end, he was utterly exhausted. On day fifteen, he made his closing speech, rallying for one final effort, and beginning with a reminder that it was 'most extraordinary' for a doctor to be accused of murdering a patient, particularly when she was dying already. He told the jury to find Dr Adams guilty only if they were sure beyond reasonable doubt: 'possibility of guilt is not enough, suspicion is not enough, probability is not enough, likelihood is not enough'.

The fact that Dr Adams had not entered the witness box, he said, should not be held against him. Think of 'the strain under which this professional man of middle years has been living for the past four or five months . . . in prison day-after-day, night-after-night, awaiting his trial . . .' Lawrence had wished to spare the doctor more 'human mental suffering' and the ordeal of being examined and cross-examined, especially since the events he would have to recall all happened so long ago. It sounded a little thin, since the opposite argument seemed a more obvious one: that after all he had endured, after the bombardment of allegations against him, the doctor would welcome his day in court, and the chance to speak in his own defence.

But, said Lawrence, there was one outstanding witness in the case, a witness 'both eloquent and unchallengeable in what he says, and that is the witness that is comprised in those eight note-books made by the nurses . . . when their memory was as fresh as paint and not trying to awaken something over which six years of oblivion had fallen'. Look at the question of the coma. The nurses remembered it. But the notebooks denied it, stating that during her last days Mrs Morrell was variously 'talkative', 'irrit-able' and 'wide awake'. The nurses had been wrong. And in a murder trial, the potential consequences of such mistakes were too terrible to contemplate. The notebooks must be trusted, not unreliable memories.

This was not about judging Dr Adams's professional compe-tence. If Dr Adams had used morphia and heroin in good faith, simply because he was an old-fashioned doctor, trained in the 1920s, then he might have been a bad doctor, the sort who were condemned by Dr Douthwaite and Dr Ashby. But that did not make him a murderer. Coming to the drug-drenched 'vital fort-night', Lawrence asked the jury to consider an old woman in the last days of her life, restless, wakeful, distressed, miserable through brain trouble. Is a doctor to say, 'I am not going to help you with any drugs'? Dr Adams, he suggested, had done the honourable thing. He did not stand back. He tried to help a distressed and dying old lady. And would a murderer have tried out variations of drugs, as Dr Adams did? Surely not – 'a murderer would have gone straight ahead with his fell purpose, would he not? – That is the dose. No need to change it. On and on and on with it. Bigger and bigger amounts. You see, you cannot make it square, can you, on evidence like that, with the suggestion that he is a murderer?'

Mrs Morrell was plainly close to death, he said, and the doctor gave her the safest hypnotic drug of all – paraldehyde. Nurse Randall had said: 'It was given to give her a good night. To give her sleep.' The object was to give Mrs Morrell a good night, not to kill her. And, according to Dr Harman, the amount Dr Adams gave her had been below the normal dose. Lawrence did not, of course, refer to the peculiarity of the missing smell.

He did spend some time on the muddled nature of Dr Douthwaite's evidence – and his on-the-hoof theory of the withdrawal and reintroduction of the morphia. The idea was 'quite mistaken and fallacious . . . an absolute absurdity'. And the other two doctors had not agreed with it, making 'his whole theory of murder come collapsing to the ground'.

As for motive: 'the prosecution have said that this was not only a murder, but it was a murder for gain. Sordid. Sordid and sinister. There has been no evidence at all to the effect that Dr Adams was short of money, but this was said to be a murder for gain.' But the motive evidence had imploded with all the talk of torn-up codicils and minor bequests, and the experts' view that Mrs Morrell was dying anyway. Murder for a legacy did not make any sense when, without bothering to kill Mrs Morrell, 'he could step back and let nature take its course'. And he urged the jury to remember the four nurses, the 'trained, experienced women who were there and under whose nose and eyes this murder was carried out'. None had been suspicious at the time. None had expressed any alarm when Mrs Morrell died. That, he thought, was one of the most significant features of the case.

He turned to Dr Adams's now-familiar words: 'easing the passing of a dying person is not all that wicked. She wanted to die. That can't be murder. It is impossible to accuse a doctor.' This comment surely supported the idea that Dr Adams had given drugs to make his dying patient comfortable, even though her life might be shortened. It was a world away from murder.

The prosecution had spoken darkly of the 'gratitude' of a patient towards a doctor who gave her morphia and heroin. At this point, Lawrence's anger infused his words. When a doctor tried to promote the comfort of a dying woman, gratitude would be completely normal. 'Are we to have all the decent emotions and responses of human relationships inverted, twisted and tainted' in support of a charge of murder?

He was nearly finished. The jury, he said, must make the right decision:

'It must be a memory that will rest with you for the rest of your lives. Let it not be a memory that will haunt your consciences that you did something wrong, or you might have done something wrong by condemning an innocent man . . . You will live with your consciences for the rest of your lives, and you will do your duty, I know.'

Lawrence had barely sat down, and Reggie Manningham-Buller was on his feet launching into an oration, pitched at 'solemn boom', and stressing 'duty' over the 'artifice of advocacy'. There were some pretty simple, straightforward questions the jury should ask themselves. Why, for instance, had Dr Adams put Mrs Morrell on a regime of morphia and heroin? Yes, she had received morphia in Cheshire, but not heroin. Even Dr Harman, who was 'an unsatisfactory witness', could suggest no reason for the heroin. So, 'why was Mrs Morrell made a drug addict by Dr Adams?' Could it have been that his intention was 'to make this elderly and rich lady, his patient, well disposed towards him with a view to benefiting under her will?'

He left the question hanging, and turned to the nurses' notebooks. Lawrence had said 'in these books lie the whole case'. But just suppose for a moment that Dr Adams 'had formed a design for murder'. If that were so, 'he would try, wouldn't he, so to arrange things that the entries in the books would not look too bad?' The nurses had never been in the room when Dr Adams gave Mrs Morrell injections. He was always alone, and the drugs he gave came from his doctor's bag. The notebooks gave no information about those injections. And whenever Dr Adams spent time alone with Mrs Morrell, he had always asked for a glass of hot water. This, according to Dr Ashby, was indicative of the use of a syringe.

Consider the 'very significant and important difference' between the doses recorded in the nurses' books and the prescriptions. *All* the prescriptions had been made up by the chemist, many had been sent to Marden Ash, and some had gone to Dr Adams at Kent Lodge. And Dr Adams had told the police 'all was given to the patient'. The evidence to be found in the notebooks was weighty enough, but the evidence based on the prescriptions was 'more weighty' and pointed conclusively to the guilt of Dr Adams.

Patrick Devlin listened to this with 'concealed amazement'. He was surprised that Reggie was still clinging to the notion that the prescriptions and not the notebooks were the vital record. There seemed no point in it. After all, Dr Douthwaite had said the doses recorded in the notebooks made death certain, so why bother with the shakier prescriptions evidence? Evidently, Reggie was wedded to the idea of presenting 'certain death' (the notebooks) and underscoring it with 'even more certain death' (the prescriptions). On this note, the court adjourned. It was a Friday night.

On Monday morning, Reggie came to the fatal fortnight, and Dr Douthwaite's first idea – that the doses administered from 8 November onwards signified an intention to kill. He had done his utmost to find an innocent explanation, but could not. Unlike Dr Harman, Dr Douthwaite was a great authority on morphia and heroin, and the members of the jury should give 'great weight' to Dr Douthwaite's opinion. He may have come up with his second idea rather late – the proposal that the 'design to murder' started on 1 November. But, Reggie stressed, Dr Douthwaite never changed his opinion as to the cause of death. The death was by drugging. The intent was to kill, whether or not that intent was formed on the 1st or 8th November. Dr Ashby had agreed that Mrs Morrell could not have survived the sedation of her last four days.

From 6 November onwards it was 'quite conclusive' that the policy was to keep Mrs Morrell drugged day and night, and the jerky spasms were due to the huge doses of heroin – both Dr

Douthwaite and Dr Ashby had said so. All the nurses had spoken of Mrs Morrell being in a coma, or semi-comatose state. The notebooks had recorded moments when Mrs Morrell woke up – but, whichever term you used, it was clear that she was generally in a 'heavily drugged sleep'. He described Mrs Morrell's last night, and Dr Adams arriving the following morning. He gave the cause of death – the immediate cause – as cerebral thrombosis. Why? When there was no indication of cerebral thrombosis?

The jury had heard all the evidence of the massive doses of heroin and morphia, of the jerky spasms and the paraldehyde just before Mrs Morrell's death. To ignore that evidence, said Reggie, and to say that death was due to natural causes would be to ignore the obvious: 'In my submission on the evidence, it is proved beyond reasonable doubt that the cause of Mrs Morrell's death was the administration of those drugs.'

Throughout the trial, the coolest head had seemed to belong to the judge, Patrick Devlin. His incisive interventions had suggested that in the tangle of medical evidence, in the morass of notebooks, prescriptions and injections, his vision was clear, his analysis sharp. In the pause before his summing up, a perfect silence settled on the room, and then he spoke.

His first directions to the jury were on matters of law. He made it clear that if Mrs Morrell was dying anyway, if her days were numbered, then it did not make murder any less of a crime: 'If her life was cut short by weeks or months it is just as much murder as if it was cut short by years.' Much discussion had taken place, he said, about whether doctors might be justified in administering drugs which would shorten life, either in the case of severe pain or helpless misery: 'It is my duty to tell you that the law knows of no special defence of this character.' No man, doctor or not, had the right to cut the thread of life. But that did not mean that a doctor attending to the dying had to calculate in minutes, or even days or weeks, the effect on a patient's life of the medicines which he administers, or else be in peril of a charge of murder. If a doctor is simply doing his job, 'he is entitled to do all that is proper and necessary to relieve pain and suffering, even if the measures he takes may incidentally shorten life'. The important word was 'incidentally'.

The second point of law was a blow for Reggie, who had fixated on 'prescriptions' over 'notebooks' to the end. Devlin told the jury they must look to the nurses' notebooks, and not the prescriptions, since there had been no evidence that the amount in the prescriptions had actually been administered (he dismissed Dr Adams's admission to Hannam as not 'true' or 'genuine'). So that was that. All Reggie's efforts on the subject had come to nothing.

For good measure, Devlin told the jury that he would have stopped the trial if the prosecution's case had depended entirely on the prescriptions, on the grounds that 'there was no evidence upon which you could properly return a verdict of guilty'. So the miraculous appearance of the notebooks, which had seemed so important to Geoffrey Lawrence and the defence, had, after all, turned out to be a lifeline for Reggie. The prosecution's case would have sunk without them.

He reminded the jury that the burden of proof should be 'beyond reasonable doubt'. Satisfaction on the balance of probabilities was not enough – which means that people 'who may probably be criminals, but cannot be shown to be beyond a reasonable doubt, go free . . .' And the jury must ask themselves 'whether it is likely that a doctor would murder his patient'. In this case, everything rested on the medical experts. For a guilty verdict, the jury should be entirely satisfied that the prosecution's medical evidence was right, and the defence's wrong.

On the facts, Devlin seemed sceptical of the prosecution's line about murder-for-money. He noted the twenty-month gap between the first heroin injections in July 1948, and Dr Adams's first attempt to get himself mentioned in Mrs Morrell's will in

March 1950. Then, after a two-year drugging campaign, all he got was 'the oak chest with the silver, value £276, compared with the £300 to the night nurse and £1,000 to the chauffeur'.

He suggested that the jury should *not* give undue weight to the whole period up until the final fortnight. Even then, the combination of Dr Adams drugging Mrs Morrell and wishing for a legacy did not necessarily make him a murderer. He might be a fraudulent rogue, but 'fraud and murder are poles apart', and the jury should be satisfied that a specific 'design for murder' was formed in the mind of the doctor. The paraldehyde, he thought, was a red herring – since, according to the prosecution, it only altered the time of death of Mrs Morrell by an hour or two.

He came to the 'essentials' in the case, and the need for the prosecution to show an act, or acts, of murder and an intention to kill. And the jury's view would have to rely on the medical evidence: 'It may be that it is very much more difficult for the Crown ever to prove that a doctor murders his patient than it is to prove other acts of murder.' None the less, the burden of proof remained the same. Devlin discouraged the jury from accepting Dr Douthwaite's theory about the dropping of the morphia, since the other doctors had disagreed with it. Dr Douthwaite and Dr Ashby, though, had agreed that the increasing doses from 8 November onwards amounted to a murderous act – this needed to be considered together with the defence argument that an old lady was dying of natural causes, and the large doses of drugs were a proper treatment. If those drugs 'eased the passing in the proper sense of the term', meaning that any acceleration of death was incidental – then that was not murder.

Dr Douthwaite was convinced that murder was the only medical explanation for the doses given to Mrs Morrell. That was clear enough. Dr Ashby was not so clear and the jury may think that he 'gave with one hand and took away with the other'. And it was with the image of Dr Ashby both giving and taking, that the day drew to a close.

The final day of the trial began with Patrick Devlin speaking of Dr Adams's state of mind. The jury would remember that Dr Douthwaite inferred from the drugs that the doctor must have intended to kill. He thought nobody could reasonably hold another view. But then Dr Harman had appeared, and said he did, in fact, disagree. So Dr Harman had destroyed Dr Douthwaite's testimony. If he could honestly disagree with the Douthwaite view, then so could Dr Adams.

Finally, 'You sit to answer one limited question: Has the prosecution satisfied you beyond reasonable doubt that Dr Adams murdered Mrs Morrell?' He made it clear that Dr Adams was within his rights to stay silent, and drew towards his close with the observation that 'this long process' was ending with the question with which it began: 'Murder? Can you prove it?' Sometimes, he said, he had told juries that he felt the prosecution's case to be strong and: 'I do not think, therefore, that I ought to hesitate to tell you in this case that here the case for the defence seems to me to be manifestly a strong one.'

But, he said, 'it is the same question in the end. It is always the same. Is the case for the Crown strong enough to carry conviction in your mind? It is your answer . . . It lies with you, the jury. Always with you.'

Patrick Devlin's summing up was in favour of an acquittal. He took the view that if the jury were to disagree with him and convict Dr Adams, their decision would not be seen as a rational outcome of the trial, but as a victory for pre-trial prejudice. While the jury deliberated, Devlin summoned Reggie Manningham-Buller and Geoffrey Lawrence to his rooms, to discuss what would happen regarding the second murder charge – the murder of Bobbie Hullett. Would Reggie and Lawrence like to proceed immediately? Devlin wrote that the Attorney-General looked 'glum' and Lawrence confessed that the strain of the trial had been very great, and he could not face another one straight away. The judge also recorded that the Lord Chief Justice, Rayner Goddard, had telephoned him to say, should Dr Adams be acquitted, he would be inclined to grant bail in respect of the second trial. Devlin was surprised – he had never heard of bail being granted in a murder case. Later, it was suggested that Rayner Goddard's view was tainted, as he had been seen dining with Roland Gwynne in Lewes in February. But, from Devlin's point of view, although bail would have been extremely unusual, it was justified.

After this short meeting, the lawyers returned to the court as, after just forty-six minutes, the jury had reached its verdict. Dr John Bodkin Adams was found not guilty of the murder of Mrs Morrell.

Patrick Devlin asked Reggie about the second indictment. 'I have most anxiously considered what course the Crown should pursue,' answered the Attorney-General. He then said that he would enter a *nolle prosequi*. Dr Adams was discharged. He was a free man.

The *nolle prosequi* was an extraordinary step. It was a legal instrument that could be used only by the Attorney-General, and was not intended for use in a court-of-law. Devlin thought Reggie was using it to cover up deficiencies in the Bobbie Hullett case, and wrote that the Attorney-General was respons-ible for an abuse of process. It left Dr Adams in a state of limbo – he had been charged with a murder that would never go to trial.

Not that he seemed to mind very much. He was free. 'Dr John Bodkin Adams stumbled from the dock of the Old Bailey yester-day with tears running down his cheeks ...' wrote Harry Longmuir of the *Daily Mirror*. 'Dr Adams stopped and pulled an apple from his pocket. He turned to the warder escorting him. "Now can I celebrate?" he asked. "Yes," said the warder. Dr Adams bit into the apple and munched, and new tears trickled down his face. He wiped his eyes and said, "I was never in any doubt about the verdict, I prayed every day . . ." [then] he ate the lunch he had ordered – lamb chops, boiled potatoes, greens and jelly. It was almost the same as the meal he ordered seventeen days ago, the day the trial began. It was the longest murder trial recorded in Britain.'

The doctor was now whisked off by Percy Hoskins of the *Daily Express* to a flat in Westgate on the north Kent coast. Another reporter and a photographer joined them, and the men spent three weeks at the flat, in secret, doing their own cooking and laundry, and spending their time recording the life story of Dr Adams, which was to be published in flashy instalments in the *Express*. This was Percy Hoskins's moment of triumph, and his reward. He had stood firm in support of the doctor, unshakeable in those moments when the rest of the press was derisive, certain of his folly. At times, his own colleagues had questioned his stand and seemed that they might ditch his line. But, in the end, the *Express* stuck by him and when the trial ended Hoskins received a telephone call from Lord Beaverbrook, with a succinct message. 'Percy,' he said, 'two men have been acquitted today. Adams and Hoskins.' On the day after the trial the *Express* printed a statement from the doctor saying: 'I feel I owe my rescue from the shadow of the gallows to three men.' These were Percy Hoskins, who had made a 'courageous stand against what must be the biggest witch-hunt in history', Edward Clarke of the Medical Defence Union, and also Geoffrey Lawrence. 'When I thanked him personally,' wrote Dr Adams, 'he said – "Your courage throughout has always enabled me to do my best."' (Lawrence said later that he never received any thanks from Dr Adams.)

These final words from the good doctor were typical of him. He was always quick to inform others of his own excellent qualities – his courage, his faith in God, his hard work, his humility. And, for those who thought him innocent, a little boasting was to be forgiven after such a shocking ordeal. But the end of the trial was not really the end of his story.

Afterwards questions were asked in the House of Commons about the role that the press had played. Politicians were critical of the lurid headlines that had suggested that Dr Adams was being investigated for 300 or even 400 deaths, the intimations that he was a Bluebeard like no other. The American magazine *Newsweek* earned particular opprobrium since in the middle of the trial it had published an article that linked the Dr Adams story with the gruesome John Haigh, the acid bath murderer, and also with John Reginald Christie. An injunction had resulted, temporarily halting the magazine's publication in Britain. The mighty *Daily Mail* and others were forced to back down and apologise to the doctor, who in the following months and years successfully brought thirteen libel cases.

On 24 April 1957, the *Medical Press* carried a long editorial lamenting the fact that the Dr Adams case had come to trial at all – based, as it seemed, on rumour alone. The consequences for patients would be greater suffering in their final days: 'Many a patient has been "kept under" at all costs to save him agony. This will, we imagine, scarcely be the case now, for every one of us will be looking over his shoulder for the smiler with the knife – somebody making notes to use against us later on.'

Questions were also asked about the Attorney-General's handling of the trial. It emerged that Reggie Manningham-Buller had not only bungled in court, he had also committed an act that left him open to charges that were worse than ineptitude. In November 1956 he had given Superintendent Hannam's highly confidential police report on Dr Adams to the secretary of the BMA – and the BMA had held on to it for several hours. Conspiracy theories were quick to grow up about the Attorney-General's action, suggesting that he was intentionally helping out the defence. It was argued that because Reggie was politically ambitious, and because he wanted the job of Lord Chief Justice, he was keen to please his political masters by placating the BMA, thus helping prevent doctors from leaving the NHS and bringing down the government. According to the theories, his misdeeds went further still – he had intentionally mismanaged the whole of Dr Adams's trial.

In truth, there was no conspiracy. Reggie was not corrupt, and the reality was that he wanted to win the trial – everything in the police and Home Office files points to that. His aim of becoming Lord Chief Justice (which he did not achieve) would have been better served by a magnificent performance at the Old Bailey than an incompetent one. And, in the files, there is to be found a perfectly believable explanation of his action, in his own words, in a letter to the Home Secretary. He thought that if the BMA saw the police files, it might be so struck by the severity of evidence against Dr Adams that it would lift its ban that prevented Eastbourne doctors from co-operating with the police. He was wrong – but his wrongheadedness was in pursuit of convicting Dr Adams, not acquitting him.

Other conspiracy theories were more ludicrous still – convoluted ideas that the doctor was let off because Harold Macmillan's wife was having an affair. She was the sister of the Duke of Devonshire who had once been the patient of Dr Adams – the suggestion being, that too close an investigation of Dr Adams would make the affair public. Another strand of thought was that the nurses' notebooks had been passed to Geoffrey Lawrence by Reggie or someone else on the prosecution's side. This is at odds with all the contemporary accounts. Dr Adams said that the notebooks had arrived anonymously at Kent Lodge in a brown paper parcel a couple of weeks after Mrs Morrell had died, and were put away in a drawer in his filing cabinet. Superintendent Hannam had failed to find them during his search on 24 November 1956, and later that night they had been recovered by Dr Adams himself, and Herbert James. Geoffrey Lawrence later told Patrick Devlin that, as he understood it, Dr Adams had actually opened the very drawer that contained the books in the presence of Superintendent Hannam, but the police officer had failed to notice them. It did not help Hannam that his warrant was to search Kent Lodge for dangerous drugs only, so he had no authority to remove anything else. Lawrence was certain that the books came to him via Herbert James.

As for Dr Adams, he had escaped a murder trial – but, none the less, it was felt that something had to be done about him. One of the first moves came from the Eastbourne Medical Society, which now threw him out on thirty-four votes to two. The sin that the Society cited was the doctor's engagement with 'unnecessary publicity' – a reference to the serialisation of his life story in the *Daily Express*. Dr Adams wrote in saying he had done his utmost to avoid publicity and had not personally benefited from it. He did not mention the £10,000 that the *Express* had paid him. On the other hand, he never spent or invested the money, which was found in an envelope, untouched, when he died.

Then, on 26 July 1957, Dr Adams appeared at the Sussex Assizes in Lewes where he was charged with a cluster of offences under the Forgery, Cremation and Dangerous Drugs Acts, including forging prescriptions and lying on cremation forms. The hearing allowed the papers one final spell of outrage. The front page of the *Daily Mirror* splashed with 'THE WEALTH OF DR ADAMS – Legacies brought him £30,000 in 10 years'. Superintendent Hannam appeared at the hearing to explain that the doctor's income from investments was around £2,000 a year with an additional £3,000 a year coming from legacies. Matters were concluded with Dr Adams being found guilty of the fourteen offences, and paying a fine of £2,400. On 10 September the Home Secretary, R. A. Butler, banned him from possessing or supplying any dangerous drugs, and on 27 November he was struck off the Medical Register by the General Medical Council.

Dr Adams, meanwhile, returned to Kent Lodge and Eastbourne life. Some said he was thick-skinned, others that he saw no reason to move. He believed himself innocent and vindicated. He regarded the forgery offences as technicalities – and at the General Medical Council his lawyer had made a spirited case that 'Dr Adams is not a wicked man. There is nothing in these charges to suggest he is.' So, self-righteous as ever and with a lot of free time to get through, he resumed his hobbies. Shooting took up much of his time, and in 1960 he shot for the English team in Belgium, though not particularly well. His shooting companions tended to regard him as a little eccentric, and not to dwell on his past 'troubles'. He travelled a good deal, sometimes taking cruises, and was a visitor to Reid's Hotel in Madeira. And he continued to keep company with elderly ladies. The author of *Doctor in the House*, Richard Gordon, once saw him in Torremolinos: 'Fat, chatty, jolly, beef-faced, moon spectacled, in a trilby hat, brim turned up all the way round, he busily organised bridge for the over-wintering widows who adored him . . . He had just been struck off, but he was having a wonderful time with the old ladies. He called them all "my dear", and they thought the world of him.'

At home, he continued to drive about in Bobbie Hullett's Rolls-Royce, and he kept his chauffeur, James White, who for several years maintained four cars as usual. But over time Dr Adams downscaled, and in the end he dispensed with the Rolls and instead made a modest Triumph Dolomite his main car. He maintained his friendship with Nora O'Hara – his former fiancée and the daughter of 'Eastbourne's wealthiest butcher'. They were often to be seen out together, at tea or dinner in Eastbourne hotels, and it was remarked upon that Nora was not the most sunny of companions, 'always telling him that he was dropping peas on the floor', or saying 'John, you're dribbling on your tie'.

Every year, Dr Adams petitioned the General Medical Council

asking to be reinstated on the register – and in 1961 he succeeded. He did not return to the NHS, but re-established a private practice that was smaller than before. The ban on his use of dangerous drugs, however, remained in force – meaning he was not allowed to prescribe morphine or heroin, though he could use his other favourite treatment – barbiturates.

They could not say so in public, but Superintendent Herbert Hannam and Detective Sergeant Charlie Hewett continued to believe that Dr Adams was a murderer who had escaped justice, and it seemed extraordinary that he was once again practising as a doctor. There was a school of thought, too, that the police had charged the doctor with the wrong offence and that a manslaughter charge would have been more successful. Many of the journalists who had covered the case agreed that, either way, the doctor should have been removed from general practice for good. Rodney Hallworth of the *Daily Mail* was one of them, and in the 1980s Hallworth joined forces with a reporter named Mark Williams to prepare the groundwork for a book about Dr Adams to be published after his death. With this in mind, Williams visited the doctor – who was now in his eighties – at Kent Lodge, on the pretext that he was writing an article about shooting (to keep his word, he did write something on the subject).

Dr Adams told Williams that he had a new 'Winchester over-and-under' gun, and said he would fetch it. When he returned, he began to demonstrate how to shoot the gun. Then, wrote Williams, 'Suddenly, he turned toward me, pointed the shotgun right between my eyes and slowly, deliberately pulled the trigger.' Why had the doctor done this extraordinary thing? Williams thought it was because he was a journalist: 'I truly believed John Bodkin Adams was capable of murder. I truly believed he had metaphorically shot me. I believed symbolically killing off all journalists, past and present.' His friends in the shooting world did not believe the reporter's story. None the less, they did repeat stories of the doctor's eccentricities – for instance, his recommendation to a friend that he perfect his shot by taking his gun to bed with him and aiming it at the picture rail.

At the age of 84 Dr Adams was frail, but still able to go clay pigeon shooting, and one day in July 1983 he was out shooting when he turned sharply and fell and broke his leg. He was taken to Eastbourne General Hospital where, three days later, he died from complications. For the press, all bets now were off – since he could no longer sue for libel – and in the week after his death all the old headlines resurfaced. 'BODKIN ADAMS: MASS KILLER OR INNOCENT?' asked Percy Hoskins's *Express* on 11 July, reporting the lawyer Melford Stevenson's comment that: 'If I had been allowed I could have successfully prosecuted Bodkin Adams for the murder of six people.' Herbert Hannam had died a few months earlier but Charlie Hewett, who had now achieved the rank of Superintendent, was still around to express his opinion, telling journalists that Dr Adams 'was as guilty as hell'.

The press turned up, en masse, at his funeral and heard Charles Aldous, a former mayor of Eastbourne, give a eulogy that drew attention to 'a vicious whispering campaign of rumour and vilification, engendered by those who had no knowledge whatsoever of the true man and his caring kindness'. The doctor's body was cremated in his home town and then his ashes were flown to Coleraine in Northern Ireland and buried at his parents' grave. Two months later, the details of his will were blasted all over the papers – Dr Adams had died an extraordinarily wealthy man. He had left more than £400,000, splitting his estate among a large number of people. The first to be mentioned was his old girlfriend Nora who, he said, could take any one possession of his that she wished to have. Nora was, in her own right, fantastically wealthy and so he did not leave her any of his fortune – which was divided between relatives and those friends who had stuck by him during his trial.

Among them was Percy Hoskins of the *Express*, who gave his legacy of £1,000 to charity – an act that was typical of the whole of the Dr Adams affair. Although in print Hoskins had been an ardent supporter, in practice he could not accept the doctor's gift. Just in case.

Afterwards

I HAVE READ the documents and written the story, and now it is time to reach a conclusion about Dr Adams. This is not an easy task and I confess this is not the final chapter that I had expected to write. I had thought that the police files would point clearly to one ending or another – mass murderer or wronged and innocent man. But that is not the case. The huge mass of evidence is of a murky, indistinct kind and I believe that it is impossible to say, beyond reasonable doubt, that Dr Adams was a prolific serial killer. In a court of law, he would most likely be acquitted not just of the murder of Edith Morrell, but of the others too – Clara Neil-Miller, Julia Bradnum, Annabella Kilgour, Harriet Hughes, Matilda Whitton, Jack and Bobbie Hullett. You could not lump them all together in a combined action – there were too many cremations and too few bodies, no damning post-mortems, and the circumstances were too variable. The Brides in the Bath approach would not work.

But, as Patrick Devlin said, the rigorous standards of the law mean that sometimes guilty men walk free. And it seems to me that, more than fifty years after all those deaths, it is sensible to judge Dr Adams by the less rigid standard generally applied to history – which is this: what do we think happened here, on a balance of probabilities, piecing together the jigsaw? And, with a view to casting my vote on that measure, I begin by consulting an expert witness of my own – Dr Richard Badcock, a psychiatrist who has thought deeply about what might drive a doctor to

kill his patients since a few years ago he spent many hours with
the infamous Dr Harold Shipman, who practised in Hyde,
Greater Manchester. It was Shipman's habit to turn up, unan-
nounced, at the home of a patient – usually an elderly woman
who thought he was attentive and kind, and who welcomed him
in. On some pretext, he would say he needed to give her an
injection, then he would inject into a vein a huge amount of
diamorphine. Death occurred within minutes, and Dr Shipman
would pack up his bag and leave. When called upon to fill in a
death certificate, his favourite cause of death was coronary
thrombosis. The evidence against him was overwhelming, and
there was no doubt at all that Shipman murdered more than 215
men and women in the decades until his arrest in 1998.

Dr Adams's relationship with morphine was different. His
sedation of patients often happened over a period of months, and
when he gave a single huge dose of morphine it was generally in
the muscle and not the vein, so would take hours rather than
minutes to have an effect. In character, though, there are striking
similarities between the two doctors. Both had preferred to work
alone, not in a team, and worked extremely long hours. Both
were dismissive and cold to nurses, and had a reputation for
being rude. Shipman's habit of turning up, out of the blue, to
check on a patient, was just like Dr Adams. Many doctors did
this from time to time, but Shipman and Dr Adams were unusual
in paying hundreds of visits to people who were perfectly well,
in no need of medical attention.

Shipman could seem to change his personality very quickly –
one minute being the kind, caring doctor, the next overbearing
and abrupt, particularly to relatives when someone had died. Dr
Adams was similar in his changes of attitude, suddenly becoming
angry if crossed, making jarring comments when someone died:
'Don't worry, you are mentioned in the will', or 'no need to
come to the funeral. She didn't want anyone there.' Shipman's
most noticeable characteristic was his supreme self-importance

and his egocentric nature. Dr Adams's arrogance was not always so blatant – but it was there all the same, thinly masked by ingratiating words and religious pronouncements. I was sure of the strength of these similarities, but less certain about their significance. So I posted my manuscript to Richard Badcock for a professional view. Then a few weeks later, on a bright November day, I took the train to Yorkshire to meet him.

He is recently retired from a post at Rampton secure hospital and now has more time for leisure pursuits, notably caravanning and Scottish country dancing. And, luckily for me, he has time to consider the case of Dr Adams. He begins by saying something that is clear and strong, and commands my full attention – namely, that he believes Dr Adams to be 'a straightforward psychopath', showing all the key characteristics of a psychopath. The doctor, he says, had a skewed conscience, demonstrated great egocentricity and did not learn from experience. From the beginning, he had an inflated sense of entitlement, encouraged by his mother and, over time, this simple quality became more complicated. Inside he was empty, and his life was being lived as though he were on the outside, looking in. 'I am pretty confident,' says Dr Badcock, 'that there was nothing inside him at all, in the ordinary human way.' He was fascinated by the lives of the well-to-do; theirs was the life he wanted for himself. But the key to Dr Adams is not money. It is social entry that drives him.

This is entirely as I would put it myself. As I have related this story, I have become convinced that the motive element drummed up by Reggie Manningham-Buller and the police was wrong. Dr Adams did not 'murder for money' and the notion that he was motivated by financial gain distorted the investigation and the trial. It made no sense for the doctor to murder someone for a legacy of £500 or £1,000. It was too big a risk for too little reward, and most of his patients were worth as much to him alive as dead. He did like the trappings of the social group that he wished to be part of – the smart clothes, the big house, the fleet of cars and the chauffeur. Above all, the Rolls-Royces – there was no better status symbol. But he could afford to buy them for himself – and when he took them from others, the reasons for his actions were complex ones.

Dr Badcock explains that a psychopath has a completely blurred boundary where possessions are concerned, and fails to distinguish between 'what is mine and what is yours'. For him, taking someone else's property is normal. This is intriguing. I have so often found Dr Adams's blatant covetousness perplexing. When he ordered that mackintosh on William Mawhood's account, it prompted the thought 'How could he do that! It's so brazen.' And the taking of Julia Thomas's typewriter when she was hours away from death made me think 'how grotesque' and how socially unacceptable to demand it, pick it up and walk off with it. There were so many examples like these of a complete disregard for social mores about ownership, for politeness, for respect for others.

There is another dimension to the taking of things – Dr Adams felt it was his right, his *due*, to have them. Actually, it went beyond that. Dr Badcock agrees that the doctor saw himself as a victim. He had a sense of grievance, and taking things helped him alleviate the associated misery. When he helped himself to William Mawhood's gold pencil, it was a small compensation for perceived injustice. The Mawhoods, he thought, should have given him *all* their money – he made that plain enough when William was dying. He was bitter and envious of the Mawhoods' lives, and wanted recompense. Similarly, when he ogled the chest of silver in Mrs Morrell's living room, it had nothing to do with desiring the chest itself – he had the money to buy a dozen of his own if he wished – and everything to do with the act of taking something from her. For a fleeting moment, he could experience the satisfaction of acquiring an element of the Morrell identity.

And taking things fits neatly with his need for an extraordinary amount of control over other people. He was endlessly telling others what to do – taking over his patients' finances, deciding where they should live, ordering them to re-write their wills. Dr Badcock interprets this sort of controlling behaviour as a way of avoiding the vulnerability and anxiety that come with normal relationships. But, he says, 'if you are permanently, successfully avoiding anxiety in this way – paradoxically, the anxiety tends to grow. The upshot is that the control needed to maintain the status quo takes on extreme forms. You have to prove to yourself that you have control.'

Of course, sedating someone into oblivion is a pretty extreme form of control, and I am reminded of the semi-comatose Margaret Pilling, whose relations tried to free her from Dr Adams's care – a challenge to his authority that resulted in a dramatic clash of wills. She must not be moved, he said. So they smuggled her out of Eastbourne without his knowledge. I think of another drugged lady, Agnes Pike. When his control was threatened by the introduction of Dr Philip Mathew, Dr Adams took the remarkable step of lunging at the patient with a syringe full of morphine with the nonsensical comment that 'she might be violent'. It was inexplicable, unless you consider the situation from the point of view of control. His command over Mrs Pike was threatened, and he reasserted it – rather desperately. I recall, also, his absolute fury in the Kenilworth Hotel when he was prevented from going upstairs to give Matilda Whitton an injection – throwing down his bag and slamming the door. And when the redoubtable Ethel Hunt said she did not need his financial advice he went berserk, slamming doors and telling her she was mentally deranged. 'Typical psychopath,' says Dr Badcock.

Anger is generally the result of some inner pain, and I read with interest an article called 'The Hidden Suffering of the Psychopath' in the *Psychiatric Times*. It is written by Dr Willem Martens, the director of the W. Kahn Institute of Theoretical Psychiatry and Neuroscience in the Netherlands, and argues that, despite their outward arrogance, psychopaths actually feel inferior and experience social isolation and loneliness. 'They believe that the whole world is against them, eventually becoming convinced that they deserve special privileges or rights to satisfy their desires.' He mentions two psychopathic serial killers – the British Dennis Nilsen and American Jeffrey Dahmer. Both killed young men, and each described 'their loneliness and social failures as unbearably painful', each was avenging experiences of rejection and humiliation. They said they did not enjoy killing for its own sake, but did it to have complete control over their victims.

People did describe Dr Adams as lonely. And it is evident from his life story that he struggled for acceptance and recognition, both at medical school where he had a breakdown and in Eastbourne where he was the outsider from Northern Ireland, never quite fitting in with the social set that he so admired. And, at the heart of his life, there was a complete absence of a sustaining relationship. No wife or partner. The only people who came close were his mother Ellen, 'the most religious woman in Ireland', who was said to be domineering and critical and, to a lesser degree, Nora O'Hara, a similar character, endlessly chastising and criticising. Dr Badcock raises another element that may have contributed to this inner misery – the moral judgement of him as a child. The story Dr Adams told of being punished by his father for refusing the offer of an apple from another boy is harsh, and makes no sense. Maybe, the whole of childhood was like that. The remedy for all of this was control. When he had it, he felt less pain. Maybe that control stopped at the heavy sedation of his patients. Or maybe it went further, and became murder.

The most thorough scrutiny of his behaviour remains that given to the Edith Morrell case and, weighing it all up, I believe this: that Dr Adams, who I now think of as a psychopath, drugged Mrs Morrell because he liked it when his old ladies, particularly the argumentative ones, were semi-comatose. His motivation was a wish to feel in control and to alleviate the pain of resentment and exclusion. He wanted Mrs Morrell's chest of silver and her Rolls-Royce because 'taking things' had become a compulsion, but these material things did not amount to a motive to kill. As time went on, he found that it took greater and greater amounts of morphine and heroin to keep the old lady under and at some point he wished to tip her over into death. There are records in the nurses' notebooks suggesting that occasional big injections may have been designed to do the job, but failed. It is quite possible, though entirely unprovable, that those last two injections, given by Nurse Randall, were not paraldehyde at all, but morphine. That would explain the mystery of the missing smell. Another doctor, Stephen Potts, has read my manuscript. 'You remember giving paraldehyde injections,' he says, 'if only for the powerful and distinctive smell of the stuff.'

Also, it seems to me that, on this lesser burden of proof, Reggie Manningham-Buller was right about the nurses' notebooks, and that they recorded the *minimum* amount of drugs that Mrs Morrell received, not the total. There was a moment in the trial when the Crown could have hammered the point home, but failed to do so. When Dr Vincent Harris was in the witness box it became clear that the notebooks failed to record at least eight of his twenty-eight visits to Mrs Morrell, so the actual visits were 40 per cent higher than the recorded ones – quite a margin of error, indicating that the notebooks were, in fact, far from being an infallible resource. And Mrs Morrell's prescriptions were all made up by the chemists of Eastbourne, all delivered to Mrs Morrell's house. Where did all that morphine and heroin end up? The nurses were not likely drug addicts and there was nothing to suggest that Dr Adams was an addict. By far the most likely recipient was Mrs Morrell. And the amount in the prescriptions was monumental, inexplicable and fatal. Doctors Douthwaite and Ashby said so. Even Dr Harman admitted that to survive those quantities would have been a 'remarkable' thing.

I consult Dr John Grenville, who was an expert witness to the Shipman Inquiry. He tells me that Dr Adams 'must have known that the amount of drugs that he prescribed for Mrs Morrell towards the end of her life would have killed her'. And, when he sees the information gathered by the police about Dr Adams's other patients, he comments that 'all this was so buried, so covered up'. The key problem with Shipman was that it never entered anybody's mind that he was behaving as he did. Had we known about the serious concern about Dr Adams's activities over twenty years 'such things might have entered people's minds a lot earlier in Shipman's career'.

As I see it, Dr Adams liked to preside over death. I think of Clara Neil-Miller, the old lady who died of pneumonia after he had her lying on a bed, naked, by an open window in February, while he sat in the room, watching and reading a book. No doctor has been able to suggest a legitimate reason for such a bizarre treatment. More likely, Dr Adams had decided that her time had come, and he was taking action to accelerate her death. I believe this. I believe too that he liked the feeling of control he had at the moment of death, and immediately afterwards. With Miss Neil-Miller, there was the collecting of his proceeds – in her case, £1,275. And he arranged her funeral and her grave, just as he had organised the funeral of her sister Hilda and dozens of other funerals. Maybe he was just very kind. But I do not think so, because there are too many examples of his explosive anger when someone rejected one of his 'acts of kindness' – declined his help with her finances, refused to move into the house he selected, did not allow him to arrange her will.

Many of Dr Adams's patients would have disagreed. They would praise him for the way in which he would turn out at any time of the day or night for a patient. They admired his willingness to give time to elderly patients who looked forward to his visits (it was the same with Harold Shipman). As Adams's great friend Herbert James had written, just before the trial: 'I have known him for thirty years and it is completely inconceivable to me that he could have done any of the acts alleged against him.' But I am struck too by the multitude of reports of malevolence – the descriptions of him as 'repulsive', 'a creeper', 'callous' and 'extremely abusive'. And, vengeful. In his earliest days in Eastbourne, he was in a rage when he prescribed 'sitting on a pail of hot water' for Elsie Muddell, because she had crossed him. By the 1950s, I believe, his vengeance had become extreme. In 1952, when Julia Thomas refused to let him manage her will and told him she would never leave him anything, he may well have smiled and kept up appearances. But within a fortnight he was giving her an injection for 'a good night's rest' after which she died. And, of course, he was taking her typewriter.

He did not think of himself as a murderer. The same was true of Shipman, whose self-image was as a superior, talented doctor. When the police confronted Shipman with the reality of his crimes, he either dismissed the evidence as wrong, or became a gibbering wreck for a brief moment, before recovering himself. In prison he resumed the role of doctor – holding surgeries for other inmates. Dr Adams's self-image was as a profoundly religious doctor. In jail he relied on religion to sustain him, speaking endlessly of God's will, consulting his Bible and praying. God, I think, helped Dr Adams's self-importance. What could be more elevated than doing God's work?

It was obvious that his show of piety was at odds with others' perception of him. Among the papers of Patrick Devlin are some notes that he made after dinner with Dr Adams's barrister, Geoffrey Lawrence, at the Savoy Grill on 26 July 1961, four years after the trial (Lawrence was now Chairman of the Bar Council). Devlin writes that Lawrence disliked Dr Adams very much and found him 'greedy, pig-headed, loquacious and dishonest'. Lawrence, according to the notes, did not call Dr Adams as a witness because of this dishonesty. Apart from anything else, he had been charging Mrs Morrell for visits he did not make. Also, his verbosity was an issue and there was a danger that he would say he had been 'easing the passing' of his patient. Patrick Devlin, in the end, thought of Dr Adams as a sort of 'mercenary mercy-killer', and considered two aspects of his personality particularly relevant – the fact that he thought lightly of the law, and his disposition to think of himself as in communication with God – a 'qualification for a certain sort of killer'. For me, 'control' remains the most potent factor.

There is one more element that, like everything else in the Dr Adams case, is highly suspicious but not conclusive. Taking a step back and looking at the long list compiled by the police of the deaths of patients in his care for the period 1946–July 1956 (see page 285), there are two outstanding features. First, the high number of deaths he put down to cerebral thrombosis or cerebral haemorrhage – 126 deaths, amounting to 42 per cent of all the deaths the doctor recorded. This is astronomical and impossible. These days about 7–8 per cent of all deaths are from those causes. And back in the late 1950s, among the elderly, the average figure would be around 14–17 per cent. Maybe the doctor was simply a poor diagnostician. Or maybe the explanation was more sinister. The pathologist, Francis Camps, regarded 163 deaths on the list as worthy of investigation – this being the very high number of patients who probably died while in a coma 'which could well be due to a narcotic or barbiturate'. It is a pity that the police were so obsessed by the motive of money and looked closely only at those cases in which Dr Adams was mentioned in a will. It might have been more fruitful to examine all those 'cerebral thrombosis' deaths. It is also worth noting that the total number of deaths was similar to that in Harold Shipman's practice – the size of the practice and the ages of their patients being alike. Maybe there are innocent reasons for the similarity of the death rates, but maybe not.

At the very least, Dr Adams was guilty of manslaughter in the case of Edith Morrell, and Bobbie Hullett too. The graver charge, of being a serial killer on an almighty scale, remains a matter of personal opinion. I think him guilty. But there is no single piece of compelling evidence. Just a mountain of suspicious circumstances.

Certifications of Death by Dr Adams, 1946–1956

1946

1.1.46
Louisa Gregory   60   Cerebral thrombosis   Home

17.1.46
Fanny Hansor   73   Myocardial failure   Home

20.1.46
Antonia Bevan-Williams 83   Myocardial failure   Home

27.1.46
John Holman   85   Chronic nephritis   Home

31.1.46
Mary Mouat   89   Cerebral thrombosis/burns of leg   Home

5.2.46
Martha Kember   72   Cerebral thrombosis   Home

17.2.46
Esther Jacobs   84   Nephritis/Diabetes   Home

18.2.46
Helen Hamilton   88   Coronary thrombosis   12 Grassington Rd

20.2.46
Ernest Sumpster   69   Cerebral thrombosis   Home

21.2.46
Rose Hunter   74   Carcinoma ventriculi   Home

9.3.46
Harriet Jones   91   Uraemia   Home

20.3.46
Emily Dawbarn   87   Gangrene of foot/   Home
                                 Senile arterial degeneration

26.3.46
William King   82   Uraemia/Nephritis   Home

3.4.46
Valerie Burnage   7 mths Acute nephritis   Home

3.4.46
Hannah Harris   77   Diabetic coma   Home

3.4.46
Kathleen Catt   55   Carcinoma of breast   Home

14.5.46
Robert Prendergast   81   Uraemia/Chronic nephritis   Home

3.6.46
Arthur Lovell   84   Myocardial failure   10 Wilmington Sq
Visitor

4.8.46
Gilbert Martin   88   Cerebral thrombosis   Home

5.8.46
Dora Turner   72   Cerebral thrombosis   Home

11.8.46
Harry Faldo   73   Cerebral thrombosis   Home

23.8.46
George Upsdell   60   Uraemia/Nephritis   12 Grassington Rd

24.8.46
Helen Walker   62   Carcinoma of uterine cervix   Home

27.9.46
Charlotte Armitage   82   Cerebral thrombosis   Home

27.9.46
Percy Cradock   73   Uraemia   Home

27.10.46
Esther Blanco   54   Uraemia/Nephritis   Home

31.10.46
Alice Thomson 94 Cerebral thrombosis 12 Grassington Rd

2.11.46
Adela Webb 75 Cerebral thrombosis Home

12.11.46
Elizabeth Hargroves 90 Myocardial failure Home

22.12.46
Emily Mortimer 75 Cerebral thrombosis Home

25.12.46
Agnes Rogers 67 Malignant ovarian cyst Esperance

1947

10.1.47
Maria Turton 87 Nephritis Home

10.1.47
Winifred Howden 79 Myocardial failure Home

23.1.47
Emma Lorden 74 Cerebral thrombosis 12 Grassington Rd

28.1.47
Julia Adams 71 Coronary thrombosis Home

10.2.47
Matilda Rendell 61 Cerebral thrombosis Home

20.2.47
Albert Fowler 74 Cerebral haemorrhage Home

20.2.47
Alice Ellison 71 Nephritis Wish Cottage, Kings Drive

23.2.47
Frederick Butler 76 Myocardial failure Home

3.3.47
Elizabeth Bucks 92 Cerebral thrombosis Highland NH

23.3.47
| Ethel Sidgreaves | 60 | Cerebral thrombosis | Landsdowne Hotel (res) |

26.4.47
| Edmund Peach | 54 | Uraemia | Home |

11.4.47
| Lily McKenzie | 72 | Cerebral thrombosis | Home |

22.4.47
| Angel Blanco | 57 | Cerebral thrombosis | 3 Upper Ave |

26.5.47
| Alexander Wilson | 67 | Myocardial failure | 12 Grassington Rd |

27.5.47
| Henry Popham | 95 | Uraemia | Home |

22.7.47
| Florence Mallett | 64 | Myocardial failure | Esperance |

8.8.47
| Annie Webster | 74 | Oedemia of lung/Nephritis | Home |

14.8.47
| Donald Middlemiss | 63 | Cerebral haemorrhage | Home |

30.8.47
| Cecilia Williams | 84 | Cerebral haemorrhage | Esperance |

26.9.47
| Arthur Starnes | 68 | Myocardial haemorrhage | Home |

23.10.47
| Minnie Marwick | 72 | Cerebral haemorrhage | Home |

4.11.47
| Arthur Stanley | 77 | Cerebral haemorrhage | Home |

8.11.47
| Jane Williams | 78 | Uraemia/Chronic nephritis | Home |

18.11.47
| William Barker | 77 | Uraemia/Acute nephritis | Home |

24.11.47
William Smith   75   Myocardial failure   Home

30.11.47
Ethel Redfern   58   Myocardial failure/   Princess Alice
Fibrotic infiltration of lung   Hospital

30.11.47
Frederick Smith   77   Carcinoma of lung   Home

7.12.47
Florence Newham   75   Cerebral haemorrhage/   Home
Cardio-vascular degeneration

15.12.47
Leslie Cockhead   86   Uraemia/Chronic nephritis   –

23.12.47
Agnes Lloyd   63   Aplastic pernicious anaemia   Esperance

1948

9.1.48
Norman Gow   69   Myocardial degeneration   Grand Hotel
Visitor

10.1.48
Ada Millard   78   Myocardial failure/   33 Jevington Gardens
Chronic nephritis

2.2.48
Ellen Reeve   76   Cerebral thrombosis   12 Grassington Rd
(res)

27.2.48
Edith Fletcher   58   Malignant ovarian cyst   Home

1.3.48
Robert Roylance   86   Uraemia/Chronic nephritis   Home

9.4.48
William Draper   55   Uraemia/Chronic nephritis   Home

14.4.48
Edith Billings   84   Pernicious anaemia   Home

14.4.48
Clare Cannon   84   Uraemia/Chronic nephritis   Home

27.4.48
Philip Christie   39   Cerebral thrombosis   Hom

11.5.48
Robert Leatham   62   Myocardial failure   Home

8.6.48
Peter Trusler   12 hrs Deformity – absence of cranial vault   Home

9.7.48
Jessie Stock   68   Cerebral haemorrhage   Esperance

20.7.48
Keble Highwood   71   Coronary thrombosis   Esperance

12.8.48
Thomas Crook   82   Carcinoma of rectum   Home

16.8.48
Jessie Bale   78   Cerebral thrombosis   Esperance

18.8.48
Olive Freebody   41   Cerebral haemorrhage   Southdown Hotel
Visitor

8.9.48
Ethel Jennings   68   Cerebral haemorrhage   Esperance

9.9.48
Stanley Katesmark   61   Myocardial failure   Home

1.10.48
Kate Williams   78   Cerebral thrombosis   Home

18.10.48
Frederick Fielding   84   Uraemia/Chronic nephritis   Home

12.11.48
Ellen Money   81   Cerebral thrombosis   12 Grassington Rd

17.11.48
Alfred Evans   78   Cerebral haemorrhage   Home

22.11.48
Mary Tite   86   Cerebral thrombosis   Home

23.11.48
Frank Strange   74   Cerebral thrombosis   Home

15.12.48
Gwendoline Price-Davies   78   Cardiac failure/   Redoubt NH
Cardio-vascular degeneration

21.12.48
Margaret Bush   85   Cerebral thrombosis   Home

24.12.48
Robert Morris   83   Myocardial failure/   Home
senile cardio-vascular degeneration

29.12.48
William Ovens   93   Uraemia/Chronic renal degeneration   Home

1949

6.1.49
Stephen Commons   40   Myocardial failure   19 Desmond Rd

13.1.49
Agnes King   77   Myocardial failure   Home

16.1.49
Edith Steward   87   Myocardial failure   Home

19.1.49
Kathleen Gilford   64   Cerebral thrombosis   Home

12.2.49
Cathreen Towner   81   Myocardial failure   31 Upland Rd

23.2.49
Ada Yates   86   Cerebral thrombosis   Home

2.3.49			
Selina Taylor	72	Cerebral haemorrhage	14 Enys Rd
8.3.49			
William Mawhood	89	Carcinoma recti	Home
17.3.49			
Marjorie Payne	63	Cerebral thrombosis	Olinda
31.3.49			
Lilian Gore	84	Myocardial failure	Home
14.4.49			
Mary Shotter	82	Cerebral thrombosis	Home
16.4.49			
Mary Cooper	85	Cerebral thrombosis	Home
18.4.49			
Guy Collier	74	Cholaemia/Fibrous degeneration of liver	Esperance
28.4.49			
Frank Cox Visitor	68	Myocardial degeneration	Queens Hotel
14.5.49			
Horatio Booty	85	Coronary thrombosis	Southdown Hotel
21.5.49			
Alexina Webb	80	Carcinoma of stomach	Olinda
2.6.49			
Albert Hollands	49	Coronary thrombosis	Cavendish Bowling Club
2.7.49			
Gladys Fawcus	62	Carcinoma of liver	Southfields
5.7.49			
Harold Braidwood	76	Cerebral thrombosis	Esperance
12.7.49			
Rebecca Shilton	80	Cardiac failure/Carcinoma of lungs/ Carcinoma of breast	Home

18.7.49
George Fielding   89   Cerebral thrombosis   Olinda

25.7.49
Fanny Grinyer   81   Cerebral haemorrhage   Home

20.8.49
Alexander Rennick   70   Uraemia/Sub acute nephritis   Olinda

28.9.49
John Bradshaw   83   Bulbar paralysis   Home

30.9.49
William Long   80   Cerebral thrombosis   Olinda

13.10.49
William Gover   86   Myocardial failure   Berrow East Home

15.10.49
Edgar Price-Jones   62   Carcinoma of caecum   Esperance

19.10.49
Annie Adams   75   Myocardial failure/Myocardial degeneration and high blood pressure   Home

22.10.49
Ruth Marshall   74   Myocardial failure   Home

25.10.49
Jane l'Anson Downs   71   Carcinoma of breast   Esperance

26.10.49
Eveline Richards   76   Cerebral thrombosis   Home

27.10.49
Edith Knight   86   Coronary thrombosis   Esperance

2.11.49
Alfred Chandler   58   Carcinoma of prostate   Home

7.11.49
Rosa Hamblin   82   Cerebral thrombosis   Tredegar

15.11.49
Ellen Thacker   82   Cerebral thrombosis   Home

19.11.49
Evelyn Pack   74   Cerebral haemorrhage   Tredegar

24.11.49
Ethel Chasey   68   Broncho pneumonia/Chronic   Home
                             bronchitis/Pulmonary fibrositis

13.12.49
Alice Jackson   86   Cerebral thrombosis   Hydro Hotel (res)

22.12.49
Andrew MacPerson   81   Coronary thrombosis   Home

24.12.49
Arthur Thompson   65   Pelvic sarcoma   Home

1950

25.1.50
Caroline Absale   83   Myocardial degeneration/Senility   Home

4.2.50
Matilda Tanner   69   Uraemia/Chronic interstitial nephritis   Home

18.2.50
Mary Price   91   Uraemia/Chronic interstitial nephritis   Home

23.2.50
Amy L'Anson Ware   76   Cerebral thrombosis/Cardio vasc degen   Home

3.3.50
Anne Molyneux   78   Cerebral thrombosis/Cardio vasc degen   Home

24.3.50
George Bristow   81   Cerebral thrombosis/Cardio vasc   Esperance
                             degen

30.3.50
Edith Eallace   78   Myocardial failure/Fibrosis of lungs/   Home
                             Phthisis

31.3.50
Eleanor Shaw   79   Cerebral thrombosis/Cardio vasc degen   Home

16.4.50
Rose Hawes   88   Cerebral thrombosis/Cardio vasc degen   Home

28.4.50
Annie Lennard   76   Cerebral thrombosis/Cardio vasc degen   Home

4.5.50
Raymond Knight   85   Myocardial failure/Cardio vasc degen   Home

20.7.50
Anne Pidgeon   57   Cerebral thrombosis   Olinda

30.7.50
Max Bickley (visitor)   86   Coronary thrombosis/   Cavendish Hotel
                                    Angina pectoris

1.8.50
Thomas Livesey   66   Uraemia/Cardio vasc degen   Olinda

8.8.50
Daniel Meakins   66   Uraemia/Chronic interstitial nephritis Home

21.8.50
Elizabeth Mesham   74   Cerebral thrombosis/Cardio vasc degen   Olinda

9.10.50
Edith Bowdler   91   Myocardial failure/Toxaemia of   Berrow
                                    gangrene foot

20.10.50
Robert Manser   81   Cerebral thrombosis   Home

29.10.50
Clara Ellison   75   Myocardial failure/Coronary   Mansion Hotel
                                    thrombosis

29.10.50
Florence Maitland   81   Cerebral haemorrhage   Esperance

13.11.50
Edith Morrell   81   Cerebral thrombosis   Home

26.11.50
Edward Cavendish,   55   Coronary thrombosis/Cardio   Home
Duke of Devonshire   vasc degen

5.12.50

| John Goulston | 77 | Uraemia/Carcinoma of prostate | Chatsworth Hotel |

13.12.50

| Dora Foster | 65 | Uraemia and cholaemia/ Carcinoma of descending colon | Home |

16.12.50

| Mary Sharp | 78 | Coronary thrombosis/Cardio vasc degen | Home |

26.12.50

| Annabella Kilgour | 89 | Cerebral thrombosis | Home |

31.12.50

| Beatrice Giles | 72 | Uraemia | Esperance |

1951

3.1.51

| Amy Manser | 82 | Uraemia/Sclerotic kidneys | Olinda |

7.1.51

| Charlotte Mendoza | 71 | Myocardial failure/Chronic bronchitis | Home |

11.1.51

| Percy Pound | 80 | Cerebral thrombosis/Cardio vasc degen | Home |

17.1.51

| Agnes Fox | 74 | Cerebral haemorrhage/Cardio vasc degen | Cumberland Hotel |

19.1.51

| William Waters | 73 | Myocardial failure/Cardio vasc degen | Home |

24.1.51

| Ethel Bates | 69 | Myocardial failure/Cardio vasc degen | Home |

5.2.51

| Dorothy Cave | 63 | Cerebral haemorrhage | Home |

6.2.51
Elizabeth Chilton   64   Pernicious anaemia   Home

13.2.51
Phoebe Wain   68   Cerebral thrombosis   47 Osborne Rd

16.2.51
Nancy Fawcitt   74   Diabetic coma   Esperance

16.2.51
Grace Levey   63   Coronary thrombosis/Cardio vasc   Home
                                 degen

19.3.51
Ellen Massey   91   Cerebral thrombosis   St Teresa

23.3.51
Olive Harrod   70   Cerebral thrombosis   Home

28.3.51
Cerise Meyer   70   Cerebral thrombosis/Paralysis   Home
                                 agitans

6.4.51
Edwin Robson   59   Coronary thrombosis   Esperance

7.4.51
Mary Prince   74   Cerebral thrombosis   Esperance

30.4.51
Richard Collings   86   Cerebral thrombosis   Home

14.5.51
Alice Lazenby   73   Myocardial failure   Home

20.5.51
Sidney Haynes   66   Myocardial failure/   Grand Hotel
                                 Fibrosis of lung   (permanent resident)

20.5.51
Theodora Hullett   67   Myocardial failure/High blood   Home
                                 pressure/Cardio vasc degen

29.6.51
Harry Hier-Davies   81   Cerebral thrombosis   Olinda

6.7.51
Adelaide Nash   69   Cerebral haemorrhage   Olinda

13.7.51
William Barrett   66   Coronary thrombosis   Sandhurst Hotel

13.7.51
William Hill   54   Carcinoma of rectum   Home

19.7.51
Laura Martindale-Vale 81   Cerebral thrombosis   Home

31.7.51
Leah Sugarman   52   Coronary thrombosis   Mansion Hotel (visitor)

12.8.51
Emily Lewin   78   Myocardial failure   Home

16.8.51
Ernest Ridpath   73   Cerebral thrombosis/   12 Grassington Rd
                              Cardio vasc degen

11.10.51
Maud Chesterman   76   Uraemia/Acute nephritis   Esperance

18.10.51
Mary Goodrich   65   Cerebral haemorrhage/   Olinda
                              Cardio vasc degen

7.11.51
Annie Bolton   70   Cerebral thrombosis/Cardio vasc degen Olinda

14.11.51
Ada Couper   85   Myocardial failure/Cardio vasc   Home
                              degen/Fractured neck

29.11.51
Harriet Hughes   66   Cerebral thrombosis/Cardio vasc degen   Home

3.12.51
Laura Brutton   78   Cerebral thrombosis/Cardio vasc   Olinda
                              degen

6.12.51
Helene Richards   66   Cholaemia/Fibrosis of liver   Home

16.12.51
Elizabeth Milsted   83   Cerebral thrombosis   Olinda

1952

2.1.52
Robert Angell   79   Coronary thrombosis   Olinda

19.1.52
Erna Kilburn   82   Carcinoma of stomach   Home

20.2.52
John Jackman   79   Coronary thrombosis/Cardio vasc degen Home

3.3.52
Henrietta Kelly   84   Uraemia/Cardiovascular   Sandhurst Hotel (res)
                             renal failure and degen

10.3.52
Bessie Day   68   Cerebral thrombosis/Cardio vasc degen Olinda

19.3.52
Edith Scott   79   Cerebral thrombosis/Cardio vasc degen Olinda

20.3.52
May Daniels   65   Carcinoma of lung/Carcinoma of breast Home

23.3.52
Cora Barr   73   Cerebral thrombosis/Cardio vasc degen Olinda

25.3.52
Susan Fletcher   86   Cerebral thrombosis/Cardio vasc degen Olinda

29.3.52
Mary Facer   82   Bulbar paralysis/Pontine haemorrhage   Berrow

10.4.52
Margaret Kite   75   Uraemia/Cardio vasc degen   Olinda

27.4.52
Alice Waters   77   Myocardial failure/Heartblock   Tredegar

10.5.52
Sarah Peerless   95   Cerebral thrombosis/Cardio vasc degen Home

Date	Name	Age	Cause	Place
27.5.52	Julia Bradnum	84	Cerebral haemorrhage/ Cardio vasc degen	Home
22.5.52	William Heap	78	Cholaemia/Primary carcinoma of liver	Home
9.6.52	Sarah Henry	51	Secondary carcinoma	Home
23.6.52	Annie Mayhew	88	Coronary thrombosis/Cardio vasc degen	Home
23.8.52	Alice Lindsay-Hogg	96	Scirrhous carcinoma of breast	Esperance
11.10.52	Edith Gower	62	Secondary carcinoma of lung/ Primary carcinoma of breast	19 Greys Rd
9.11.52	Annie Norton Dowding	79	Toxaemia/Carcinoma of sigmoid colon	Esperance
22.11.52	Julia Thomas	72	Cerebral thrombosis	Home
25.11.52	Ida Eatough	55	Myocardial failure/Cholaemia	Olinda
27.11.52	Annie Greem	90	Cerebral thrombosis	Home
28.11.52	Mary Macdonald	96	Cerebral thrombosis	Home
2.12.52	Sarah Tilley	97	Cerebral thrombosis	Home
12.12.52	Gertrude Clogg	74	Cerebral thrombosis	Olinda

1953

3.1.53
Brian Boehm   17   Acute myocarditis/Septic influensal   Home
                                     septicaemia

4.3.53
Harold Cooper   64   Cerebral haemorrhage/   Grand Hotel
                                     Cardio vasc degen

8.1.53
Annie Clemence   97   Myocardial failure/uraemia/   Manor Hall
                                     general arteric sclerosis

15.1.53
Hilda Neil-Miller   86   Cerebral thrombosis   Home

23.1.53
William Cooper   80   Myocardial failure/Cardio vasc degen   Home

21.1.53
Helen Soden   64   Uraemia/Chronic nephritis   Esperance

26.1.53
Clifford Lawrence   62   Cerebral haemorrhage   Victoria Court Hotel

9.2.53
John Haggar   81   Cerebral thrombosis   Home

9.2.53
Anne Macdonald   72   Coronary thrombosis   Olinda

15.2.53
Margaretta Armour   69   Coronary thrombosis   Home

19.2.53
Alice Richardson   80   Myocardial failure   Home

22.2.53
Robert Middleton   70   Myocardial failure/Cardio vasc degen   Home

27.2.53
Adelaide Nash   44   Acute and severe malsena/   4 Beslow Rd
                                     Sprue and macrocytic anaemia

23.3.53
Robert James   74   Uraemia/Renal sclerosis   Esperance

24.3.53
Florence Avann   66   Carcinoma of stomach   Home

11.5.53
Henry Clifford   86   Myocardial failure   4 Kings Ave

16.5.53
John Dear   82   Uraemia/Acute pyelitis   Home

19.7.53
Percy Morgan-Jones   79   Cerebral thrombosis/   Esperance
                                 Cardio vasc degen/Prostatectomy

20.7.53
Amelia Cawdron   77   Cerebral haemorrhage/   Edgehill
                                 Cardio vasc degen

5.8.53
Edward Dodd   56   Cerebral thrombosis/Cardio vasc   Olinda
                                 degen

12.8.53
Sarah Meade   74   Cerebral thrombosis/Cardio vasc degen Olinda

26.8.53
Louise Devis   62   Myocardial failure/Operation for   Esperance
                                 acute intestinal obstruction

28.8.53
John Anderson   82   Myocardial failure/Cardio vasc degen   Home

27.10.53
John Stephens   69   Myocardial failure/Chronic   Victoria Court
                                 bronchitis and asthma   Hotel

26.12.53
Constance Brierley   80   Uraemic coma/Chronic   Grand Hotel (res)
                                 nephritis and pyelitis

29.12.53
Clara Boles   85   Cerebral haemorrhage/   Manor Hall
                                 Cardio vasc degen

1954

21.1.54
Edgar Thomas   84   Cerebral thrombosis/   Chatsworth Hotel (res)
Cardio vasc degen

24.1.54
Daisy Gore-Browne   79   Cerebral thrombosis/   Esperance
Cardio vasc degen

9.2.54
Gertrude Nottidge   84   Cerebral thrombosis/Cardio vasc degen   Olinda

22.2.54
Clara Neil-Miller   87   Coronary thrombosis/Myocardial degen   Home

9.2.54
Harry Blagrove   74   Uraemia/Carcinoma of prostate   Home

25.2.54
William Hacker   74   Uraemia/Renal congestion/   Home
Cardio vasc degen

5.3.54
Cicely Hill   74   Cerebral haemorrhage   Esperance

8.4.54
Laura Haggar   77   Coronary thrombosis   Home

27.4.54
Ada Reader   85   Cerebral thrombosis   Home

9.5.54
Florence Cavill   86   Cerebral haemorrhage/Rupture of   Home
atherosclerotic blood vessel and
nephrosclerosis

3.6.54
Samuel Clark   87   Myocardial failure/Operation for   Esperance
acute intestinal obstruction

1.8.54
Jane Smith   78   Coronary thrombosis/Cardio vasc   Home
degen

2.8.54
Evelyn Tomlinson 75 Uraemia and cardio vasc degen/ Tredegar
Fracture of neck of femur

26.8.54
Walter Tomlinson 77 Coronary thrombosis/Cardio vasc degen Home

3.11.54
Edward Couper 93 Myocardial failure/Cardio vasc degen Home

18.11.54
Alan Gillies 68 Cholaemia/Fibrositis of liver Esperance

21.12.54
Sidney Prince 85 Cerebral thrombosis Home

22.12.54
Edith Holton 62 Diffuse carcinomatosis/Primary Esperance
in breast

31.12.54
Ellen Attfield 70 Cerebral haemorrhage/ Home
Cardio vasc degen

1955

6.1.55
Blanche Pechin 81 Diffuse carcinomatosis/ Hydro Hotel
Carcinoma left breast

13.1.55
George Osborn 82 Cerebral thrombosis/Cardio vasc degen Home

17.1.55
Florence Lennard 75 Coronary thrombosis/ Tredagar
Cardio vasc degen

14.2.55
Frank Avann 60 Cerebral haemorrhage/ Edgehill
Cardio vasc degen

19.2.55
Mary Edwards 86 Cerebral haemorrhage Home

9.4.55
George Blunt   Cerebral thrombosis/Atheosclerosis   Home

13.4.55
Mary Jackson   83   Cerebral thrombosis/Cardio vasc degen   Home

30.5.55
James Priestley Downs   88   Cerebral thrombosis/   Esperance
                                      Cardio vasc degen

2.5.55
Leslie Woolrych   69   Oedema of lung/Cerebral thrombosis   Home

6.7.55
George Smith   73   Coronary thrombosis   Esperance

16.7.55
Lily Wintle   70   Cerebral thrombosis/Cardio vasc degen   Home

24.7.55
Frances Payne   90   Cerebral thrombosis   Esperance

25.7.55
Annie Tanner   73   Coronary thrombosis   Home

27.7.55
John Tansley   91   Cerebral haemorrhage   Home

5.8.55
Dora Harris   91   Myocardial failure/Carcinoma of rectum Home

13.8.55
Arthur Dixon   82   Coronary thrombosis   Esperance

22.8.55
Edith Inman   67   Anaemia and asthenia/   Southfields
                                      Carcinoma of ovary

6.10.55
Mary Wheale   52   Coronary thrombosis   Southfields

24.11.55
Emily Dawson   78   Uraemia/Renal degen   Southfields

24.11.55
Roland Speed   68   Myocardial failure/Cardio vasc degen Tredegar

17.12.55
Constance Luard   74   Severe haematemesis/   Manor Hall
                                 cirrhosis of liver/cholaemia

25.12.55
Lionel Swift   78   Myocardial failure/   Highland Lodge
                                 Cardio vasc degen

1956

4.1.56
Henrietta Butler   82   Broncho-pneumonia/   Home
                                 Myocardial infarction/Advanced
                                 atherosclerosis and gallstones

6.1.56
Frederick Williams   88   Cerebral thrombosis/Cardio vasc   Home
                                 degen

13.1.56
Edward Henley   84   Uraemia/Cardio vasc degen   Manor Hall

4.2.56
Frank Stacey   73   Cerebral thrombosis   Home

8.2.56
Emily Goldsmith   82   Cerebral haemorrhage/   Home
                                 Cardio vasc degen

10.3.56
George Pearce   82   Cerebral thrombosis   Home

13.3.56
Ann Starr   84   Cerebral haemorrhage   Home

14.3.56
Alfred (Jack) Hullett   71   Cerebral haemorrhage   Home

15.3.56
Louisa Morgan-Jones   80   Cerebral thrombosis   Home

27.3.56
Henry Stokes   87   Uraemia coma/Renal degeneration   Home

24.4.56
Lilian Powell   70   Coronary thrombosis   Sandhurst Hotel

24.4.56
Margaret Smith   83   Cerebral thrombosis   Esperance

28.4.56
Joseph Cofman-Nicoresti 85   Coronary thrombosis   Home

21.6.56
Kate Wager   64   Coronary thrombosis   4 Southfields Rd

14.7.56
Constance Smith   82   Myocardial failure/   Chatsworth Hotel
                                      Carcinoma of descending colon

23.7.56
Gertrude (Bobbie) Hullett 50   Barbitone poisoning/suicide   Home

Acknowledgements

I WOULD LIKE to thank all the people who helped with the research for this book. The staff at the National Archives, the Newspaper Library at Colindale and the British Library were of great assistance, as were Jennifer Nash and her colleagues at the East Sussex Record Office.

I was granted permission to consult the archives of Dr Adams's solicitor and great friend, Herbert James, and I am particularly grateful for that. Also, I would like to thank Sarah Lutyens for allowing me to quote from Sybille Bedford's book *The Best We Can Do*. SB Publications of Seaford, East Sussex, kindly allowed me to quote from John Surtees's book *The Strange Case of Dr Bodkin Adams*. Extract from *Easing the Passing: The Trial of Dr John Bodkin Adams*, by Patrick Devlin, published by The Bodley Head. Copyright © Timothy and Matthew Devlin Trustees 1985. Reproduced by permission of Sheil Land Associates Ltd.

Special thanks go to Judith Hibbert, whose research skills are second to none and who traced numerous documents and people connected with the Dr Adams story. I would also like to thank Bobbie Hullett's daughter, Patricia Piper, and granddaughter, Judi Piper-Dadswell, for their help and their interest, and Iain Hannam for sharing memories of his grandfather, Herbert.

I am indebted to Francis FitzGibbon QC, who took the time to read my account of Dr Adams's trial, and to discuss it, and to the Home Office forensic pathologist Stuart Hamilton, who helped me understand the exhumation reports written by Francis

Camps. I am grateful to Dr John Grenville, medical expert for the Shipman Inquiry, who was happy to meet me to discuss Dr Adams's treatment of, and prescriptions for, his patients. Another expert, Dr Richard Badcock, was most generous with his time, and I was fascinated by his observations about both Harold Shipman and Dr Adams. Dr Stephen Potts of Edinburgh Royal Infirmary kindly read my manuscript, checking the medical details and sharing his interesting thoughts about Dr Adams's activities. In the early stages of my research Dr Raj Persaud shared some stimulating reflections on Dr Adams's character.

In the spring of 2011 Kate, Joan and Murray Stuart-Smith hosted a lunch to discuss Dr Adams, and invited Paul and Virginia Kennedy. Virginia is Patrick Devlin's daughter, and I am grateful for her invitation to visit Pewsey to see Lord Devlin's papers relating to the Dr Adams trial.

I would like to thank my agent Natasha Fairweather, and my editor Roland Philipps. Eleanor Birne at John Murray was the first champion of the Dr Adams proposal, and Juliet Brightmore sourced the pictures. Also, Caroline Westmore and Becky Walsh.

Boadicea Meath-Baker transcribed vast amounts of archive material, and Lucy Kellaway was a brilliant reader of my many drafts. Her ideas and suggestions were always right.

At home, Agnieszka Makar kept the show on the road, while Paula Sothern and Andy Banks provided a wonderful room in which to write. Carol Robins and her family were as supportive and inspirational as ever. And dear Tom McMahon was fabulous.

Photographic Sources

Getty Images: 3 below, 5 above, 8. Mirrorpix: 4 above. Rex Features: 4 below, 6 above and below left, 7 above and below right. TopFoto: 1 below, 2 below, 3 above, 5 centre and below, 6 below right, 7 below left. Private Collections: 1 above, 2 above, 3 above left.

Notes

Introduction

1 'unless it be the judge on his bench'. *The Lancet*, 25 March 1950. 'General Practice in England Today', Joseph S. Collings.

1 'economic destiny of other people'. Ibid.

Chapter 1

5 'wrap people around her little finger'. Interview Patricia Piper.

5 Family fortune had been sunk into mines in South Africa and lost there. Ibid.

7 'was absolutely like a person demented'. SPA 4/8/11, statement of Dr John Bodkin Adams, 26 July 1956.

8 'a flight from undue stress into unconsciousness'. *The Lancet*, 6 May 1922.

8 'vomiting usually ceases immediately and recovery quickly follows'. *The Lancet*, 8 April 1922.

9 'Another baby, rather than a new wireless, if it can be afforded, may effect a permanent cure'. *The Lancet*, 26 March 1938.

9 'utterly ashamed by the publicity, [and] broke down with jangled nerves'. *Daily Mirror*, 2 January 1950.

9 end of the holiday, she was 'wonderfully well'. MEPO 2/9785/2, further statements, statement of the Revd Harry Copsey, 24 July 1956.

11 a solarium and a terrace that had a fabulous view over the sea. Hoskins, p. 11.

10 was reputed to earn more than £60,000 a year. Hoskins, p. 15.

10 'Both Mr and Mrs Hullett thought there was nobody like him'. MEPO 2/9784, statement of Nellie Caton.

11 at the Grand Hotel on Saturday nights. SPA 4/8/11, statement of Dr John Bodkin Adams, 26 July 1956.

11 'There is no reason why you shouldn't go together'. Ibid.

11 'I shall probably shock Eastbourne, but I don't care'. MEPO 2/9785/2, further statements, statement of Hugh Hubbard Ford, 29 July 1956.

11 though she found Jack an odd old man. Interview Patricia Piper.

11 'South Africa the next year, New Zealand another year . . .' MEPO 2/9785/2, further statements, statement of Hugh Ford, 29 July 1956.

11 'He said: "That's true, you are right"'. SPA 4/8/11, statement of Dr John Bodkin Adams, 26 July 1956.

12 'and I treated him for various functional nervous illnesses'. Ibid.

12 '"why didn't you get a London man?"'. Ibid.

13 'These doctors have murdered me!' MEPO 2/9785/2, further statements, statement of Hugh Ford, 29 July 1956.

13 'we got him through and out of danger'. SPA 4/8/11, statement of Dr John Bodkin Adams, 26 July 1956.

13 also for falling asleep during operations. Surtees, p. 19.

13 'a great state of agitation – half hysterics'. SPA 4/8/11, statement of Dr John Bodkin Adams, 26 July 1956.

14 'as she seemed so relieved at every sign of recovering good health'. MEPO 2/9785/2, further statements, statement of Hugh Ford, 29 July 1956.

14 and repeated high doses of barbiturates, as well as morphine and heroin. MEPO 2/9785/2, extracts from chemists registers.

14 such a rebuff from the doctor that she never asked him again. MEPO 2/9784, report of Superintendent Hannam, 16 October 1956.

15 'I am too full of dope to say anything sensible'. MEPO 2/9785/2, further statements, statement of Hugh Ford, 29 July 1956.

15 He could die suddenly, at any time. MEPO 2/9785/2, further statements, statement of Roy Campbell Price.

15 insinuated strongly that it had been brought on by Dr Adams. MEPO 2/9784, report of Superintendent Hannam, 16 October 1956.

16 'a type which contains a highly-concentrated form of morphia . . .' MEPO 2/9785/2, statement of Gladys Miller, 11 September 1956.

16 '"He complained of a headache last night"'. MEPO 2/9785/2. Ibid.

16 'I thought his death was unusual'. MEPO 2/9785/2. Ibid.

17 'Then she became quite impossible'. SPA 4/8/11, statement of Dr John Bodkin Adams, 26 July 1956.

17 parlourmaid Mary Mayo told the housemaid Teresa Yogna. MEPO 2/9785/2, further statements, statement of Teresa Yogna, 16 March 1957.

17 'in bed, prostrate'. MEPO 2/9784, statement of Harriet Martha Henson, 6 August 1956.

17 but Bobbie was too distressed to attend. Ibid.

17 'She looked awful and gradually, from March, got so thin'. MEPO 2/9785/2, further statements, statement of Evelyn Patricia Tomlinson, 26 July 1956.

17 'She seemed to be holding herself in'. MEPO 2/9785/2, further statements, statement of Kathleen Durrant.

18 'she was in a very distressed frame of mind'. MEPO 2/9785/2, further statements, statement of Hugh Hubbard Ford, 29 July 1956.

18 she was in an 'overwrought and nervous state'. SPA 4/8/11, statement of John Sherwood Dodd, 24 July 1956.

18 'How strange she was in her behaviour and what an anxiety it was to him . . .' MEPO 2/9785/2, further statements, statement of Hugh Hubbard Ford, 29 July 1956.

18 'she seemed to be under the influence of some sort of drug'. Ibid.

18 he tried reducing the dose to two 5-grain tablets, or sometimes 6. SPA 4/8/11, statement of Dr John Bodkin Adams, 26 July 1956.

18 sometimes she gave herself injections. MEPO 2/9784, statement of Harriet Martha Henson, 6 August 1956.

19 Bobbie told him that he had given her an injection. MEPO 2/9785/2, further statements, statement of William Galloway, 28 December 1956.

19 no 'ampules, cotton wool or anything that I expected to see . . .' MEPO 2/9785/2, further statements, statements of Teresa Yogna and Celia Mary Mayo.

19 'she felt as if the floor was coming up to her'. MEPO 2/9785/2, further statements, statement of Evelyn Patricia Tomlinson, 26 July 1956.

19 shortly afterwards she 'became pale and shrunken'. MEPO 2/9785/2, further statements, statement of the Revd Harry Copsey, 24 July 1956.

19 The Bishop, who knew Bobbie, 'was very distressed at her condition'. Ibid.

19 'leaning against the wall for support'. MEPO 9/9785/2, further statements, statement of Teresa Yogna, 16 March 1957.

20 Bobbie should get away from Eastbourne, and from the care of Dr Adams. MEPO 2/9785/2, further statements, statements of Teresa Yogna, Celia Mary Mayo and Kathleen Durrant, MEPO 2/9784, statement of Harriet Martha Henson, 6 August 1956.

20 'gossip in Eastbourne that Mrs Hullett was being drugged'. MEPO 2/9784, statement of Harriet Martha Henson, 6 August 1956.

20 'she became rather absent minded and . . . was forgetting things'. MEPO 2/9785/2, further statements, statement of Teresa Yogna, 16 March 1957.

20 'she was rather heavily doped for the occasion'. MEPO 2/9785/2, further statements, statement of Hugh Hubbard Ford, 29 July 1956.

20 'appeared as well as I have ever known her'. MEPO 2/9785/2, further statements, statement of the Revd Harry Copsey, 24 July 1956.

20 'She had no interest at all in life'. MEPO 2/9785/2, further statements, statement of Gertrude Patty Leefe.

21 But Bobbie would not listen. Interview Patricia Piper.

21 'I wasn't very effective in my arguments'. MEPO 2/9785/2, statement of Hugh Hubbard Ford, 29 July 1956.

21 'put me out of the way'. MEPO 2/9785/2, further statements, statement of the Revd Harry Copsey, 24 July 1956.

21 'pull yourself together'. SPA 4/8/11, statement of Dr John Bodkin Adams, 26 July 1956.

22 'that was the only one she thought of'. Ibid.

22 'she was more cheerful and more natural'. SPA 4/8/11, statement of John Sherwood Dodd, 24 July 1956.

22 Rolls-Royce Silver Dawn, worth close to £3,000. MEPO 2/9785/2, further statements, statement of Reginald Matthews, 8 March 1957.

22 describe her condition as a 'nerve storm'. SPA 4/8/11, statement of Dr John Bodkin Adams, 26 July 1956.

22 she appeared 'cheerful and natural' again. SPA 4/8/11, statement of John Sherwood Dodd, 24 July 1956.

22 'a person who has come to a decision about something'. MEPO 2/9785/2, further statements, statement of Percy Robert Handscomb, 24 July 1956.

23 wrote him a cheque for £1,000. MEPO 2/9784, report of Superintendent Hannam, 16 October 1956.

23 'This lady is not long for this world'. Surtees, p. 49.

23 'her rotting body coming in about four days after'. SPA 4/8/11, statement of Dr John Bodkin Adams, 26 July 1956.

24 reassured her that she would look after Bobbie. MEPO 2/9785/2, further statements, statement of Kathleen Reed, 17 March 1957. Interview Patricia Piper.

24 'she took nothing with it. No tablet or anything'. MEPO 2/9785/2, further statements, statement of Celia Mary Mayo.

25 the two women decided to telephone the doctor. MEPO 2/9785/2, further statements, statement of Celia Mary Mayo and Kathleen Reed.

26 It was she and Kathleen Reed who suggested that a locum come. Ibid.

26 Dr Adams said that it was *his* suggestion. SPA 4/8/11, statement of Dr John Bodkin Adams, 26 July 1956.

26 nothing wrong with her breathing or circulation. MEPO 2/9785/2, further statements, statement of Dr Ronald Vincent Harris, 29 July 1956.

26 she understood that Bobbie received sleeping tablets from Dr Adams. Ibid.

27 'I don't know where she got them from and I am not touching anything'. MEPO 2/9785/2, statement of Kathleen Reed, 17 March 1957.

27 her respiration being 'regular and normal'. SPA 4/8/11, statement of Dr John Bodkin Adams, 26 July 1956.

28 'she had been so miserable and unhappy'. MEPO 2/9785/2, further statements, statement of Evelyn Patricia Tomlinson, 26 July 1956.

28 she completely trusted him. Interview Patricia Piper.

28 she must not be moved 'because of her heart condition'. SPA 4/8/11, statement of Agnes Higgins, 27 July 1956.

29 a stimulant that could be used to counteract the effects of barbiturates. Ibid.

29 then 'there would be little chance of recovery'. SPA 4/8/11, statement of John Dodd, 24 July 1956.

29 her chances of survival, overall, were fifty-fifty. MEPO 2/9785/2, further statements, statement of Hugh Hubbard Ford, 29 July 1956.

29 'Never remove me to Esperance [Nursing Home] or hospital whatever may be my condition'. SPA 4/8/11, statement of Dr John Bodkin Adams, 26 July 1956.

29 it was not urgent, and said 'Monday will do'. MEPO 2/9785/2, further statements, statement of Albert Newman, 2 January 1957. MEPO 2/9785/2, further statements, statement of Reginald Hudson, 11 January 1957.

30 'very slowly in doses of 10 ml every five minutes'. MEPO 2/9785/2, further statements, statement of Dr Peter Cook, 11 January 1957.

30 the weekend at the Princess Alice, but she never came. Surtees, p. 50.

30 gave Bobbie 10 ml of the Megimide intravenously, and then no more. SPA 4/8/11, statement of Dr John Bodkin Adams, 26 July 1956.

30 'It must be because of the temperature'. SPA 4/8/11, statement of Agnes Higgins, 27 July 1956.

30 she and Dr Adams both thought she would die that day. Ibid.

31 and notify the coroner's office then. MEPO 2/9785/2, further statements, statement of Angus Sommerville, 8 January 1957.

31 oxygen had no effect, and Bobbie deteriorated further. SPA 4/8/11, statement of Agnes Higgins, 27 July 1956.

31 'I realised then that I had expected it really in a way since Friday'. MEPO 2/9785/2, further statements, statement by Evelyn Patricia Tomlinson, 26 July 1956.

Chapter 2

33 cheerful, prayerful, honest, fearless, determined? Hoskins, p. 7.

33 'One Day, One Step'. Ibid.

34 'then it would have had a grave influence on my future life'. *Daily Express*, 15 April 1957.

34 'the most religious woman in Ireland'. *Sunday Express*, 10 October 1965.

34 'very popular and was known to be a good man'. Hallworth, p. 18.

34 'with fine views over Loch Neagh to the mountains beyond'. Ibid.

35 that John was 'a wee bit mean'. Ibid., p. 19.

35 'gambling in every form knowing this to be the wishes of my father and mother . . .' *Daily Express*, 15 April 1957.

36 first with one group and then another. Hallworth, p. 21.

36 'virulent septic infection'. *Daily Express*, 15 April 1957.

36 they advised that he give up medicine altogether. Ibid.

38 'in the spring of 1922 – I went to Eastbourne'. Ibid.

39 the composer Edward Elgar, and the aviator Amy Johnson. Pugh, pp. 82–3.

39 'and made a full recovery'. Surtees, p. 12.

40 he set up the Eastbourne branch of the Young Crusaders Bible Class. Hoskins, p. 7.

40 'gardens, park and woodlands'. Prospectus for the sale of Ratton, 1923.

41 it never mended properly despite three operations on it. SPA 4/8/11, statement of Edith May Mawhood, 4 September 1956.

42 'The servants always provided tea for all of them'. Ibid.

42 she loaned him some of her husband's pyjamas. Ibid.

43 he did the same thing again – this time with a new pair of boots. Ibid.

43 specially customised chassis for carrying medical equipment. Hoskins, p. 8.

43 'frequently changing the make of cars he used'. SPA 4/8/11–51, statement of David George Jenkins, 29 September 1956.

44 owned a Daimler car and had her own chauffeur. Ibid.

44 his fishing rods, golf clubs and cameras. Hoskins, p. 8, MEPO 2/9784, report of Superintendent Hannam, 16 October 1956.

44 he did, in this case, pay up what was owed to her. SPA 4/8/11, statement of Edith May Mawhood, 4 September 1956.

44 'I always put people against Dr Adams whenever I could'. SPA 4/8/11, 35 Notes of Detective Sergeant Sellors's conversation with Elsie Margaret Muddell, 27 August 1956.

45 'he still persisted and continued to make the arrangements . . .' SPA 4/8/11-24, statement of Mrs Eva Hope Carlyle, 20 September 1956.

46 and found that his efforts had been frustrated, he became 'very annoyed'. SPA 4/8/11-34, statement of Elsie Orange Randall, 20 September 1956, MEPO 2/9784, report of Superintendent Hannam, 16 October 1956.

46 *The Financial Times*, Rand Mines and Imperial Tobacco. ACC 6011, papers relating to Matilda Whitton.

46 Northampton on business trips or to see her friends there. MEPO 2/9784, report of Superintendent Hannam, 16 October 1956.

47 she had given it to the doctor as a gift. Ibid.

47 a second car – this one brand new. SPA 4/8/11, statement of Beryl Dorothea Buck, 5 September 1956.

47 'many days, and sometimes weeks, in bed'. MEPO 2/9784, report of Superintendent Hannam, 16 October 1956.

47 'holding the patient's hand or with his hand on her knees'. Ibid.

47 'she thought Dr Adams would marry her'. SPA 4/8/11, statement of Beryl Dorothea Buck, 4 September 1956.

47 'arranging her affairs and helping with her investments'. Ibid.

48 she signed the new will. ACC 6011, papers relating to Matilda Whitton.

48 'would be up most of the time'. SPA 4/8/11, statement of Elsie Gander, 29 August 1956.

48 'whether she was ill in Northampton'. MEPO 2/9784, statement of Lucy Maud Atkins, 7 September 1956.

48 prescriptions were of a 'hypnotic sedative type'. MEPO 2/9784, report of Superintendent Hannam, 16 October 1956.

48 'she thought the injections upset her'. SPA 4/8/11, statement of Beryl Dorothea Buck, 4 September 1956.

49 'he grabbed his coat, went out and really slammed the door'. Ibid., MEPO 2/9784, report of Superintendent Hannam, 16 October 1956.

49 he replied that she had no relatives. MEPO 2/9784, report of Superintendent Hannam, 16 October 1956.

50 'notified the doctor, but before he arrived she was dead'. MEPO 2/9784, statement of Bridget Monnolly, 13 December 1956.

50 'high blood pressure, renal insufficiency'. Hoskins, p. 11, MEPO 2/9784, report of Superintendent Hannam, 16 October 1956.

50 a bottle of Mrs Whitton's pills in his pocket. SPA 4/8/11, statement of Elsie Gander, 29 August 1956.

50 and told her to keep the death quiet. Ibid.

50 along with a small attaché case. MEPO 2/9784, statement of
Bridget Monnolly, 13 December 1956.

50 five massage treatments and seven electrical treatments. ACC
6011, papers relating to Matilda Whitton.

51 was soon sold off by Dr Adams. MEPO 2/9784, statement of
Emma Benson, 27 October 1956.

51 He tore it up and threw it in the wastepaper basket. Hoskins,
p. 10.

Chapter 3

52 Charbonnel et Walker of Old Bond Street in London. ACC
6011, accounts of Dr John Bodkin Adams.

53 sometimes he accompanied him on holidays. MEPO 2/9784,
report of Superintendent Hannam, 16 October 1956.

53 'daughter of Eastbourne's wealthiest butcher'. Hallworth,
p. 24.

53 a house in Carew Road, Eastbourne. ACC 6011, papers relating
the sale of 42 Carew Road.

53 rent out his chauffeur to her at 10 shillings a time. ACC 6011,
accounts of Dr John Bodkin Adams.

54 'do not feel in a position to issue a death certificate'. Surtees,
p. 52.

55 'to obtain the aid of Dr Camps'. MEPO 2/9785/2, further
statements, statement of Angus Sommerville, 8 January
1957.

55 'some suspicious circumstances'. MEPO 2/9784, letter from
Detective Sergeant, H. Grieves, 7 August 1956.

55 'pills sent her nearly mad and through them she died'.
Hallworth, p. 11.

56 'to await the results of a post-mortem examination'. Hoskins,
p. 24.

56 'it's about time somebody caught up with that bloody doctor'.
Ibid.

56 'she might have been the cause of her own death'. MEPO 2/9785/2, further statements, statement by Evelyn Patricia Tomlinson, 26 July 1956.

56 'the whole thing was a planned suicide'. MEPO 2/9785/2, further statements, statement of Hugh Hubbard Ford, 29 July 1956.

57 'in any way addicted to drugs of any sort'. MEPO 2/9785/2, further statements, statement of Percy Robert Handscomb, 24 July 1956.

57 was trying to 'shield, if possible, my dearest friend Mrs Hullett'. MEPO 2/9785/2, further statements, statement of Percy Robert Handscomb, 27 July 1956.

58 Dr Adams, with Dr Harris at his side, had failed to take. MEPO 2/9785/2, further statements, Francis Camps memo relating to Bobbie Hullett.

58 'he had never had such a large dose before'. MEPO 2/9785/2, further statements, letter from Francis Camps.

59 death of the widow of a rich retired Lloyd's underwriter, he said. Hoskins, p. 25.

59 'Immediate destination, James Donne's office. Then the police station'. Ibid., p. 26.

60 his officers were now trying to get at the truth. Ibid.

60 'Rich Widow Drama: CID Act'. *Daily Sketch*, 26 July 1956.

60 'who owns three motor cars and has an extensive practice'. *Daily Mail*, 26 July 1956.

61 'a sumptuous boudoir of silks and brocades'. Hallworth, p. 12.

61 'The seams, I was told, were reinforced . . .' *Daily Mirror*, 8 August 1956.

62 in the presence of a dozen paparazzi with cameras. *Daily Mirror*, 21 August 1956.

65 the jury concluded that Bobbie Hullett had committed suicide. MEPO 9785/1, transcript of the Bobbie Hullett inquest.

65 'it was all over they might have a champagne party'. Hoskins, p. 33.

66 'My conscience is clear,' he informed the reporters. Hoskins, p. 34.

Chapter 4

67 yellow gloves and to carry a smart umbrella. Hallworth, p. 37.

67 and renounced spats for good. Ibid., p. 36.

68 His nickname – The Count. Interview Iain Hannam.

69 'a rather nasty type of pretentious bore'. Quoted in Russell Taylor, p. 44.

69 'who did not wish to see *Look Back in Anger*'. *The Observer*, 13 May 1956.

71 'plastic bag containing toilet requisites and negatives'. MEPO 2/9537

72 'The general prognosis is very poor indeed . . .' Ibid.

72 forever throwing them about in the garden. Ibid.

73 'with the back edge of the chopper'. Ibid.

73 'which made things very sinister . . .' *Law Society Gazette*, 2 June 2005. 'Murder Most Foul', by James Morton.

74 'Put that bloody chopper away it haunts yer . . .' MEPO 2/9537.

75 'immaculate man with the broad shoulders . . .' *Daily Express*, 29 October 1953.

75 'gave his evidence in a grave and solemn manner'. Rawlinson, p. 53.

75 'a terrible one and is absolutely untrue'. *The Times*, 29 October 1953.

76 a bruising one. He never forgot it. *Law Society Gazette*, 2 June 2005. 'Murder Most Foul', by James Morton.

76 'I couldn't kill you but I could do the next best thing . . .' MEPO 2/9537.

Chapter 5

77 the doctor had delivered Pugh's children. Hallworth, p. 36.

77 'Dr Adams was interested in their financial affairs'. SPA 4/8/11, statement of Edith Grace Easter.

78 'and would turn out at any time of the night'. SPA 4/8/11, statement of Helen McSweeney.

78 sometimes to hold her hand. SPA 4/8/11, statement of Kathleen May, 13 September 1956.

78 'far too friendly', and unlike that of any other doctor. SPA 4/8/11, statement of Nurse Marjorie Savage, 14 September 1956.

78 'for money and all he can get'. SPA 4/8/11, statement of Eunice Hitch, 30 August 1956.

79 'I felt I could not do this with Dr Adams . . .' SPA 4/8/11, statement of Minnie Sheperdess Carey, 28 September 1956.

79 not to work with Dr Adams again. SPA 4/8/11, statement of Grace Osgood, 15 September 1956.

79 'there's plenty of money there'. SPA 4/8/11, statement of Blanche Goacher, 13 September 1956.

79 'and he would have them collected'. SPA 4/8/11, statement of Nurse Marjorie Savage, 14 September 1956.

80 and 'a disgrace to the profession'. Hallworth, p. 27.

80 'menace in their midst' who should be removed. MEPO 2/9784, report of Superintendent Hannam, 16 October 1956.

80 84 per cent of GPs had voted against it. Loudon, p. 1.

81 'Dr Adams's activities became greatly restricted'. MEPO 2/9784, report of Superintendent Hannam, 16 October 1956.

81 drawing cheques on her bank account. Ibid.

82 'the technique which this gentleman will adopt'. Ibid.

82 so badly that she was left unconscious. MEPO 2/9785/2, further statements, statement of Gladys Parker, 29 January 1957.

82 the founder of a local camera club. Surtees, p. 16.

82 he was abrupt and refused to tell her. MEPO 2/9785/2, further statements, statement of Edna Baldock, 26 January 1957.

83 sit at her bedside and stare at her. Ibid.

83 'best of my recollections contained hypnotics'. SPA 4/8/11, statement of Philip Walter Mathew, 10 September 1956.

83 'deeply under the influence of drugs'. Ibid.

84 'that she came from New Zealand'. Ibid.

84 'ulterior in its method of medical treatment'. MEPO 2/9784, report of Superintendent Hannam, 16 October 1956.

84 diamonds and pearls, and expensive furniture. ACC 6011, papers relating to Irene Herbert.

85 a 'rapid decline in good health'. MEPO 2/9785/2, further statements, statement of Gladys Parker, 29 January 1957.

85 who understood her condition. Ibid.

85 returned her to the care of her doctor. Ibid.

85 'all his kindness, which I can never repay'. MEPO 2/9784, report of Superintendent Hannam, 16 October 1956.

85 arranged for the storage of her many furs. ACC 6011, papers relating to Irene Herbert.

85 chauffeur available to her, at £2 a time. Ibid.

86 'Dr Adams tried to induce her to sell the car to him'. MEPO 2/9784, report of Superintendent Hannam, 16 October 1956.

86 apart from her burns, and was mentally alert. SPA 4/8/11, statement of Marian Richards, 15 September 1956.

87 'I couldn't sign the paper for the doctor this morning'. Ibid.

87 'A callous remark I thought, at such a time'. SPA 4/8/11, statement of Olga Mouat Smith, 3 September 1956.

87 he decided not to take the case further. MEPO 2/9784, report of Superintendent Hannam, 16 October 1956.

87 not the heart condition for which she was being treated. MEPO 2/9785/2, extracts from chemists' registers, MEPO 2/9784, report of Superintendent Hannam, 16 October 1956.

87 a large medical bill, some £234. ACC 6011, papers relating to John Bodkin Adams.

88 threatened to report him to the General Medical Council. MEPO 2/9784, report of Superintendent Hannam, 16 October 1956.

88 and kept the proceeds, £12. Ibid.

89 included Dr Adams in her will – but now she cut him out again. Ibid.

89 'why, I do not know'. SPA 4/8/11, letter from Irene Pearce Myott, 24 August 1956.

90 'a little reminder of the dear patient'. Ibid.

90 'and hoped my affairs were in good hands'. SPA 4/8/11, statement of Ethel Helen Hunt, 5 September 1956.

90 'my financial position was not attractive'. Ibid.

91 and the door of his car as he went. Ibid.

91 the doctor as 'a real scrounger'. MEPO 2/9784, report of Superintendent Hannam, 16 October 1956.

91 he cut him out altogether. SPA 4/8/11, statement of Christopher Rippon, solicitor, 14 September 1956.

92 'Dr Adams drove off in his car'. Ibid.

92 and had enquired about William's will. Ibid.

92 'something of my husband's and took it away with him'. Ibid.

92 the executors decided to pay him £876. SPA 4/8/11, statement of Christopher Rippon, solicitor, 14 September 1956.

Chapter 6

94 nickname 'Scotland Yard's Dr Watson'. Hoskins, p. 37.

94 call Percy, even before you called your lawyer. 'Murder, We Wrote', Victor Davis in *British Journalism Review*, vol. 15, no. 1, 2004, p. 58.

95 Eastbourne 'seemed to be getting out of hand'. Hoskins, p. 38.

95 waiting for him at the station. Hoskins, p. 38.

95 and the 'wild rumours'. Hoskins, p. 2.

95 'like lava from Etna in eruption'. Hoskins, p. 45.

95 'and ready for the scaffold as John Bodkin Adams'. Hoskins, p. 1.

96 'this ugly competition is the *Daily Mail* . . .' *Tribune*, 31 August 1956.

96 'A clever manipulation . . .' Hoskins, p. 48.

97 'most senior officers at Scotland Yard'. Hoskins, p. 35.

97 'the rivals were playing it double fortissimo'. Hoskins, p. 36.

97 'a million pounds was involved. Untrue'. Ibid.

97 the national average 11.7. Hoskins, p. 5.

98 'professional head on the chopping block'. Hoskins, p. 43.

98 'clear to me that his unconcern was genuine'. Hoskins, p. 1.

98 If found guilty, he might hang. Ibid.

98 'never mentioned them to me. They stayed loyal to me'. *Daily Express*, 16 April 1957.

99 'gratitude for considerable kindness'. MEPO 2/9784, report of Superintendent Hannam, 16 October 1956.

100 'both to his mother, his other relatives, and to me,' she said. MEPO 2/9784, statement of Sara Emily Watson, 27 October 1956.

101 'particularly the manner in which she died'. MEPO 2/9784, report of Superintendent Hannam, 16 October 1956.

101 similar bequest – the dining room clock, and £200. ACC 6011, papers relating to Annabella Kilgour.

102 unless the clearest credible facts support it. MEPO 2/9784, report of Superintendent Hannam, 16 October 1956.

102 'as she was always partly unconscious'. MEPO 2/9784, statement of Elaine Wilson, 28 August 1956.

103 The nurse saw no symptoms of influenza. SPA 4/8/11, statement of Clara Brierley, 12 September 1956.

103 Mrs Pilling was 'under the influence of drugs'. Ibid.

103 'she would otherwise be in great pain'. MEPO 2/9784, statement of Elaine Wilson, 28 August 1956.

103 Mrs Pilling's condition did not improve. SPA 4/8/11, statement of Clara Brierley, 12 September 1956.

103 thoroughly enjoy the trip in the ambulance. Ibid.

103 all of which were now thrown away. Ibid.

104 'I have never been able to account for'. Ibid.

105 his solicitor, Herbert James, at her bedside to help her. MEPO 2/9784, report of Superintendent Hannam, 16 October 1956.

105 'a. cerebral thrombosis, and b. cardio vascular degeneration'. Ibid.

105 'to share out part of the proceeds of a dying woman'. Ibid.

106 'a peculiar-tempered lady'. SPA 4/8/11, statement of Elizabeth Bryant, 10 September 1956.

106 and always gave him chocolates. Ibid.

106 'and became wandering in her mind'. Ibid.

106 typewriter – worth £27 – as a keepsake. MEPO 2/9784, statement of Alfred John Michael Maidlow Davis, 25 October 1956, MEPO 2/9784, statement of Gwendoline Werge, 27 November 1956.

107 'hypodermic syringe to inject Mrs Thomas'. SPA 4/8/11, statement of Elizabeth Ellen Bryant, 10 September 1956.

107 'went to bed and had the injection'. MEPO 2/9784, statement of Alfred John Michael Maidlow Davis, 25 October 1956.

107 'and walked off with it'. Ibid.

108 'One of his hobbies is photography'. MEPO 2/9784, report of Superintendent Hannam, 16 October 1956.

108 'seemed to be having medicine of some kind'. SPA 4/8/11, statement of Florence Sankey, 8 September 1956.

109 'The doctor will advise me what to do'. Ibid.

109 she 'simply adored him'. SPA 4/8/11, statement of Gertrude Boston, 14 September 1956.

109 'you will see me riding in my Rolls'. SPA 4/8/11, statement of Nurse Gwendoline Marion Stuart-Hemsley, 13 September 1956.

109 meringues and drinking tea. Surtees, p. 32.

109 'my husband his compliments and out he went'. SPA 4/8/11, statement of Nurse Gwendoline Marion Stuart-Hemsley, 13 September 1956.

110 'Not so very long after that she died'. Ibid.

110 Mrs Norton-Dowding was 'slowly slipping away'. SPA 4/8/11, statement of Eva Barham, 23 August 1956.

110 to give her injections in her arm. SPA 4/8/11, statement of Gertrude Boston, 14 September 1956.

110 'I'll meet you at the airport'. Ibid.

111 they should not be informed of her condition. Ibid.

111 and Dr Adams received £500. MEPO 2/9784, report of Superintendent Hannam, 16 October 1956.

115 'so many of this doctor's cases'. MEPO 2/9784, communication from Derby Borough Police, MEPO 2/9784, report of

Superintendent Hannam, 5 December 1956, SPA 4/8/11, statements of Nurses Gladys Miller and Annie Sweeney.

Chapter 7

116 a coachman when they married in 1890. ACC 6011, papers relating to Julia Bradnum.

117 *News from Afar* and *Christian World*. Ibid.

117 'called to higher service'. Illustration in Hallworth.

117 her wages 'in payment for her upbringing'. ACC 6011, papers relating to Julia Bradnum, letter from Bertie Love, 17 June 1952.

117 as laying carpets and fixing curtains. Ibid.

118 her washing and drying in her bedroom. ACC 6011, papers relating to Julia Bradnum, letter from Bertie Love, 18 July 1952.

119 'Auntie told him all her troubles'. SPA 4/8/11, statement of Lily Overall Love, 16 August 1956.

119 'and holding her hand'. MEPO 2/9784, report of Superintendent Hannam, 16 October 1956.

119 'thought there was nobody like him'. MEPO 2/9784, statement of Frank Potter, 27 August 1956.

119 'opened the door and ushered me out'. Hallworth, p. 51.

120 'someone was trying to force her to'. MEPO 2/9784, report of Superintendent Hannam, 16 October 1956.

120 divided among 'those that she loved'. SPA 4/8/11, statement of Lily Overall Love, 16 August 1956.

120 garden and chatting to her neighbours. Ibid.

120 'Miss Worthington thought she had not recognised her'. MEPO 2/9784, report of Superintendent Hannam, 16 October 1956.

121 she could contact him quickly. Hallworth, p. 51.

121 very quickly, with Dr Adams by her side. Ibid.

121 'been out of the house for about a half-hour'. Ibid.

121 flabbergasted at the news and couldn't understand it. MEPO 2/9784, report of Superintendent Hannam, 16 October 1956.

122 visit his aunt's bank, to make inquiries. ACC 6011, papers relating to Julia Bradnum.

122 no legal force, since it had not been witnessed. MEPO 2/9784, report of Superintendent Hannam, 16 October 1956.

122 'bad state of repair and decoration'. ACC 6011, papers relating to Julia Bradnum.

123 and Hannam's thoughts turned to exhumation. MEPO 2/9784, report of Superintendent Hannam, 16 October 1956.

123 decorated with imitation cherries and flowers. Hallworth, p. 1.

124 'kept them in that dazed and doped condition'. SPA 4/8/11, report of Superintendent Hannam, 28 August 1956.

124 'condition was due to sedatives'. SPA 4/8/11, statement of Phyllis Mary Owen, 1 October 1956.

124 pills were to stop. After that she got better. SPA 4/8/11, statement of Isabel Neil-Miller, 1 September 1956.

125 'to confide in me but was unsuccessful'. Ibid.

125 a family friend who lived in Eastbourne. Ibid.

126 the funeral and the burial site at the cemetery. MEPO 2/9784, report of Superintendent Hannam, 16 October 1956.

126 'appeared to be under the influence of drugs'. Ibid.

127 His hands were 'very comforting to her'. Ibid.

127 'so much about their personal and financial backgrounds'. Hallworth, p. 5.

128 'had to be dragged out of her'. MEPO 2/9784, report of Superintendent Hannam, 16 October 1956.

128 this one for £500 and payable to Dr Adams. Ibid.

128 'been February, perhaps the coldest of the year'. MEPO 2/9784, report of Superintendent Hannam, 5 December 1956.

129 'the whole circumstances of her death are unsatisfactory'. MEPO 2/9784, report of Superintendent Hannam, 16 October 1956.

Chapter 8

130 three hundred thousand head of cattle. Cheever, p. viii.

130 'a wicked piece of work'. Surtees, p. 18.

131 'too deep in War work to have any time for me'. ACC 6011, papers relating to Edith Morrell.

131 'This country is riddled with them . . .' Ibid.

132 'in the same year can stand anything!' Ibid.

132 'ensure by all means that my life is extinct'. Ibid.

133 'we will just leave things as they are'. Ibid.

133 'to attend to her comforts generally'. MEPO 2/9784, statement of Rosaleen Spray, 28 November 1956.

134 'a feeling of utter contempt for him'. Ibid.

134 silver candlesticks as a Christmas present. Ibid.

134 'stop and admire it and its pieces'. MEPO 2/9784, report of Superintendent Hannam, 16 October 1956.

134 'a technique to get Mrs Morrell to give it to him'. Ibid.

134 'there was nothing left – all the service had gone'. MEPO 2/9784, statement of Thomas Henry Price, 25 November 1956.

135 'and every day as he did when he had a rich patient'. SPA 4/8/11, statement of Nurse Agnes White, 31 August 1956.

135 he was 'very kind and attentive'. MEPO 2/9785/2, statement of Annie Mason Ellis, 28 August 1956, MEPO 2/9785/2, statement of Caroline Randall, 27 August 1956.

135 and told her to give it more thought. MEPO 2/9784, report of Superintendent Hannam, 16 October 1956.

136 take his instructions from Mrs Morrell in person. Ibid.

136 generally of drugs that he had in his bag. MEPO 2/9784, statement of Harry Gibson, 27 November 1956, statement of Thomas Price, 25 November 1956, statement of Helen Stronach, 25 November 1956.

136 'played up a good deal and was a very trying patient'. MEPO 2/9784, statement of Helen Stronach, 25 November 1956.

136 'neither of us abused the privilege'. MEPO 2/9784, statement of Bessie Woodward, 28 November 1956.

136 'dead if we had the same. This old lady is tough'. Ibid.

137 'a very difficult patient with a violent temper'. MEPO 2/9784, statement of Brenda Doreen Hughes (previously Bartlett), 30 November 1956.

137 'the quantity was slowly increased and oftener'. MEPO 2/9785/2, statement of Caroline Randall, 27 August 1956.

137 'unsolicited advice of the nurse on those matters'. Ibid.

137 before flying back to Scotland. MEPO 2/9784, report of Superintendent Hannam, 16 October 1956.

138 She tore up the codicil. Transcript of trial of Dr Adams.

138 further injections, with drugs that he took from his bag. MEPO 2/9784, further statement of Caroline Randall, 25 November 1956.

138 'if I was unduly worried to ring him again'. MEPO 2/9784, statement of Brenda Hughes, 30 November 1956.

139 'That's a beautiful car'. MEPO 2/9785/2, statement of James Dean, 27 August 1956.

139 had no idea what was in the injection. MEPO 2/9784, further statement of Caroline Randall, 25 November 1956.

139 in a coma for two hours before she died. MEPO 2/9784, report of Superintendent Hannam, 16 October 1956.

139 took away with him Mrs Morrell's infra-red lamp. MEPO 2/9784, statement of Brenda Hughes, 30 November 1956.

140 enough to buy another Rolls-Royce, had he wanted to. Hallworth, p. 50.

140 'in possession of a fatal supply and hope for the best'. MEPO 2/9785/2, letter from L. C. Nickolls to Superintendent Hannam, 11 September 1956.

141 'in the amount shown without some peculiar intent'. Ibid.

Chapter 9

143 and he asked Hannam to do all he could to dispel the gossip. MEPO 2/9784, report of Superintendent Hannam, 16 October 1956.

143 on a shooting holiday to Scotland. Ibid.

144 'it is all God's plan to teach me a new lesson'. SPA 4/8/11, statement of Superintendent Hannam, 2 October 1956.

145 'Good night, and thank you very much for your kindness'. Ibid.

146 'would resemble clinical narcotic poisoning'. MEPO 2/9784, report of Superintendent Hannam, 16 October 1956.

146 a post-mortem could be performed. Ibid.

147 'The whole thing looks odd to me'. Ibid.

147 Jack Hullett's death was 'extremely doubtful'. Ibid.

147 'to include him as a beneficiary under their wills.' Ibid.

150 could 'never be proved'. Ibid.

150 further investigation, if the Director of Public Prosecutions recommended it. MEPO 2/9785/2, note from Commander 'C', 22 October 1956.

150 'I think I could have said he killed more'. Hallworth, p. 42.

151 'She's cracking, Charlie. We'll have it next time.' Hallworth, p. 6.

151 'like so many of the cases, left us without a body'. Hallworth, p. 7.

151 'What a shock,' said the doctor. MEPO 2/9784, report of Superintendent Hannam, 26 November 1956, report of Charlie Hewett, MEPO 2/9784, 26 November 1956, report of Brynley Pugh, 27 November 1956.

152 'I haven't any. I very seldom ever use them'. Ibid.

152 the account of what happened next came from Hannam's memory. MEPO 2/9784, Superintendent Hannam's statement of 26 November 1956, MEPO 2/9784, Superintendent Hannam's report of 5 December 1956.

152 was corroborated by his loyal aide, Charlie Hewett. MEPO 2/9784, Charlie Hewett's statement of 26 November 1956.

152 'No, none. All was given to the patient'. Ibid.

156 officially with the forgery and cremation form offences. Ibid.

157 '5,000 pheno-barbitone tablets for use in his practice'. MEPO 2/9784, report of Superintendent Hannam, 5 December 1956.

157 the drugs should be sent to Kent Lodge. Ibid.

157 Dr Estcourt 'has no direct evidence of any actual case'. MEPO 2/9784, report of Superintendent Hannam, 16 October 1956.

158 'That can't be murder. It is impossible to accuse a doctor'.

MEPO 2/9784, report of Superintendent Hannam, 5 December 1956.

158 'charge Adams with the murder of Mrs Morrell!' Hallworth, p. 58.

158 preferred to pursue a more recent death, with a body. Ibid.

159 'we were engaged there for some twenty minutes'. MEPO 2/9784, report of Superintendent Hannam, 4 January 1957.

159 'I didn't think you could prove murder, she was dying in any event'. Ibid.

159 'I will see you in heaven,' said Dr Adams. MEPO 2/9/9785, additional statement of Superintendent Hannam, 20 December 1956.

Chapter 10

160 keep prices down, cutting profits if necessary. *Daily Express*, 11 December 1956.

160 declaring that he was 'absolutely fit'. *Daily Express*, 15 December 1956.

162 'You lose your individuality and become just another number'. *Daily Express*, 17 April 1957.

162 'to adapt myself to the prison routine without asking any special favours'. Hoskins, p. 56.

163 'assured me there was nothing that he lacked'. ACC 6011, letter from Leigh Taylor, Hempsons to Herbert James.

163 but also a supply of chocolate pineapples from Joseph Terry. ACC 6011, papers relating to the accounts of Dr Adams.

163 someone whose wages were a mere £4 a week. Ibid.

164 'inconceivable to me that he could have done any of the acts alleged against him'. ACC 6011, letter from Herbert James to Leigh Taylor, 26 January 1957.

164 Dr Adams wrote to him, in praise of 'such a wonderful friend'. ACC 6011, letter from Dr Adams, date unclear.

164 'She never ceased to send me words of encouragement,' he told Percy Hoskins. Hoskins, p. 56.

164 'that he did not think he could be in any way helpful'. ACC 6011, diary of activities of Herbert James, 12 January 1957.

165 too eager to oppose Simpson in court. Simpson, pp. 230–52.

166 nothing useful could be said about drugs in either case. MEPO 2/9784, papers relating to exhumations, MEPO 2/9785/2, papers relating to Francis Camps.

166 the most significant since that of John Christie. *New York Times*, 16–17 January 1957.

167 'enjoyed by most of the Bar and not so much by the litigants'. Devlin, p. 38.

168 'we say that was a fatal dose and a dose meant to kill'. *Daily Express*, 15 January 1957.

168 'We say it was because Dr Adams knew quite well that Mrs Hullett was going to die that weekend'. Ibid.

169 'the public saw only the back of his florid neck and bald head'. *New York Times*, 17 January 1957.

169 'puckish, mousy little man with a mind as orderly as a calculating machine'. *Time*, 22 April 1957.

169 'polysyllables such as "cerebral" and "respiratory" sound like something out of Keats'. Hounsome, p. 183.

169 often out of doors, yachting, swimming or playing cricket. *Oxford Dictionary of National Biography*.

170 Dr Adams would be tried at the Old Bailey for the murder of Edith Morrell. *Daily Express*, *Daily Mirror*, 25 January 1957.

170 but he could not now remember why he had done so. MEPO 2/9785/2, further statements, additional statement of Dr Ronald Vincent Harris.

171 'under no circumstances would he ever see Dr Adams again'. MEPO 2/9785/2, statement of Superintendent Hannam, 4 February 1957.

171 circulated widely in the town, under the title 'Adams and Eves'. ACC 6011, letter to Leigh Taylor of Hempsons from Herbert James.

172 He also considered an action for contempt of court. Ibid.

173 'the game was worth the candle: if you asked yourself that, you were finished'. Devlin, pp. 39–40.

173 'most of his convictions were wrong-headed, he was ineluctably a do-badder'. Ibid.

173 'Reggie's climb in real life appeared to his contemporaries'. Ibid.

174 or might not, go ahead with the Bobbie Hullett indictment. Devlin, p. 43.

174 'he was obviously and deeply disturbed'. Devlin, p. 44.

Chapter 11

175 'crime in England does seem to have a specially fascinating aura'. *New York Times*, 3 March 1957.

176 'another thing in blue heels. I find that a fascinating bit of information'. Spoto, p. 32.

176 become *Vertigo* – starring James Stewart and Kim Novak. McGilligan, pp. 545–7.

177 'to suggest that the doctor's therapeutic batting average seemed to be slipping badly'. *New York Times*, 3 March 1957.

178 'false names and stolen cars, belongs essentially to a war period,' he wrote. Ibid.

179 'easily filled with any or all of the patients who during that time had died'. Devlin, p. 25.

180 'upholstered in blue serge, red-faced, bald, facing the Judge, facing this day'. Bedford, p. 17.

180 'A loquacious man, then,' she observed, correctly. Bedford, p. 18.

180 'as some might say, impressive, or as others, ponderous'. Devlin, p. 2.

180 A 'somewhat massive figure' in the courtroom. Bedford, p. 19

181 'had kept near to the maximum in morphia but exceeded it in heroin by about 75 per cent'. Devlin, p. 3.

184 'and at once he reveals both grasp and charm'. Bedford, p. 27.

Chapter 12

186 in Patrick Devlin's words, 'girlish and zestful'. Devlin, p. 55.
186 'blurred features except for a narrow mouth and strong jaw'.
Bedford, p. 30.
189 'He goes on,' wrote Bedford, 'treading very lightly'. Bedford, p. 34.
192 'the heartland of the prosecution and taking command of it'.
Devlin, p. 61.
192 'Mr Lawrence must get full marks for audacity'. Bedford, p. 37.
199 'The sequence and control of details, the moods of tone'.
Bedford, p. 41.
199 'doesn't mean the old lady didn't get plenty of dope from
whoever it was'. Ibid.
200 'a thin, rather pale, tallish, fairish woman, dressed in beige,
apparently not strong'. Bedford, p. 44.
201 hurried down the steps of the dock. *Daily Mirror*, 20 March
1957.

Chapter 13

202 'hysterical, wanting to die and weeping'. *Daily Mirror*, 20 March
1957.
202 'astute in cross-examination and a suave advocate'. *Daily
Express*, 20 March 1957.
203 'Mr Lawrence was fully armed'. Devlin, p. 78.
207 buzzing with 'compressed energy'. Bedford, p. 58.
209 'Greek chorus to Lawrence's rendering of the notebooks'.
Devlin, p. 82.
210 'the charge of the Imperial Guard at Waterloo'. Devlin, p. 83.

Chapter 14

216 he would probably 'throw in his hand'. Devlin, pp. 90–1.
217 spoke 'with the voice of doom'. Ibid.

219 'after two years of prescribing was too much to swallow', Devlin, pp. 97–8.

219 'chest out, chin in, as a tenor might go forward for his aria'. Bedford, p. 96.

224 Dr Harris 'blossomed'. Bedford, p. 117.

Chapter 15

225 'my duodenal ulcer, please arrange my admission'. *British Medical Journal*, 1996; 312:1264 (18 May).

225 'gives the impression that his head touches the canopy'. Bedford, p. 123.

225 'things either were or they were not'. Devlin, p. 107.

226 'an expression of obstinate mortification on his face . . .' Bedford, p. 124.

229 the journalists now said, 'it's a walkover'. Ibid., p. 131.

232 'Good gracious me!' Bedford, p. 134.

236 'Douthwaite was artless in not trying to make one'. Devlin, p. 115.

242 'an exercise to bring the word "boggle" briefly into its own'. Devlin, p. 122.

242 this was 'euthanasia with a taint of legacy hunting'. Devlin, p. 123.

242 'to leave a puzzled jury and a puzzled jury may not be a good jury'. Devlin, p. 124.

Chapter 16

245 'both high-strung and controlled'. Bedford, p. 164.

249 'stumbling over benches and each other to run the news to a telephone'. Bedford, p. 184.

249 'the unexpected sacrifice of the queen' in a game of chess. Devlin, p. 142.

251 'has his own brand of certainty'. Bedford, p. 185.

Chapter 17

259 an oration, pitched at 'solemn boom'. Bedford, p. 212.

264 but as a victory for pre-trial prejudice. Devlin, p. 177.

265 he had been seen dining with Roland Gwynne in Lewes in February. Cullen, p. 633.

265 although bail would have been extremely unusual, it was justified. Devlin, p. 178.

265 responsible for an abuse of process. Devlin, pp. 181–2.

266 'the longest murder trial recorded in Britain'. *Daily Mirror*, 10 April 1957.

266 'two men have been acquitted today. Adams and Hoskins'. Hoskins, p. 196.

266 'courage throughout has always enabled me to do my best'. Hoskins, p. 200.

267 successfully brought thirteen libel cases. Hoskins, p. 213.

268 prevented Eastbourne doctors co-operating with the police. HO 287/253.

269 the police officer had failed to notice them. Private papers of Patrick Devlin.

269 threw him out on thirty-four votes to two. Surtees, p. 124.

269 had not personally benefited from it. Ibid.

269 found in an envelope, untouched, when he died. Hoskins, p. 216.

270 'There is nothing in these charges to suggest he is'. *Daily Mirror*, 28 November 1957.

270 English team in Belgium, though not particularly well. Surtees, p. 130.

270 '"my dear", and they thought the world of him'. Cited in Surtees, p. 126.

270 'John, you're dribbling on your tie'. Surtees, pp. 133–4.

271 'killing off all journalists, past and present'. Hallworth, pp. 239–40.

272 his gun to bed with him and aiming it at the picture rail. Surtees, pp. 134–5.

272 Dr Adams 'was as guilty as hell'. *Daily Express*, 11 July 1985.

272 'the true man and his caring kindness'. Hoskins, p. 215.

Afterwards

279 'rights to satisfy their desires'. *Psychiatric Times*, January 2002, vol. XIX, issue 1.

282 'the acts alleged against him'. ACC 6011, letter from H. V. James, 26 January 1957.

283 a 'qualification for a certain sort of killer'. Devlin, p. 199.

283 figure would be around 14–17 per cent. http://www.ons.gov.uk, http://www.mortality-trends.org

283 'could well be due to a narcotic or barbiturate'. DPP 2/2572

Bibliography

ARCHIVES

National Archive (NA), Kew

ASSI 36/220
CRIM 8/26
DPP 2/2570–2576
HO 287/240
HO 287/253
HO 287/259
HO 287/273

MEPO 2/9537
MEPO 2/9752
MEPO 2/9784
MEPO 2/9785/1–2
MEPO 2/9786–9790

MH 135/156

Files that remain closed:

MEPO 2/9889
Investigation into missing documents

LO 2/144
Relating to conduct of police and parliamentary questions

East Sussex Record Office

ACC 6011
SPA 4/8/10–36

NEWSPAPERS AND MAGAZINES

Daily Express
Daily Mail
Daily Mirror
Daily Sketch
Eastbourne Gazette
Eastbourne Herald Chronicle
Newsweek
New York Times
Paris Match
The Observer
The Times
Time Magazine
Tribune

JOURNALS

British Journalism Review
British Medical Journal
The Lancet
Law Society Gazette
Psychiatric Times

WEBSITES

Oxford Dictionary of National Biography http://www.oxforddnb.com
Office for National Statistics http://www.ons.gov.uk
Mortality Trends http://www.mortality-trends.org

GPs threaten to resign from the NHS 1957:
http://www.bbc.co.uk/archive/nhs/5140.shtml
Auction of some of Dr Adams's possessions:
http://www.liveauctioneers.com/catalog/19096/page5

BOOKS

Bedford, Sybille, *The Best We Can Do: An Account of the Trial of John Bodkin Adams*, Collins, 1958

Cheever, Lawrence Oakley, *The House of Morrell*, The Torch Press, 1948

Cullen, Pamela, *A Stranger in Blood. The Case Files on Dr John Bodkin Adams*, Elliott & Thompson, 2006

Dawes, Frank, *Not in Front of the Servants: Domestic Service in England 1850–1939*, Wayland Publishers, 1973

Devlin, Patrick, *Easing the Passing: The Trial of Dr John Bodkin Adams*, Faber and Faber, 1986

Douglas-Home, Jessica, *Violet, the Lives and Loves of Violet Gordon Woodhouse*, The Harvill Press, 1997

Farson, Daniel, *Soho in the Fifties*, Michael Joseph, 1988

Firth, Violet M., *The Psychology of the Servant Problem*, The C W Daniel Co, 1925

Gibson, Ronald, *The Family Doctor*, Allen & Unwin, 1981

Hallworth, Rodney and Williams, Mark, *Where There's a Will: The Sensational Life of Dr John Bodkin Adams*, The Capstan Press, 1983

Horne, Alistair, *Macmillan, Vol 2: 1957–1986*, Macmillan, 1988

Hoskins, Percy, *Two Men were Acquitted, The Trial and Acquittal of Dr John Bodkin Adams*, Secker & Warburg, 1984

Hounsome, Robert, *The Very Nearly Man*, Matador, 2006

Jackson, Arnold S., MD, *The Answer is . . . Your Nerves*, Windmill Press, 1947

Jackson, Robert, *Francis Camps: Famous Case Histories of the Celebrated Pathologist*, Hart-Davis MacGibbon, 1975

Jesse, F. Tennyson, *Murder and its Motives*, Harrap, 1952

Kynaston, David, *Family Britain 1951–57*, Bloomsbury, 2009

Lamb, Richard, *The Macmillan Years: 1957–63*, John Murray, 1995

Loudon, Irvine, Horder, John and Webster, Charles, eds, *General Practice Under the National Health Service 1948–1997*, Clarendon Press, 1998

McGilligan, Patrick, *Alfred Hitchcock – A Life in Darkness and Light*, Wiley, 2003

Osborne, John, *Look Back in Anger*, Bantam Books, 1965

Peters, Carole, *Harold Shipman: Mind Set on Murder*, Andre Deutsch, 2006

Pugh, Peter, *Grand Hotel*, The Grand Hotel, 1987

Rawlinson, Peter, *A Price Too High. An Autobiography*, Weidenfeld & Nicolson, 1989

Rivett, Geoffrey, *From Cradle to Grave: Fifty Years of the NHS*, King's Fund, 1998

Russell Taylor, John, ed., *John Osborne, Look Back in Anger. A Casebook*, Macmillan, 1968

Simpson, Keith, *Forty Years of Murder*, Granada, 1978

Spoto, Donald, *The Life of Alfred Hitchcock*, Collins, 1983

Surtees, John, *The Strange Case of Dr Bodkin Adams*, S B Publications, 2000

Ussher, Jane M., *Women's Madness: Misogyny or Mental Illness?*, Harvester Wheatsheaf, 1991

Whittle, Brian and Ritchie, Jean, *Harold Shipman: Prescription for Murder*, Sphere, 2007

Index